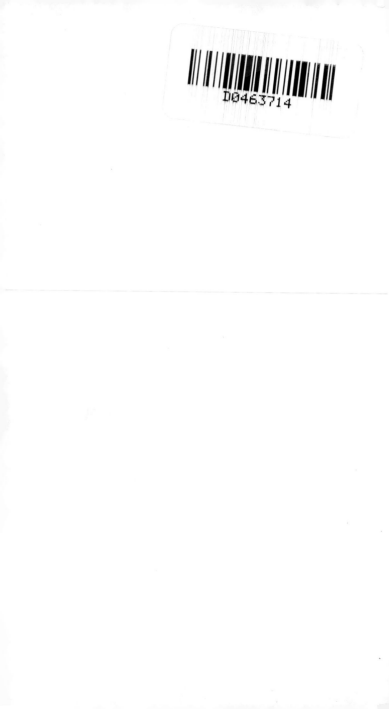

HOME HEALTH
Nursing
Care Plans

HOME HEALTH
Nursing
Care Plans

MARIE S. JAFFE, R.N., M.S.

Formerly Nursing Faculty,
University of Texas at El Paso,
College of Nursing and Allied Health,
El Paso, Texas

LINDA SKIDMORE-ROTH, R.N., M.S.N., N.P.

Formerly Nursing Faculty,
New Mexico State University,
Las Cruces, New Mexico;
Formerly Nursing Faculty,
El Paso Community College,
El Paso, Texas

Second Edition

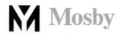

St. Louis Baltimore Boston Chicago London Philadelphia Sydney Toronto

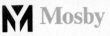
Mosby

Dedicated to Publishing Excellence

Executive editor: N. Darlene Como
Developmental editor: Laurie Sparks
Project manager: Mark Spann
Production editor: Stephen C. Hetager
Cover designer: Liz Fett
Cover illustration by Rip Kastaris

Second Edition

Printed in the United States of America

Mosby–Year Book, Inc.
11830 Westline Industrial Drive
St. Louis, Missouri 63146

Library of Congress Cataloging-in-Publication Data

Jaffe, Marie S.
    Home health nursing care plans / Marie S. Jaffe, Linda Skidmore
–Roth. —2nd ed.
        p.   cm.
    Includes bibliographical references and index.
    ISBN 0-8016-6699-6
    1. Home nursing—Planning.   2. Nursing care plans.   I. Skidmore
–Roth, Linda.   II. Title
    [DNLM: 1. Home Care Services—handbooks. 2. Nursing Assessment–
–handbooks.   3. Patient Care Planning--handbooks.   WY 39 J23h]
RT120.H65J34   1993
362. 1'4—dc20
DNLM/DLC   **174135**
for Library of Congress   92-48860
                                                                      CIP

95 96 97   UG/D   9 8 7 6 5 4 3

◣ *Preface*

This second edition of *Home Health Nursing Care Plans* has been developed to assist those providing home nursing services with a guide to appropriate interdisciplinary approaches for all aspects of care necessary to achieve an overall goal of optimal health and function of the homebound client. At the same time, it serves to recognize and reflect agency and insurance requirements related to providing nursing care in the home setting.

Nursing care provided in the home generally focuses on treatment of diseases and associated conditions and on client teaching for self-care, since reimbursement is generally available only for these services; however, nurses continue to be forerunners in health promotion and disease prevention. These concepts are integrated throughout the book to assist nurses to promote health while providing treatment-oriented care. Community health nurses, nursing students, and home health ancillary personnel in public and privately owned agencies, as well as clinics and newly emerging home health care divisions in hospitals, will benefit from this small, compact, easily carried reference with its comprehensive home care–specific content and nursing process format.

The most pronounced difference from the first edition is the deliberate but appropriate removal of hospital-oriented interventions and the elaboration of more specific and realistic home interventions for the nurse and client/family. Acute care problems are still addressed, however, for those clients discharged from the hospital with needs that require more complex care in the home and for those with long-term illnesses. An outstanding feature of the revision is an emphasis on the assessment and teaching functions of the nurse with each nursing diagnosis listed for a care plan.

The conditions selected for inclusion are identified by medical diagnoses and have been chosen on the basis of their relevance to the population of clients served in the home setting. It is important to note that conditions that may be cared for in the home vary in different regions of the country.

Appropriate care planning and documentation are required

by government and third-party payors to justify payment for care given in the home and the future care needs of clients. It is hoped that this second edition will better benefit those giving home care to clients and ultimately will allow them to continue to receive care in a familiar and less threatening environment.

Marie S. Jaffe
Linda Skidmore-Roth

◣ Guidelines For Using This Book

The following outline presents an overview of the book's contents, with an explanation of each section and suggestions for use.

1. *Assessments* are guides to be used as resources for collection of data that will be incorporated into the interventions on the basis of specific problem identification in the nursing diagnosis. Offered are guides that are related to body systems, body functions, psychosocial concerns, family concerns, and environmental considerations. The guides are referred to in most care plans and are to be used as comprehensive tools by which the nurse may view the client by utilizing those items pertinent to a particular problem or condition. The guides may also be used for interventions that are not referred to if the nurse desires to do so, since a complete nursing assessment is usually required for all clients cared for in the home.

2. *Care Plans* are grouped under major body systems in alphabetical order and reflect general practice rather than specialty practice in home nursing care. The organization and content of each plan follow a logical progression and include the following:

   a. An introductory paragraph defining and describing the condition and concluding with the reason and goals for home care.

   b. Nursing diagnoses related to the illness (one to five may be developed), which are taken from the most recent available (1992) approved list of the North American Nursing Diagnosis Association (NANDA). Those that relate to an individual client may be used, and additional diagnoses may be added from the list offered in the Appendixes if needed.

   c. Related or risk factors for each nursing diagnosis follow. One or more may be given that may or may not be used, but the possibility of using other relationships based on specific client problems should not be precluded.

d. Defining characteristics (which are new to this edition) are signs and symptoms or possible observations that are related to a particular nursing diagnostic stem and its related factors. The nursing diagnosis, related factors, and defining characteristics provide a valuable background for each problem in the care plan.

e. Outcome criteria include a short-term goal and a long-term goal that are expected to be achieved to solve a specific problem area identified by the nursing diagnosis. They are offered as an aid for the nurse to develop goals with the client and include the behaviors and physical evidence that one would expect to suggest goal achievement. As with the nursing diagnosis material, the outcome criteria may be used as they are or supplemented by client-specific and mutually developed goals and their associated observations. Each short-term or long-term goal includes a time frame for outcomes, which, at best, is an estimate and may be longer or shorter as a client's individual condition would warrant. The time frames serve only as a guide for the nurse to determine what is realistic and workable for a client.

f. Interventions are divided into nurse and client/family actions for each nursing diagnosis. This organization assists in determining who is responsible for what actions to implement the plan of care and is home care user friendly to the extent that it is meant to include any caretaker in the home. The nursing interventions are primarily oriented toward assessments, tasks, and instruction/information to be performed by the nurse; the client/family/caretaker interventions are listed as the actions to be performed after the nurse performs the instruction/information component of the care plan. Other interventions for the nurse or client may be added as needed. Each nursing intervention includes visit time frames for implementation, which are intended to be suggestions; they are flexible enough to accommodate changes appropriate to individual client needs and agency policy. A special effort has been made to include referral to other disciplines in the interventions, whether these are available within or outside the agency.

3. *Appendixes* contain material that may be used to supplement the care plans. They include a listing of all NANDA-approved nursing diagnoses, a listing of psychosocial nursing diagnoses with possible related factors, procedures for universal precautions and medication administration, insurance payment guidelines, tips on documentation, guidelines for client self-determination, a selection of common laboratory values, and a listing of selected home care resources.

A most important thought and suggestion that the authors would like to leave with the user of the care plans is to modify and/or supplement any material that has been offered to better suit the identified needs of a specific client or family/care-taker.

◢ Contents

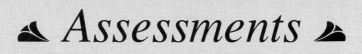

Assessments

◣ *Health History/ Medications*

IDENTIFYING INFORMATION

Age, sex, race, ethnicity, marital status, children and ages
Religious practices, cultural influences
Occupation
Educational level
Health insurance
Residence
Source of information

PAST HISTORY

Statement about general health
Other medical conditions and dates of onset or occurrence
Surgeries and injuries and dates
Hospitalizations for injuries and medical problems
Immunizations and dates
Military history, travel, and dates
Childhood diseases and ages at which they occurred
Psychiatric illness and treatment
Usual health care patterns and kind of practitioner used
Use of rehabilitative/support personnel
Life-style patterns and personal habits in sleep, nutrition, fluid
  intake, urinary and bowel elimination, activity, sexual behav-
  ior, personal hygiene, others

MEDICATIONS/TREATMENTS

Oxygen use
Street or recreational drug use
Homeotherapy
Over-the-counter drugs: type, frequency, dosage, length of
  use, side effects, desired effect, and condition(s) being treated
Prescribed drugs: name, dosage, frequency, route, length of
  use, side effects, desired effect, condition(s) being treated,
  how taken, drug form and contraindications
Potential for toxicity
Aids used to ensure safe, correct administration

Effect of client's age on absorption and excretion
Treatment for adverse effects

PRESENT HISTORY

Chief complaint (in client's words if possible)
Onset and development of problems, where took place, what was done
Signs and symptoms, location, severity, duration, frequency; changes and effect on client; meaning of disease to client
Factors that alleviated or aggravated symptoms
Client's knowledge of disease, procedures, and planned therapy
Client's adaptation to disorder if chronic
Laboratory and diagnostic tests done during hospitalization
Medications and treatments since discharge
Homebound status

PSYCHOSOCIAL HISTORY

Consumption of coffee, alcohol, tobacco; amount, frequency, type
General appearance
Living arrangements, significant persons and relations with them
Occupation and income, ability to pay for health care (Medicare, Medicaid, CHAMPUS, private insurance, Workman's Compensation)
Education, degrees, profession if applicable
Recreation and interests; retirement if applicable
Friends, community involvement, church activities
English as a second language or no English spoken
Emergency contact and telephone number

FAMILY HISTORY

Health status of parents, spouse, siblings, children, including deaths with ages and causes
Health status of grandparents and other blood relatives
Roles and responsibilities of family members and whether they work outside the home
Relationships with family members, activities, response to stress or crisis
History of abuse by family members or relatives
Marital relationship
Family members' history of heart conditions, diabetes, cancer, or other diseases
Adaptation of family members to care of client in the home

REVIEW OF SYSTEMS

Height, Weight, Vital Signs, Temperature

Pulmonary System
- Chronic obstructive pulmonary disease (COPD); pneumonia; upper respiratory infection; influenza; throat infections; pain in throat, nose, chest; congestion of or discharge from nose; epistaxis; hemoptysis; cough and sputum with characteristics; dyspnea with or without exertion; wheezing; abnormal breath sounds

Cardiovascular System
- Chest pain; arm, throat or jaw pain; edema; dyspnea; palpitations; hypertension; phlebitis; diminished circulation to extremities; heart condition; claudication; paresthesia

Neurologic System
- Headaches; fainting; seizures; tremors; dizziness; paralysis; changes in sensory perception (touch, taste, smell, vision, hearing), mentation changes; use of glasses, contact lens, hearing aid; motor changes (gait, coordination); sleep/rest patterns; speech

Gastrointestinal System
- Hepatitis; diverticulosis; gallstones; peptic ulcer; colitis; ostomy; cirrhosis; abdominal pain; nausea; vomiting; diarrhea; constipation; hemorrhoids; indigestion; swallowing; anorexia, excessive flatus, belching, or eructation; changes in stool color, consistency, or frequency; chewing problems; presence of dentures and fit; 24-hour dietary intake; special diets

Endocrine System
- Diabetes, thyroid condition, polyuria, polydipsia, appetite, tolerance of heat or cold, Cushing's syndrome

Hematologic System
- Anemia; skin hemorrhages, bruising, petechiae; previous transfusions; bleeding from any site; weakness; pallor; night sweats

Musculoskeletal System
- Fractures; arthritis; osteoporosis; pain or stiffness in joints; redness, swelling, heat in joints; limited range of motion (ROM); fatigue; weakness, pain in muscles; assistive devices; ability to perform activities of daily living

Renal/Urinary Systems
- Difficulty in urination, dysuria, dribbling, incontinence, urgency, frequency, retention, hematuria, calculi, urinary tract infections (UTI), glomerulonephritis, prostatic hypertrophy, chronic renal failure; fluid intake/output for 24 hours

Integumentary System
- Rash; pruritis; lesions; change in skin color, nails, or hair; scar tissue; dryness; oiliness

Reproductive System
- Lesions on or drainage from penis or vuiva; rashes or irritations on penis or vulva; vaginal infections; sexually transmitted disease; infertility; use of birth control; sexual pattern and satisfaction or difficulties; age at menarche and menopause; abnormal vaginal bleeding or menstrual irregularity; number of pregnancies, live births, abortions; complications of pregnancy; impotence; last menstrual period (LMP); last Pap smear, mammogram, and breast examination; lumps or pain in breasts; discharge from breasts; penile implant

Psychiatric
- Depression, nervousness, chronic anxiety or worry; mood swings; decreased self-concept; effect of stress; thoughts of suicide; hallucinations, delusions, paranoid manifestations

◣ *Pulmonary System Assessment*

PAST HISTORY

Lung and Airway Disorders
- Bronchitis
- Asthma
- Emphysema
- Tuberculosis
- Pneumonia
- Pleurisy, pleural effusion
- Lung malignancy
- Influenza, colds, and frequency
- Chest surgery or injury

Signs and Symptoms of Respiratory Distress
- Dyspnea with or without exertion, breathlessness
- Coughing and sneezing: amount and frequency
- Sputum: amount, consistency, color
- Chest pain
- Wheezing

Family History
- Respiratory disorders: acute and chronic
- Allergies, eczema

Allergies
- Plants
- Animals
- Foods
- Drugs
- Environmental pollutants

Immunizations
- Pneumonia
- Influenza

Activities of Daily Living (ADL)
- Position during sleep for optimal breathing
- Amount of exercise and effects on breathing
- Abilities for personal self-care and/or ADL
- Homebound status

Psychosocial History
- Tobacco consumption: amount and duration of use
- Alcohol consumption
- Personality traits, anxiety
- Home environment and exposure to irritants (odors, smoke, sprays, allergens, air conditioning, humidity)
- Adaptation to illness or chronic condition

Past Treatments and Diagnostic Procedures
- Desensitization therapy
- Medications (prescribed and OTC) taken for respiratory or other condition
- Breathing treatments (nebulizer, physiotherapy, breathing exercises)
- Lung biopsy, thoracentesis, bronchoscopy
- Chest x-ray studies, pulmonary function studies, sputum culture, laboratory tests for drug levels and arterial blood gas levels (ABGs)
- Past or recent hospitalizations

PRESENT HISTORY

Chief Complaint, Including Onset and Length of Time Present

Signs and Symptoms
- Respiratory rate, ease, depth; factors precipitating increases or other changes
- Dyspnea, orthopnea, tachypnea
- Chest pain
- Fatigue, activity intolerance
- Cyanosis, pallor
- Productive or nonproductive cough and characteristics (amount, color, consistency)
- Use of accessory muscles

Knowledge of Disease and Planned Home Therapy

Present Treatments and Diagnostic Procedures
- Laboratory and diagnostic tests and results
- Use of oxygen
- Medications (oral, inhalants)
    Bronchodilators
    Sedatives
    Steroids
    Tranquilizers
    Others

PHYSICAL EXAMINATION

Inspection
- Symmetry of chest (shape, expansion, movement)
- Color of lips, ears, nails
- Breathing pattern using mouth, diaphragm, chest, abdomen; use of accessory muscles
- Nail bed capillary refill
- Clubbing of fingers
- Confusion
- Fatigue
- Restlessness
- Diaphoresis

Palpation
- Chest for pain or masses
- Skin for warmth, dryness, smoothness
- Intercostal muscles for firmness, smoothness, bulging, retraction

- Vocal and tactile fremitus and location of increases or decreases
- Symmetry of anterior and posterior chest expansion

Percussion
- Lung field resonance: hyperresonance, dull sound, flatness, tympany
- Pitch, intensity, duration (anteriorly and posteriorly with bilateral comparison)

Auscultation
- Voice sounds for intensity at airways and periphery
- Adventitious sounds such as rales, rhonchi, wheezes, stridor; note position in lungs (½, ¼, bases)
- Normal breath sounds such as bronchial, tracheal, vesicular, bronchovesicular, and whether diminished or absent and location
- Breath sounds heard in areas where not expected (abnormal)

◣ *Cardiovascular System Assessment*

PAST HISTORY

Cardiovascular Disorders
- Hypertension
- Congestive heart failure
- Stroke
- Coronary artery disease
- Myocardial Infarction
- Thrombophlebitis
- Leg ulcer, varicose veins
- Arterial insufficiency
- Heart surgery (bypass, valvular)

Signs and Symptoms of Cardiac or Vascular Distress
- Pain in chest, arms, throat, jaw or extremities
- Heart palpitations
- Dyspnea, orthopnea, cough
- Neck vein distention

- Edema
- Cold, numbness, or tingling of extremities
- Discoloration of extremities
- Dizziness, weakness

Family History
- Heart or vascular condition; acute or chronic
- Hypertension
- Coronary heart disease
- Diabetes mellitus
- Asthma
- Stroke
- Obesity

Allergies
- Medications
- Foods

Activities of Daily Living (ADL)
- Sleeping with head elevated
- Abilities for personal self-care, and/or ADL
- Exercising and effect on pulse and respiration
- Homebound status
- Special diet: low-cholesterol/fat, low-sodium, low-calorie

Psychosocial History
- Tobacco, caffeine, and alcohol consumption; daily and over period of years
- Personality traits
- Occupation and work-related stress
- Adaptation to illness or chronic condition

Past Treatments and Diagnostic Procedures
- Pacemaker insertion
- Holter monitor
- Medications (prescribed and OTC) taken for heart or other condition
- Cardiac rehabilitation
- Electrocardiogram, echocardiogram, angiogram, cardiac catheterization, x-ray studies, stress test
- Laboratory tests for enzymes, lipid panel, electrolytes, pro-thrombin time
- Cardiac or vascular surgery
- Angioplasty, laser treatments
- Past or recent hospitalizations

PRESENT HISTORY

Chief Complaint, Including Onset and Length of Time Present

Signs and Symptoms
- Blood pressure; pulse rate (beats/min) and regularity; apical pulse; factors that cause changes in baselines; changes with position or posture (sitting, standing, lying)
- Onset, duration, precipitating factors if any, alleviating factors if relevant
- Chest, arm, throat, jaw pain; aching in legs; pain in leg calf; edema and/or redness
- Dyspnea, orthopnea
- Palpitations
- Edema, weight gain
- Changes in pulse rate (slow or rapid), and regularity
- Change in mentation; headache
- Insomnia, restlessness, fatigue
- Changes in skin color (pallor, redness, cyanosis)

Knowledge of Disease and Planned Home Therapy

Present Treatments and Diagnostic Procedures
- Laboratory and diagnostic tests and results
- Use of oxygen
- Medications (oral, sublingual)
    Antihypertensives
    Vasodilators
    Cardiotonics
    Diuretics
    Anticoagulants
    Aspirin
    Nitrates
    Others

PHYSICAL EXAMINATION

Inspection
- Symmetry of chest, legs, and arms
- Pulsations in the aortic area, pulmonary area, right-ventricular area, apical or left-ventricular area
- Skin of arms, hands, legs, and feet for color and texture (pink, warm, smooth, dry); color change in extremities when dangling or elevated (should return to normal in 10 seconds)
- Hair distribution on legs and arms; clubbing of fingers

- Rashes, scars, ulcers, and exudate and discoloration (brownish color, eschar, irregular shape of ulcer, chronic venous stasis)
- Veins flush with skin surface or venous enlargement
- Capillary refill of nail beds of less than 3 seconds

Palpation
- Skin of extremities smooth, dry, warm to touch
- Masses in extremities or chest
- Pain or tenderness in chest or extremities
- Veins smooth and full or dilated and tortuous
- Cardiac thrills (pulsations of the heart that feel like the throat of a purring cat)
- Radial pulse rate and characteristics
- Femoral, popliteal, carotid, temporal, and dorsalis pedis pulse rates and characteristics
- Apical pulse, point of maximum impulse (PMI), and other areas of pulsations of the heart
- Edema in legs: dependent or pitting
- Calf for signs of phlebitis (tenderness, tension)
- Homans' sign: present or absent

Auscultation
- Apical and radial pulses, noting rate, regularity, and pulse deficit
- Apical pulse, noting rate, regularity, intensity
- Blood pressure, using brachial artery and noting Korotkoff signs and pulse pressure
- Heart sounds (S_1 and S_2), extra heart sounds (S_3 and S_4)
- Murmur, noting timing, location, sound distribution
- Clicks and snaps, noting timing, intensity, and pitch
- Friction rub
- Carotid artery for bruits

◣ *Neurologic System Assessment*

PAST HISTORY
Neurologic Motor and Sensory Disorders
- Multiple sclerosis
- Muscular dystrophy

- Cerebrovascular accident (CVA)
- Seizure disorder
- Head trauma
- Spinal cord injury
- Motor or sensory aberrations
- Parkinson's disease
- Hearing, vision, speech impairments
- Surgeries (craniotomy, laminectomy)

Signs and Symptoms of Neurologic Disease
- Headaches
- Tremors
- Paralysis
- Gait disturbance
- Mental retardation
- Behavioral changes (confusion, disorientation, mood, affect)
- Speech changes
- Mentation changes
- Seizure activity

Family History
- Neurologic disorders; acute or chronic
- Hypertension
- Stroke
- Epilepsy
- Alzheimer's disease/dementia
- Huntington's chorea
- Diabetes mellitus

Allergies
- Medications

Activities of Daily Living (ADL)
- Abilities for personal self care and/or ADL
- Amount of independence or dependence
- Rest/sleep/nap patterns (hours/24 hours; frequency; times; length; use and effect of sleeping aids, prescribed or OTC; factors that promote or prevent sleep)
- Homebound status

Psychosocial History
- Drug, alcohol, tobacco consumption, daily and over period of years
- Occupational exposure to toxic agents that affect mental functioning

- Personality traits
- Adaptation to illness or chronic condition

Past Treatments and Diagnostic Procedures
- Medications (prescribed or OTC) taken for neurologic or other condition
- Cerebral angiogram, lumbar puncture, scans, myogram, ocular studies, blood flow studies, magnetic resonance imaging (MRI), electroencephalogram (EEG), skull or spinal x-ray studies
- Laboratory tests for electrolyte panel, cultures (cerebrospinal fluid, blood)
- Cranial or spinal surgery
- Past or recent hospitalizations

PRESENT HISTORY

Chief Complaint, Including Onset, Length of Time Present, and Precipitating Factors

Signs and Symptoms
- Anxiety
- Sleep pattern changes, insomnia
- Headaches, back pain, dizziness
- Memory deficits; changes in level of consciousness and behavior
- Sensory problems (paresthesias)
- Motor problems (imbalance, paralysis, tic)
- Quadriplegia, paraplegia
- Fatigue; mood and communication problems
- Aggressive behavior

Knowledge of Disease and Planned Home Therapy

Present Treatments and Diagnostic Procedures
- Laboratory and diagnostic tests and results
- Medications (oral)
    Sedatives
    Hypnotics
    Narcotic and nonnarcotic analgesics
    Tranquilizers
    Antidepressants
    Anticonvulsants
    Others

PHYSICAL EXAMINATION

Inspection

- Vital signs, including temperature
- Motor function (gait; coordination; balance; tremors during rest or intentional; ataxia; speech difficulty; dysphagia; symmetry of muscle size; loss of muscle mass; muscle tone for spasticity, flaccidity; muscle strength in upper and lower extremities; involuntary muscle movements; range of motion in all joints)
- Sensory function (touch, pain, proprioception, vision, hearing, discriminatory sensation, temperature)
- Mental function (level of consciousness; orientation to time, place, and person; memory; attention span; ability to make judgments and problem solve; ability to communicate; anger; agitation; euphoria; depression; lability)
- General appearance (posture, personal hygiene, facial expression)

Spinal Nerve Innervation

C-4: Motor function from neck downward
C-5: Raising of arms
C-5 through C-6: Flexion of elbow
C-6: Dorsiflexion of wrist
C-7: Extension of elbow
C-8: Flexion of finger
T-1: Abduction of finger
T-1 through T-8: Movement of thoracic musculature
T-6 through T-12: Movement of abdominal musculature
L-1 through L-3: Flexion of hip
L-2 through L-4: Extension of knee
L-4 through L-5: Dorsiflexion of ankle
L-5 through S-1: Extension of great toe
S-1 through S-2: Plantar flexion of ankle
S-3 through S-5: Movement of perianal muscle

Cranial Nerve Innervation

   I. Olfactory (sensory—smell): Odor identification, such as coffee, spice, or alcohol
  II. Optic (sensory—vision): Snellen chart for visual acuity; gross confrontation test; periphery test of four visual-field quadrants
 III. Oculomotor (motor—pupil constriction; eyelid and extraocular movements): Use penlight for pupil constric-

tion; size and shape; ptosis of eyelid; accommodation to finger moving toward nose

IV. Trochlear (motor—eye movement inward and downward): Convergence of eyes inward when finger moves toward nose

V. Trigeminal (motor—temporal, masseter muscles and lateral jaw movement; sensory—maxillary, mandibular facial and ophthalmic sensitivity): Movement of jaw and mastication muscles and ability to open and close jaws; sensitivity to sharp and dull object applied to each area with eyes closed; sensitivity of cornea to application of cotton wisp

VI. Abducent (motor—eye abduction): Eye muscle movement for disconjugate gaze; eyes not moving together

VII. Facial (motor—facial expressions; sensory—taste): Face and scalp muscle movement; grimacing; closing eyes tightly; discriminating salty and sweet tastes

VIII. Acoustic (sensory—hearing with cochlear division and balance with vestibular division): Weber's and Rinne's tests for auditory acuity; balance testing done by physician

IX. Glossopharyngeal (motor—pharynx; sensory—taste and pharyngeal sensation): Swallowing ability and gag reflex; rise of uvula when saying *ah;* taste sensation at posterior tongue; hoarseness

X. Vagus (motor—pharynx, larynx, palate; sensory—pharynx, larynx): Ability to speak, phonation; swallowing and gag reflex with nerve IX

XI. Spinal accessory (motor—sternocleidomastoid and trapezius muscle movements): Shoulder shrugging and turning head against resistance

XII. Hypoglossal (motor—tongue): Tongue protrusion, deviation, and strength

Palpation
- Symmetry, shape, masses, depressions of head and muscles
- Carotid and temporal pulses, comparing strength and quality bilaterally
- Muscles for tone, shape, size, and atrophy
- Skeletal muscle reflexes
    Biceps and brachioradial (C-5, C-6)
    Triceps (C-6, C-7, C-8)

Patellar (L-2, L-3, L-4)
Achilles (S-1, S-2)
Upper abdominal (T-8, T-9, T-10)
Lower abdominal (T-10, T-11, T-12)
Perineal or anal (S-3, S-4, S-5)
Cremasteric (L-1, L-2)

Auscultation
- Blood pressure
- Bruits over eyes, temples, mastoid processes

Gastrointestinal System Assessment

PAST HISTORY

Gastrointestinal Disorders
- Peptic ulcer
- Inflammatory bowel disease
- Diverticulosis
- Hepatitis
- Cirrhosis
- Enteritis
- Gallbladder disease
- Hemorrhoids
- Hernia
- Esophageal varices
- Gastrointestinal hemorrhage or surgery

Signs and Symptoms of Gastrointestinal Distress
- Nausea, vomiting
- Weight changes
- Anorexia
- Indigestion/heartburn
- Dysphagia
- Constipation
- Diarrhea
- Blood in vomitus or stool
- Abdominal pain/distention

Family History
- Gastrointestinal disorders: acute and chronic
- Ulcers
- Hemorrhoids
- Colorectal malignancies
- Hepatitis
- Obesity

Allergies
- Foods
- Medications

Patterns of Bowel Elimination and Nutrition Intake
- Characteristics, frequency, color, and amount of stool
- Increased flatus
- Laxatives or enemas used; type and frequency
- Food likes and dislikes, appetite, amount, frequency, ability to chew, dentures and denture pain
- Caloric intake (24-hour intake)
- Cultural influences
- Weight loss or gain/ideal body weight

Activities of Daily Living
- Abilities for self-care (feeding and toileting)
- Special diet; low or high calorie
- Homebound status

Psychosocial History
- Tobacco, caffeine, alcohol use: daily and over period of years
- Personality traits
- Stress, anxiety, and effect on elimination and nutrition
- Adaptation to illness or chronic condition

Past Treatments and Diagnostic Procedures
- Presence of bowel diversion: type, care, and response
- Medications (prescribed and OTC) taken for gastrointestinal or other conditions
- Proctoscopy, gastroscopy, colonscopy, scans, magnetic resonance imaging (MRI), stomach and bowel x-ray studies, gallbladder x-ray studies, liver biopsy
- Stool for occult blood, ova, parasites, toxins, culture
- Gastrointestinal or mouth surgery
- Past or recent hospitalizations

PRESENT HISTORY

Chief Complaint, Including Onset and Length of Time Present and Severity

Signs and Symptoms
- Pain and characteristics
- Anorexia, nausea, vomiting
- Heartburn, flatulence, eructation
- Constipation, diarrhea, absence of bowel movements
- Weight changes
- Jaundice, pruritis
- Blood in vomitus or stool; black, tarry or chalky stool; coffee-ground vomitus

Knowledge of Disease and Planned Home Therapy

Present Treatment
- Diagnostic procedures and results
- Results of complete blood counts, electrolytes, blood urea nitrogen, bilirubin, lipase, amylase, and other laboratory tests
- Nasogastric tube feedings, total parenteral nutrition
- Gastric decompression, suctioning
- Enemas, bowel irrigation
- Medications (oral, rectal)
    - Vitamins
    - Antacids
    - Antiemetics
    - Antidiarrheals
    - H_2 antagonists
    - Laxatives, stool softeners, suppositories
    - Others

PHYSICAL EXAMINATION

Inspection
- Body contour, abdomen, umbilicus (shape, protrusion, size)
- Height and weight, noting amount over or under normal for age, size, sex, and frame
- Skin: rash, smoothness, scars, edema, color
- Drainage from nasogastric tube or ostomy
- Stool and vomitus for abnormal constituents or consistency
- Mouth for pain, caries, dentures, stomatitis, lesions, bleeding, odor
- Anus for pain, itching, inflammation, bleeding, hemorrhoids
- Jaundice of skin, sclera, and mucous membranes

Auscultation
- Absence of bowel sounds for 5 minutes in four quadrants
- Presence of bowel sounds in four quadrants, including frequency, pitch, loudness, rushing, swishing, gurgling

Percussion
- Abdominal distention for dull, tympanic, or wavelike sounds
- Bladder distention for dull sounds

Palpation
- Abdominal masses, pain, nodes, distention, tautness, warmth or coldness
- Skin turgor

◣ *Endocrine System Assessment*

PAST HISTORY

Endocrine Disorders
- Diabetes mellitus
- Diabetes insipidus
- Addison's disease
- Hyperthyroidism or hypothyroidism
- Pituitary tumor
- Surgery (thyroidectomy)

Signs and Symptoms
- Weight changes, appetite and hydration changes
- Mentation, visual disturbances
- Libido, menstrual disorders
- Weakness, fatigue, changes in muscle activity
- Changes in respiration, pulse, temperature; presence of dyspnea, palpitations
- Changes in elimination patterns (bowel and urinary)
- Frequent infections

Family History
- Endocrine disorders: acute and chronic
- Diabetes mellitus
- Thyroid disease

- Hypertension
- Obesity

Allergies
- Foods
- Medications
- Iodine

Patterns of Diabetes Mellitus Care
- Years disease present
- Insulin/hypoglycemic therapy
- Special dietary control

Activities of Daily Living
- Abilities for self-care and/or ADL
- Ability to follow regimen for diabetes mellitus
- Special diet: diabetic, low calorie, low fat
- Exercise requirements
- Homebound status

Psychosocial History
- Tobacco, alcohol use; daily and over periods of years
- Personality traits
- Stress from occupation or chronic condition
- Adaptation to illness or chronic condition
- Cultural preferences in diet

Past Treatments and Diagostic Procedures
- Medications (prescribed or OTC) taken for endocrine or other conditions
- Ultrasonograms, scans, x-ray studies of skull
- Laboratory tests: complete blood counts, glucose, thyroid function, electrolytes
- Exposure to or treatment with radiation
- Surgery of any gland
- Past or recent hospitalizations

PRESENT HISTORY

Chief Complaint, Including Onset and Duration, Severity

Signs and Symptoms
- Weakness, fatigue, muscle weakness, twitching, spasms, numbness, tingling, cramping, tremors, wasting, reduced strength
- Bone pain, aching
- Nervousness, irritability, drowsiness, confusion
- Libido changes

- Anxiety, depression, apathy, syncope
- Pruritis
- Headache, malaise
- Anorexia, nausea, vomiting
- Polyuria, polydipsia

Knowledge of Disease and Planned Home Therapy

Present Treatments and Diagnostic Procedures
- Diagnostic procedures and test results
- Medications (oral, parenteral)
    Insulin
    Hypoglycemics
    Steroids
    Thyroid preparation
    Male/female sex hormones

PHYSICAL EXAMINATION

Inspection
- Vital signs, height and weight
- Symmetry of extremities, edema (location, type, grade)
- Skin color, turgor, dryness, oiliness, texture, edema, distribution of fat
- Nail texture; hair amount, distribution, texture
- Moon face, protruding eyeballs, thickening of tongue, hoarseness, breath odor

Palpation
- Decreased deep reflexes or absence of reflexes
- Thyroid enlargement, hardness, nodules or asymmetry (thyroid normally not palpable)

◣ Hematologic System Assessment

PAST HISTORY

Blood Disorders and Disorders of Blood-Forming Organs
- Anemias
- Leukemia, lymphoma

- Immune disorders
- Hemophilia
- Other blood dyscrasias
- Surgery (splenectomy)

Signs and Symptoms of Hematologic Diseases
- Weight loss
- Fatigue, weakness, pallor, shortness of breath
- Pain in bones or joints
- Bleeding from any site, bruising on body parts
- Enlarged nodes

Family History
- Hematologic disorders: acute and chronic
- Anemias
- Hemophilia
- Sickle cell trait
- Allergies
- Malignancies

Allergies
- Foods
- Medications
- Chemicals

Activities of Daily Living (ADL)
- Abilities for self-care and/or ADL
- Special diet; high iron, folic acid
- Homebound status

Psychosocial History
- Personality traits
- Life-style, including drug habits and sexual preference
- Occupation and exposure to chemicals, lead, other toxic agents or environmental pollutants
- Alcohol consumption: amount and duration
- Adaptation to illness or chronic condition

Past Treatments and Diagnostic Procedures
- Transfusions of blood or blood products and response
- Bone marrow transplant
- Medications (prescribed and OTC) taken for hematologic or other condition
- Bone marrow puncture, scans, node biopsy
- Laboratory tests: complete blood count, platelets, reticulo-cytes, prothrombin time, iron level

- Past or recent hospitalization
- Surgery of any kind

PRESENT HISTORY

Chief Complaint, Including Onset and Length of Time Present

Signs and Symptoms
- Change in behavior, level of consciousness
- Fatigue, weakness, dizziness, headache, pallor, shortness of breath
- Pain in bones or joints, mouth or tongue
- Anorexia, nausea, emaciation
- Night sweats
- Small or large hemorrhages on skin
- Bleeding from any site (prolonged or excessive)

Knowledge of Disease and Planned Home Therapy

Present Treatments and Diagnostic Procedures
- Laboratory and diagnostic tests and results
- Medications (oral, parenteral)
    Antiinfectives
    Antiinflammatories
    Immunosuppressives
    Antineoplastics
    Tranquilizers
    Antituberculins
    Iron, folic acid
    Vitamin B_{12}
    Others

PHYSICAL EXAMINATION

Inspection
- Vital signs, height and weight
- Ecchymoses or petechiae
- Buccal cavity for edema, redness, bleeding, ulceration
- Skin color, texture, pruritis
- General appearance for dehydration, cachexia

Palpation
- Size of liver, spleen
- Lymph nodes: enlargement, tenderness, movement, size, and consistency in neck, axilla, and inguinal areas
- Joint swelling

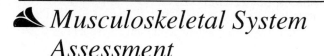 *Musculoskeletal System Assessment*

PAST HISTORY

Muscle, Bone and Joint Disorders
- Arthritis and type
- Bursitis
- Fractures
- Gout
- Low back syndrome
- Osteoporosis
- Paget's disease
- Ruptured disk
- Bone malignancy
- Neuromuscular disease
- Musculoskeletal surgery or injury (amputation, hip/knee replacement, laminectomy)

Signs and Symptoms of Musculoskeletal Disorders
- Pain, swelling in joints
- Muscle weakness, twitching or deterioration
- Poor coordination or balance in walking or other movements
- Changes in range of motion (ROM) and activity and mobility
- Presence of cast or splint or use of traction for fracture or to provide support
- Paralysis
- Burning, numbness, tingling in extremities
- Contracture(s), abnormal body alignment
- Pathologic fractures

Family History
- Joint or bone disorders: acute and chronic
- Neurologic motor deficits
- Neuromuscular disease
- Musculoskeletal disease

Allergies
- Foods
- Medications
- Chemicals

Activities of Daily Living (ADL)
- Abilities for self-care and/or ADL
- Use of aids for eating, toileting, dressing, personal hygiene/care
- Ability to use hands and fingers to grasp, hold objects
- Ability to walk; energy and endurance and effect on joints
- Special diet: low uric acid, high calcium, low calorie
- Homebound status

Psychosocial History
- Tobacco, alcohol, and chemical consumption; daily and over period of years
- Personality traits
- Occupation and need for mobility and dexterity; proneness to accidents
- Adaptation to disability or chronic illness

Past Treatments and Diagnostic Procedures
- Medications (prescribed and OTC) taken for bone, muscle, or joint disease
- Physical and occupational therapy and rehabilitation
- Cold or heat applications
- X-ray studies, scans, electromyogram, myelogram
- Laboratory tests for electrolytes, uric acid, sedimentation rate, rheumatoid factor, complete blood count, alkaline phosphatase
- Use of TENS stimulator
- Bone or joint surgery, use of cast or traction
- Past or recent hospitalizations

PRESENT HISTORY

Chief Complaint, Including Onset and Length of Time Present

Signs and Symptoms
- Pain in affected area
- Redness, swelling, warmth in affected area
- Weakness, fatigue
- Loss of mobility, coordination or balance, or weight-bearing ability
- Limited ROM
- Loss of sensation in extremity
- Muscle spasms, reduced muscle strength and mass

- Diminished peripheral pulse in extremities, delayed capillary refill

Knowledge of Disease and Planned Home Therapy

Present Treatments and Diagnostic Procedures
- Laboratory and diagnostic tests and results
- Use of trapeze, cast, brace, traction, aids for ADL
- Presence of limb prosthesis
- Bed rest, chair, amount of activity allowed
- Medications (oral)

    Analgesics
    Antirheumatics
    Antiinflammatories (steroid and nonsteroid)
    Muscle relaxants
    Antibiotics
    Stool softeners
    Vitamin and mineral supplement (calcium and vitamin D)
    Others

PHYSICAL EXAMINATION

Inspection
- Symmetry of legs and arms, shoulders, clavicles, scapulae, musculature
- Full ROM of all joints; degree of motion
- Ability to sit, lie, get up, stand, walk; posture
- Deformities or contractures, deviations, changes in contour
- Presence of scoliosis, kyphosis, lordosis, hammer toe
- Gait, coordination, balance, and endurance
- Body alignment in supine, prone, side-lying positions
- Amputation
- Presence of enforced immobilization
- Skin of casted extremity or body part (pink, warm, dry with sensation present, peripheral pulse felt)
- Ability to move toes/fingers on casted part

Palpation
- Warmth and pain at joint(s) or injury
- Crepitus from joint motion
- Muscles for strength, mass, tone
- Reflexes for presence
- Tenderness on pressure or movement
- Thickening, bony enlargement around joints

◣ *Renal/Urinary System Assessment*

PAST HISTORY

Kidney and Bladder Disorders
- Renal failure
- Pyelonephritis, glomerulonephritis
- Calculi
- Urinary tract infection
- Neurogenic bladder
- Prostatic hypertrophy
- Hypertension
- Kidney transplant
- Renal or bladder surgery

Signs and Symptoms of Renal/Urinary Disorders
- Pain in kidney or bladder area
- Urinary incontinence, bladder distention
- Retention, hesitancy, dribbling, urgency, frequency, burning, dysuria, nocturia
- Urine amount, color, odor, sedimentation, hematuria, pus, mucus, clarity and odor
- Polyuria, oliguria, anuria
- Weight gain
- Type and amount of fluid intake and output for 24 hours
- Edema, distention, fever, bruising, restlessness, insomnia
- Skin: dryness, itching, poor turgor; dry lips and mucous membranes
- Mentation changes

Family History
- Renal or bladder disorders: acute and chronic
- Congenital or familial renal or urinary conditions
- Hypertension
- Connective tissue disorder
- Diabetes mellitus

Allergies
- Foods
- Medications

Activities of Daily Living
- Abilities for self-care (toileting)
- Special diet: low in salt, potassium, calcium, or protein

Psychosocial History
- Tobacco, caffeine, alcohol use; daily and over period of years
- Personality traits
- Sexually transmitted diseases
- Exposure to environmental or occupational nephrotoxic substance (heavy metals, carbon tetrachloride, phenols, pesticides)
- Adaptation to illness or chronic condition

Past Treatments and Diagnostic Procedures
- Presence of urinary diversion: type, care, and response
- Medications (prescribed and OTC) taken for renal/urinary or other conditions
- Ultrasonogram; scans; intravenous pyelogram; x-ray studies of kidney, ureter, and bladder; cystoscopy; kidney biopsy
- Laboratory tests for blood urea nitrogen, creatinine, urinalysis, urine culture, others
- Surgeries, trauma, or use of instruments in manipulation of tract during procedures
- Past or recent hospitalizations

PRESENT HISTORY

Chief Complaint, Including Onset, Duration, Precipitating Factors, Alleviating Factors If Relevant

Signs and Symptoms
- Pain
- Weight gain, edema
- Changes in urinary pattern
- Changes in urinary characteristics
- Anorexia, nausea, vomiting
- Thirst, dry skin, poor turgor
- Weakness, muscle cramping
- Pruritis, visual changes
- Fluid imbalance
- Electrolyte imbalance

Knowledge of Disease and Planned Home Therapy

Present Treatments and Diagnostic Procedures
- Diagnostic procedures and laboratory results
- Current fluid requirements, restrictions
- Use of urinary drainage devices or catheterizations
- Hemodialysis or peritoneal dialysis
- Dietary restrictions
- Medications (oral)
  Analgesics
  Diuretics
  Antiinfectives
  Steroids
  Anticoagulants
  Others

PHYSICAL EXAMINATION

Inspection
- Blood pressure elevation
- Skin color, pruritis, petichiae, ecchymoses, dryness, urate crystals
- Oral mucous membranes dry, redness, ulcerations
- Edema of hands, feet, sacral region, legs; abdominal distention; neck vein distention
- Urinary output and characteristics with or without indwelling catheter
- Behavior changes in regard to alertness, confusion, cognitive ability, level of consciousness
- Fruity or urine odor to breath, foul odor to urine
- Condition of urinary diversion site, dialysis shunt or abdominal site, urinary catheter site

Palpation
- Size and movement of kidneys
- Pain in kidney, bladder area
- Bladder distention, abdominal distention

Percussion
- Dullness over bladder if distended

◣ *Integumentary System Assessment*

PAST HISTORY

Skin Disorders
- Dermatitis
- Acne
- Eczema
- Infestations, scabies, lice
- Infections of skin, nails, scalp
- Skin malignancy
- Integumentary surgery (graft, cosmetic)

Signs and Symptoms of Integumentary Disorders
- Alopecia
- Dandruff
- Itching, breaks in skin
- Brittleness, ridging, redness, swelling of nails and cuticles
- Tendency to have infections, herpes simplex
- Sensitivity to sun, soaps, deodorants, perfumes, others
- Dryness, oiliness, excessive moisture, body odor
- Skin color changes
- Lumps or growths on the skin
- Bruising, delayed healing
- Ulcerations on extremity

Family History
- Integumentary disorders: acute and chronic
- Allergies, eczema

Allergies
- Foods
- Medications
- Cosmetics
- Environmental contacts

Activities of Daily Living
- Pattern of bathing, with frequency and time, soap used, toothpaste, shaving cream, and razor used, lotions and powders used
- Pattern of hair and nail care, with shampoo, rinse, nail pol-

ish used, hair tint used, cuticle trimming of toenails and fingernails
- Ability to perform personal self-care
- Homebound status

Psychosocial History
- Personality traits, anxiety
- Effect on body image if dermatitis or scarring present
- Occupational exposure to irritants such as dyes, sprays, perfumes, allergens
- Home environment exposure to allergens or irritants
- Adaptation to skin condition and effect on self-concept

Past Treatments and Diagnostic Procedures
- Desensitization therapy
- Medications (prescribed and OTC) taken for skin, hair, and nail conditions
- Skin biopsy
- Past or recent hospitalization

PRESENT HISTORY

Chief Complaint, Including Onset and Length of Time Present

Signs and Symptoms
- Changes in skin color, eruptions, breaks, and precipitating factors
- Hair loss and precipitating factors
- Nail changes and precipitating factors
- Injury from burns, with degree of damage to skin and pain

Knowledge of Disease and Planned Home Therapy

Present Treatments and Diagnostic Procedures
- Laboratory and diagnostic tests and results
- Medications (oral, topical)
    Antiinflammatories
    Antipruritics
    Antianxiety agents
    Antibiotics
    Antiacne agents
    Others

PHYSICAL EXAMINATION

Inspection
- Skin color for cyanosis, redness, jaundice, pallor, pigmentation
- Bleeding, bruising

- Presence of striae, rashes, urticaria, bites
- Skin dryness, oiliness, sweating, peeling, scaling, crusting
- Pruritis, odor, exudate, cleanliness
- Presence of edema, pain, breaks, or incision
- Lesions, lipomas, keloids, warts, nevi, with location and distribution
- Blisters, cellulitis, superficial infections
- Nail cleanliness, texture, thickness, angle, ingrown nails or hangnails, presence of infection
- Hair cleanliness, quantity, texture, distribution, color, odors, brittleness, oiliness or dryness; dandruff; baldness
- Scalp infestation, lesions

Palpation
- Skin temperature (hot or cool), texture (rough, bumpy, smooth, thin, thick)
- Skin turgor, elasticity, moisture, motility
- Tumors, cysts, or any elevation or lumps on skin or scalp
- Capillary return in nails and movement of nail plate when pressed

◣ *Reproductive System Assessment*

FEMALE

Past History

Reproductive Disorders
- Sexually transmitted diseases
- Tubal pregnancy
- Abortions
- Pelvic inflammatory disease (PID)
- Infertility
- Menstrual disorders
- Endometriosis
- Breast, uterus, ovarian, vaginal malignancy
- Surgery (mastectomy, hysterectomy)

Signs and Symptoms of Reproductive Organ Disorders
- Breast pain, tenderness, discharge; change in nipple
- Dyspareunia

- Rashes or irritations of genitalia with pruritis
- Discharge from meatus, vagina
- Dysuria, urinary frequency, retention, incontinence
- Dysmenorrhea, amenorrhea

Family History
- Breast or reproductive malignancy (ovary, uterus)
- Reproductive disorders: acute or chronic

Allergies
- Scented feminine powders, pads, tampons

Activities of Daily Living
- Birth control use and effectiveness
- Breast self-examination and frequency, pap smear, mammogram
- Ability for toileting and genitalia hygiene
- Presence of indwelling catheter and ability for care
- Homebound status

Psychosocial Status
- Personality traits
- Number of children, pregnancies
- Age at menarche; frequency, duration, regularity of periods; amount of pain, bleeding between periods; last menstrual period
- Date or age of menopause, hot flashes, discharge, pain
- Intercourse frequency if active; satisfaction level
- Sexual orientation; multiple partners if appropriate
- Ability to carry out role function to satisfaction
- Adaptation to infertility or other chronic condition

Past Treatments and Diagnostic Procedures
- Intrauterine device, birth control implant
- Medications (prescribed and OTC) taken for gynecologic disorder
- Ultrasound, diagnostic dilatation and curettage, mammogram, laparoscopy, amniocentesis, breast or endometrial biopsy
- Laboratory tests for pregnancy, complete blood count, typing and Rh factor
- Surgeries such as mastectomy (simple or radical), hysterectomy, salpingectomy, oophorectomy, cystocele or rectocele repair, tubal sterilization
- Past or recent hospitalizations

Present History

Chief Complaint, Including Onset and Length of Time Present

Signs and Symptoms
- Abdominal pain, dysmenorrhea, amenorrhea
- Abnormal vaginal bleeding or discharge
- Genital pruritis, irritation
- Infertility
- Dyspareunia
- Dysuria

Knowledge of Disease and Planned Home Therapy

Present Treatments and Diagnostic Procedures
- Laboratory and diagnostic tests and results
- Use of birth control devices
- Radiation or chemotherapy
- Presence of urinary catheter
- Medications (oral, vaginal)
    Hormones
    Antibiotics
    Antiinflammatories
    Analgesics
    Fertility therapy
    Others

Physical Examination

Inspection (as appropriate)
- External genitalia for discharge, redness, swelling, ulcerations or lesions, inflammation
- Bulging of vaginal walls
- Pediculosis pubis
- Cervical color, position, ulceration, bleeding, discharge, masses
- Vaginal mucosa color, inflammation, ulcers, masses
- Breast size, symmetry, contour, moles, dimpling, rash, edema, venous pattern, color
- Nipple size, shape, discharge, rash, ulcers, induration

Palpation
- Vaginal muscle tone, nodules, tenderness
- Cervical position, shape, mobility, consistency, tenderness
- Uterine size, shape, consistency, motility, tenderness, masses
- Breast elasticity, fullness, tenderness, nodosity

- Nipple elasticity, discharge with pressure
- Axillary nodes
- Masses in breasts: size, shape, location, consistency, motility, and tenderness

MALE

Past History

Reproductive Disorders
- Sexually transmitted diseases
- Hernia
- Prostatitis
- Hydrocele
- Epididymitis
- Prostatic hypertrophy
- Surgery (prostatectomy, penile implant, orchiectomy)

Signs and Symptoms of Reproductive Organ Disorders
- Pain in scrota, testes
- Discharge from penis
- Lesions on penis
- Impotence
- Urinary difficulty with urgency, frequency, weak stream; difficulty starting or stopping; incontinence; inability to empty bladder

Family History
- Reproductive disorders: acute or chronic

Activities of Daily Living
- Scrotal self-examination and frequency
- Ability for toileting and genitalia hygiene
- Presence of indwelling catheter and ability for care
- Homebound status

Psychosocial Status
- Personality traits
- Intercourse frequency if active; satisfaction level
- Sexual orientation; multiple partners if appropriate
- Ability to carry out role functions to satisfaction
- Effect of impotence on self-concept
- Adaptation to illness, impotence, or other chronic condition

Past Treatments and Diagnostic Procedures
- Penile device or implant
- Medications (prescribed and OTC) taken for reproductive disorders

- Cystoscopy, prostate biopsy
- Laboratory tests for urinary culture, complete blood count, enzymes
- Surgeries such as vasectomy, prostatectomy, herniorrhaphy, orchiectomy, penile implantation
- Past or recent hospitalizations

Present History

Chief Complaint, Including Onset and Length of Time Present

Signs and Symptoms
- Urinary abnormalities
- Pain in area
- Bleeding or discharge from penis
- Genital pruritis, irritation
- Penile lesions, ulcers, soreness

Knowledge of Disease and Planned Home Therapy

Present Treatments and Diagnostic Procedures
- Laboratory and diagnostic tests and results
- Use of aids/device for impotence
- Radiation or chemotherapy
- Presence of urinary catheter
- Medications (oral)
    Analgesics
    Antibiotics
    Antispasmodics
    Antiinflammatories
    Hormones
    Others

Physical Examination

Inspection
- Penis, meatus, and scrotum for ulcers, scars, rashes, nodules, discharge, swelling
- Circumcision and cleanliness
- Pediculosis pubis
- Urethral meatus position
- Size and shape of penis for age
- Contour of scrota; testes in place
- Breast and nipple symmetry, lesions, drainage, induration

Palpation
- Penile shaft for masses, tenderness, induration
- Testes for size, shape, consistency, tenderness, symmetry

- Prostate (rectal examination) softness, swelling, tenderness
- Hernia (via inguinal canal)
- Breasts or nipples for masses, tenderness, discharge on pressure

---

◣ *Eye, Ear, Nose, and Throat Assessment*

PAST HISTORY

Eye, Ear, Nose, and Throat Disorders
- Infections
- Glaucoma
- Cataracts
- Retinal detachment
- Tonsillitis
- Deviated septum, nasal polyps
- Allergic rhinitis
- Presbyopia, presbycusis
- Macular degeneration
- Surgery or injury (tonsillectomy, enucleation, cataract, keratoplasty)

Signs and Symptoms of Eye, Ear, Nose, or Throat Disorders
- Eye, ear, nose, or throat pain
- Discharge from eye, ear, nose
- Multiple colds
- Halitosis
- Buzzing or roaring in the ears
- Loss of equilibrium, vertigo
- Headaches
- Difficulty in swallowing
- Runny or stuffy nose, epistaxis
- Hoarseness
- Changes in visual, auditory acuity

Family History
- Eye, ear, nose, and throat disorders: acute and chronic
- Allergies

Foods
Medications
Environmental pollutants
Animals
Chemicals
Other

Activities of Daily Living

- Effects of visual or auditory impairment
- Use of glasses or contact lenses, eye prosthesis
- Use of hearing aid, lip reading, signing
- Loss of teeth and use of partial or full dentures
- Changes in sense of smell or taste
- Ability to perform self-care and care of glasses, contacts, prosthesis, dentures, hearing aid; ability to instill eye drops
- Response to hair sprays, noise levels, use of cotton swabs to clean ears, mouthwash
- Homebound status

Psychosocial History

- Effect of impairment on self-concept and occupation
- Personality traits, anxiety or depression
- Home environment exposure to allergens and irritants
- Effects of age and emotions on impairment or disease
- Adaptation to illness or impairment

Past Treatments and Diagnostic Procedures

- Densensitization therapy
- Medications (prescribed and OTC) taken for ear, eye, nose, or throat conditions or other conditions
- Last visit to dentist
- Date of most recent hearing or vision testing
- Laboratory tests for complete blood count, throat and nasal culture
- Skull x-ray studies, ocular procedures, laser procedure
- Surgeries such as tonsillectomy; cataract, corneal or retinal surgery; stapedectomy; mastoidectomy; submucous resection; polypectomy
- Past or recent hospitalization

PRESENT HISTORY

*Chief Complaint, Including Onset and Length of Time
Present*

Signs and Symptoms
- Pain or soreness in area
- Onset, duration, precipitating factors if any
- Dysphagia, difficulty in chewing
- Discharge from eye, ear, nose, throat
- Redness, swelling of eye, throat, nasal mucosa
- Epistaxis
- Changes in sensory perception and acuity
- Temperature elevation
- Hoarseness, loss of voice

Knowledge of Disease and Planned Home Therapy

Present Treatments and Diagnostic Procedures
- Laboratory and diagnostic tests and results
- Nasal packing, eye covering and dressing
- Eye, ear, throat irrigations
- Medications (oral, drops, topical)
     Analgesics
     Antibiotics
     Antiinflammatories
     Antiglaucoma agents
     Decongestants
     Others

PHYSICAL EXAMINATION

Inspection
- Symmetry of eyes, lids, brows, ears
- Lids: color, structure, edema, lesions
- Conjunctival and scleral color; opacities, markings of iris
- Pupils: size, shape, equality, reaction
- Intactness of extraocular movements
- Round, intact lacrimal glands; moisture or dryness of eyes
- External ears and auricles for lesions, deformities
- External ears and auricles for color, size, and position
- Canals and tympanic membranes, drainage
- Nose deformities, shape, symmetry, color, edema, drainage, bleeding, septal alignment
- Lips: color, dryness, cracking, edema, ulcers

- Gums, buccal cavity, and throat: color, swelling, bleeding, inflammation
- Tonsils (if present) for redness, swelling, pus

Palpation
- Pinnae for firmness, masses, elasticity, pain
- Structure of nose
- Tenderness in frontal or maxillary sinuses

◤ *Psychosocial Assessment*

MENTAL/COGNITIVE/LEARNING

Past History
- Educational level, educational achievements
- Attitude toward learning, ambition
- Difficulties in achieving educational or vocational goals
- Learning disabilities
- Interest in and willingness to learn about care and procedures
- Ability to listen, comprehend information given
- Ability to read and follow written instructions
- Vocabulary level and attention span
- Memory and ability to recall events
- Hearing, visual impairments
- English spoken or English as a second language

Present History
- Knowledge and understanding of illness and prognosis
- Cerebral function, including orientation, memory, recall, concentration, level of consciousness, communication pattern
- Sensory function, including vision, hearing
- Physical ability, strength for self-care
- Ability to think rationally, make judgments, problem solve
- Ability to express needs and maintain record of care and procedures

PSYCHIATRIC

Past History
- Psychiatric treatments, therapist
- Institution, including discharge dates

- Attitude toward treatments
- Medications prescribed, street or recreational drugs used
- Alcohol intake, amounts and length of time
- Suicide potential and precipitating factors
- Family history of mental disorders
- Relationships with family members and feelings about family

Present History

- Personal appearance: hygiene, clothing, physical characteristics, posture, mannerisms, facial expression, gestures
- Communication: tone, quality, flow, speed, use of associative looseness, flight of ideas, blocking, mutism, circumstantiality, word salad, echolalia
- Mood, affect
- Orientation to time, place, and person
- Delusions, hallucinations, illusions
- Coping ability and skills
- Stressors present
- Presence of chronic anxiety, worry, depression, insomnia
- Lives alone, isolation, support of significant others
- Lives with others but isolates self
- Participation in social interactions and activities

ADVANCE DIRECTIVES

- Awareness of Patient Self-Determination Act and its requirements and need for written information about advance directives
- Presence of an advance directive or form for health care:
    Living will
    Durable power of attorney for health care
- Family understanding of and conflicts about client's directives
- Knowledge of rights of autonomy and consent to or refusal of care in home
- Location of the advance directive or a copy

SPIRITUAL

- Religious beliefs and practices
- Feelings about a supreme being and how this view deals with illness
- Feelings about what will happen during illness
- Specific people helpful in religious life
- Religious symbols of importance (Bible, prayer, rosary, literature)

- Rituals of importance (communion, lighting Sabbath candles, Sacrament of the Sick)
- Religious restrictions (dietary laws, fasting, blood transfusion, medical treatment, birth control, abortion)
- Need for church attendance, priest, minister, or rabbi
- Identified spiritual leader

OCCUPATIONAL/RECREATIONAL

Past History
- Type of past employment
- Feelings about past employment
- Effects on health
- Reasons for leaving or changing vocation
- Presence of occupational hazards
- Hobbies and avocational activities

Present History
- Type of present employment/retirement
- Feelings about work/retirement
- Activity involved in work
- Effect of work environment on health (stress, chemicals, allergens)
- Plans for returning to work
- Housekeeping tasks (amount, kind, and participation)
- Need for more education or wish for vocational retraining
- Type, frequency, and degree of participation in play and recreation
- Effect of illness on recreational interests/hobbies
- Alternative interests and activities while illness is present
- Need to change recreational activities permanently
- Adaptation to retirement and role changes

◣ *Functional Assessment*

GENERAL
- Homebound status, complete bed rest, activity restrictions
- Independence or dependence in self-care and activities of daily living and desire and willingness to perform and adapt to limitations

- Degree of disability or handicap
- Presence of artificial limb
- Rehabilitation therapy by physical and/or occupational therapist

BATHING/GROOMING

- Ability to wash body (shower, tub bath, sponge bath)
- Use of aids to bathe (long handles for sponge, mitt on hand, bars in tub or shower, skid-proof tub, stool in tub or shower stall)
- Ability to brush teeth, hair (brushing, soaking, comb, dryer)
- Use of aids to brush teeth, hair (long and built-up handles, extension handles, mounted dryer or brush with suction cup, squeeze bottles for shampoo and toothpaste)
- Ability to shave or apply makeup (electric or safety razor, makeup kit)
- Use of aids to shave and apply makeup (shaving cream, mirror mounted with suction cups, built-up handles, hanging mirror around neck)

DRESSING/UNDRESSING

- Type of clothing easy to put on and remove (loose fitting; elastic at waist; closures with zipper, Velcro; shoes with Velcro closures; wide openings to slip over head or slip on with front open)
- Ability to dress and undress (buttons, zipper, tie laces, apply shoes and hose)
- Use of aids for dressing (hooks, zippers, long handles for hose and shoes)

TOILETING

- Ability to use bathroom, commode, bedpan, urinal
- Use of aids for toileting (grab bars; mounted toilet seat with side arms; tongs or mounting for toilet tissue)

FEEDING

- Ability to feed self; partial or total assistance; ability to prepare meal
- Use of aids for eating (china and flatware with suction cups; flatware with swivel; extension handles on flatware; bumper guard on dishes; bib for droppings; cuff to hold utensils)
- Use of aids for drinking (grippers on cup or glass; large handles; long, bending straws; suction cups for cup or glass)

MOBILITY

- Ability to walk, sit, stand, or lie down; amount of assistance needed
- Use of aids for mobility and movement (wheelchair, walker, crutches, cane, brace, elevated chair, adjustable seat or ejector chair, footstool, trapeze, holding rails, mechanical lift), hospital bed (electric or semielectric)

GENERAL ACTIVITIES

- Book holder; tilted table; clipboard; holder for pencil; card or pad holder; mounts on chair for radio, books; remote control for electric appliances
- Cars with special modifications, use of vans or buses with wheelchair lift
- Magnifiers, large print reading materials and telephone, amplifier on phone; special wiring for turning lights on or to alert client if deaf
- Automatic dialer and speaker phone attachment

◢ *Environmental Assessment*

HOME MODIFICATIONS

- Call bell, water, tissues, wastebasket, telephone within reach
- Space for equipment and supplies near client
- Space for storage of extra equipment and supplies
- Door wide enough to accommodate wheelchair, commode
- Laundry facilities for clothing, linens, supplies
- Bathroom, commode within access for use
- Hot and cold running water or means to heat water
- Ramp or other access to home
- Room on first floor (if possible or if client is unable to use stairway) with window, ventilation, temperature control
- Scales for weight in bathroom or near bed
- Hospital bed, trapeze connection
- Chair to assist client to standing position

SAFETY FACTORS

- Client's feeling of safety in home
- Cleanliness of home, disorder, noise, waste disposal

- Safety bars and aids for ambulation and activities of daily living (ADL)
- Refrigeration for foods, medications, supplies
- Proper lighting, arrangement of furniture, clear pathways
- Frayed or loose wiring or electrical connections, grounding of equipment
- Pathways dry and not slippery
- Side rails up or bed in low position if client using hospital bed
- Ability to perform ADL independently or amount of assistance needed
- Isolation or protective isolation procedures carried out
- Proper body alignment and positioning if client is on bed rest
- Use of restraints; smoking and precautions taken
- Presence of allergens, dust, animals, plants, sprays
- Use of aids for ADL and to prevent falls
- Available emergency numbers to call
- Proper cleansing and disinfection of reusable supplies
- Proper administration of medications and use of aids to ensure accuracy
- Proper hand washing procedure when required
- Presence of indoor plumbing vs drawn water and adequate storage for water
- Woodstove/kerosene heater safety and use and ability to fuel fire

◤ *Family Assessment*

PAST AND PRESENT PHYSICAL HISTORY

- Chronic illness of family members
- Functional abilities or disabilities
- Health practices
- Types of practitioners used
- Medications taken by family members
- Energy levels of family members
- Physical strength and ability to perform procedures

PAST AND PRESENT PSYCHOSOCIAL HISTORY

Emotional Status/Mental Abilities

- Changes in family life caused by client needs
- Willingness to perform procedures and care for client

- Support of client by member most likely to become caretaker
- Family attitude toward illness or disability
- Ability of family members to adapt
- Ability of family to set goals, problem solve
- Decision maker in the family
- Family stressors and ability to cope
- Relationship of client and family members
- Family arguments, separations, divorces

Psychiatric Disorders

- Chronic anxiety in family
- Depression of family member
- Behavior disorder of family member
- General mental health of family
- Presence of alcoholism, family violence, suicides, drug abuse

Cultural Influences

- Spiritual beliefs
- Language barriers, English as second language
- Beliefs regarding health care and health professionals
- General values and ethnic identity of family

Economic Assessment

FINANCIAL RESOURCES

- Ability to perform financial responsibilities and handle money
- Occupation; effect of illness on work and ability to continue with same occupation
- Retirement income/effect of illness on limited income
- Ability to purchase or rent equipment, supplies, and services used in the home
- Possible number of home visits and cost
- Programs available to assist:
  Foundations
  Churches
  Voluntary agencies and support groups
  National associations
  Government grants

- Qualification for Medicaid
- Third-party payors:
    Medicare, CHAMPUS
    Private insurance
    Veterans administration
    Public aid

RESOURCES FOR EQUIPMENT AND SUPPLIES

- Pharmacy and supply companies
- Home health agencies
- Home infusion and supply companies
- Durable equipment companies (purchase or rental)
- Medical supplies companies (disposable and reusable)
- Community organizations that offer medical supplies, financial assistance

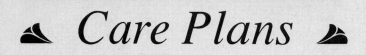

Care Plans

Pulmonary system

▲ Asthma

Asthma is an airway-reacting, obstructive pulmonary disease characterized by an irritation and constriction of the bronchi and bronchioles, resulting in bronchospasms, excessive mucus production, dyspnea, and frequently wheezing, especially in acute episodes. The causes may be extrinsic (associated with allergic responses) or instrinsic (associated with stress, activity or exercise, or respiratory infection) or a combination of these.

Home care is primarily concerned with the teaching of medication regimens to prevent or control attacks, prevention of upper and lower pulmonary and sinus infections, and assistance in reducing stressors.

Nursing diagnosis

Anxiety

Related factors: Threat of death; threat to or change in health status

Defining characteristics: Dyspnea, fear of suffocation, apprehension regarding recurrence of attacks, feelings of helplessness and tension, change in life-style needed to control breathing

OUTCOME CRITERIA

Short-term
Reduction in anxiety, as evidenced by verbalization of fear and concern, relaxed posture, respirations slower and more quiet, statements that client feels better, is less anxious, able to sleep better (expected within 2 to 7 days)

Long-term
Anxiety reduced to optimal coping capabilities, as evidenced by avoidance of physical and emotional stressors, compliance with treatment regimen with positive responses, control of

anxiety during dyspneic episodes (expected within 2 weeks and ongoing)

NURSING INTERVENTIONS/INSTRUCTIONS

1. Assess mental and emotional status and effect of stressors on breathing (see Psychosocial Assessment, p. 41, for guidelines) (first visit).
2. Establish rapport and exhibit a caring, accepting attitude while client expresses fears and concerns about the condition, its symptomatology, chronicity, and any perceived disability (each visit).
3. Assess client's inner personal resources and coping abilities; note reactions and responses to instructions and various treatment modalities (first visit).
4. Assist client in identification of stressors and realistic adaptation in avoiding them (first and second visits).
5. Instruct client in guided imagery and relaxation techniques and in music therapy (first and second visits).
6. Instruct client in the importance of a measured, paced routine for all activities of daily living (ADL) and to avoid those that cause fear and uncertainty (first visit).
7. Provide continuing information about client's condition, tests, treatments, and progress; anwser all questions honestly. Set up a telephone appointment to respond to these questions if information is not immediately available (each visit).
8. Initiate referral to self-help or support groups or to counseling if indicated (any visit).

CLIENT AND FAMILY/CARETAKER INTERVENTIONS

1. Attempt to prevent or discourage stressful situations and noxious stimuli.
2. Practice guided imagery and visualization techniques during stressful and nonstressful episodes.
3. Identify present coping skills and refine or develop more effective ones to decrease anxiety.
4. Have someone present during attack so client is not alone; have telephone numbers for emergency assistance nearby and available.
5. Ask questions about condition and reason for treatments if needed.

6. Consult physician if you are unable to control anxiety and respirations are affected.
7. Consult psychological couselor to control breathing pattern and reduce anxiety if necessary.

Nursing diagnosis

Ineffective airway clearance

Related factors: Tracheobronchial secretions, obstruction

Defining characteristics: Altered breath sounds (wheezing), changes in rate or depth of respirations, cough with or without sputum, excessive mucus, dyspnea

OUTCOME CRITERIA

Short-term
Adequate oxygenation, as evidenced by respiratory rate, depth, and ease within baseline determinations; usual speech pattern; absence of dyspnea, cough, or wheezing; absence of complaints of chest tightness, pressure, or feelings of suffocation; pulse and blood pressure within preestablished baselines; airway clear of mucus, with chest clear and with normal breath sounds and air movement; skin pink, warm, and dry (expected within 1 to 2 days)

Long-term
Adequate respiratory functioning, as evidenced by breathing with optimal level of ease necessary to maintain desired or limited life-style (expected within 1 to 2 weeks)

NURSING INTERVENTIONS/INSTRUCTIONS

1. Assess respiratory status, rate, depth, and ease; wheezing that is more pronounced on expiration; dyspnea; difficulty in speaking; use of accessory muscles; hyperinflated appearance of chest; cough; tachycardia; diaphoresis; and factors that precipitate these signs and symptoms (see Pulmonary System Assessment, p. 6) (each visit).
2. Instruct client to take own respirations and pulse and record in log; allow for return demonstration (first visit).
3. Instruct client to avoid known allergens, noxious stimuli, emotional stressors, and environmental temperature changes (first visit).

4. Assess effect of activity on respiratory status and energy level; reinforce need to exercise moderately and regularly and to maintain activity tolerance. Instruct client to pace activities and rest if breathing is affected (first visit).

5. Instruct client in positioning during rest or sleep, generally semi-Fowler's (first visit).

6. Instruct client in breathing exercises (first and second visits).

7. Instruct client to drink 2 to 3 liters (2 to 3 quarts or 10 to 12 glasses) of fluid daily unless restricted (first visit).

8. Administer oxygen by nasal cannula at 2 L/min as ordered, using compressed cylinder, concentrator, or liquid system; instruct in self-administration, safety precautions, and care of equipment (each visit).

9. Instruct client in use of humidifier, incentive spirometer, nebulizer, and hand-held inhaler (first visit).

10. Instruct client in use of prophylactic cromolyn sodium, bronchodilators (oral and inhalation), steroids, mucolytics, and expectorants; include dosage, time, frequency, food and drug interactions, method of administration, and side effects. Instruct client to stop drug and call physician if side effects occur (first visit; reinstruct on second visit).

11. Initiate referral to respiratory therapist and durable equipment company as indicated (first visit).

CLIENT AND FAMILY/CARETAKER INTERVENTIONS

1. Take and record rate and depth of respirations twice daily and log any changes in breathing pattern.

2. Perform deep breathing and physical exercise regimen daily.

3. Use humidifier and breathing apparatus as ordered.

4. Safely administer oxygen by cannula when needed.

5. Maintain predetermined fluid intake over 24 hours.

6. Administer medications correctly by proper route; avoid taking any other drugs unless approved by physician; report any adverse effects of medication to physician; carry bronchodilator inhaler at all times.

7. Have laboratory tests for theophylline level when ordered.

8. Avoid exposure to allergens and irritants, including house dust, dirty heating or air conditioning filters, dog or cat hair, molds, pollens, and environmental pollutants; elimi-

nate offending foods, odors, passive smoking, and other known irritants.
9. Wear identification bracelet or carry card with information about condition, medications, and allergies.
10. Refer to American Lung Association and self-help groups for information and support.

Nursing diagnosis

High risk for infection

Related factors: Inadequate primary defenses (decrease in ciliary action, stasis of body fluids); chronic disease; increased environmental exposure to infectious agents

Defining characteristics: Inability to mobilize and remove secretions, change in sputum color and breathing pattern, temperature elevation, chest pain

OUTCOME CRITERIA

Short-term

Prevention of respiratory infection, as evidenced by normal range of temperature; sputum clear, thin, and easily coughed up and removed (expected with daily assessment)

Long-term

Maintenance of a pulmonary system free of acute infection (acute bronchitis, pneumonia, influenza) (expected to be ongoing).

NURSING INTERVENTIONS/INSTRUCTIONS

1. Assess temperature for elevation; note amount and characteristics of sputum and compare with tenacious, yellowish or green or brown sputum of infectious process (each visit).
2. Instruct client to avoid exposure to infection potential (first visit).
3. Instruct client in administration of antiinfectives, including dose, frequency, method, route, food and drug interactions, and side effects (first visit).

CLIENT AND FAMILY/CARETAKER INTERVENTIONS

1. Take temperature if client is feeling chilled or complains of malaise or if sputum changes color, and report to physician.

2. Avoid exposure to persons with upper respiratory or pulmonary infections.
3. Maintain an environment that is free of irritants, well ventilated, and of optimal temperature and humidity.
4. Cover mouth and nose when sneezing and coughing. Dispose of tissues and contaminated articles in a waterproof bag; seal and dispose of properly.
5. Wash hands frequently and when necessary to prevent transmission of infectious agents.
6. Disinfect reusable equipment and supplies; air dry and store in clean plastic bag.
7. Administer prescribed antiinfectives correctly; take full course of medication, and report responses

Nursing diagnosis

Ineffective management of therapeutic regimen (individual)

Related factors: Excessive demands made on individual; decisional conflicts

Defining characteristics: Inappropriate choices of daily living for meeting the goals of a treatment or prevention program; verbalization that client did not take actions to include treatment regimens in daily routines or take actions to reduce risk factors for exacerbation of illness

OUTCOME CRITERIA

Short-term
Performance of health behaviors consistent with therapeutic regimen, as evidenced by verbalization of specific behaviors needed for optimal health and prevention of complications or exacerbation of symptoms (expected within 1 week)

Long-term
Compliance with management of therapeutic regimen, as evidenced by active participation in therapy, demonstration of health behaviors consistent with goals of therapy, and dealing with social situations that oppose or present a conflict with regimen (expected within 1 month and ongoing)

NURSING INTERVENTIONS/INSTRUCTIONS

1. Provide client with detailed written instructions and a plan for specific behavior, such as medications via oral and

inhalation routes, control of activity and environment, respiratory exercises, foods and other allergens to avoid, and other measures specific to client (first visit).
2. Inform client to use reminders or clues to perform or change a behavior (first visit).
3. Instruct client in monitoring behavior(s) regularly and recording for analysis and in need for alternative behavior(s) or strengthening behavior(s) (first and second visits).
4. Instruct client in use of a structured method of performing aspects of therapeutic regimen, such as a checklist, calendar or pill dispenser (first visit and reinforce second visit).
5. Encourage client to seek out ongoing support groups for long-term opportunities to reinforce behavior(s) and comply with regimen (any visit).

CLIENT AND FAMILY/CARETAKER INTERVENTIONS

1. Demonstrate accurate performance of specific health behavior(s) consistent with goals of therapeutic regimen.
2. Engage in activities that assist in compliance with therapeutic regimen and strengthen coping ability.
3. Use alternative resources and support groups.
4. Verbalize plan to deal with situations that oppose therapeutic goals and exacerbate condition.
5. Verbalize, plan, and perform specific health-related activity, with recording and analysis of behavior(s) to modify.

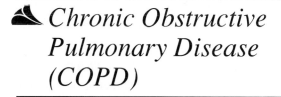

Chronic Obstructive Pulmonary Disease (COPD)

Chronic obstructive pulmonary disease is a progressive disorder of the lungs and airways. It includes diseases such as emphysema and chronic bronchitis. The disorder is characterized by long-term destruction of the walls of the alveoli, which affects oxygen and carbon dioxide gas exchange, and chronic inflammation and narrowing of the bronchioles, affecting air outflow. COPD is caused by smoking, air and chemical pollutants, α-antitrypsin deficiency, and the aging process. Changes in the respiratory system, such as loss of elasticity, decreased vital capacity, and increased residual air, associated with the aging process contribute to the prevalence and severity of the disorder.

Home care is primarily concerned with the teaching of medication regimens, which involve various routes, depending on the progression and severity of the disease; the maintenance of daily well-being as the disease progresses to the end stage; and the use of assistive mechanical ventilation. Emphasis is also placed on infection protection and control.

Nursing diagnosis

Anxiety

Related factors: Threat of death; change in health status

Defining characteristics: Apprehension, uncertainty about outcome, fear of suffocation, increased helplessness and tension

OUTCOME CRITERIA

Short-term
Reduction in anxiety level, evidenced by verbalization of fear and concerns and their causes; anxiety reduced and within manageable level during dyspneic episodes (expected within 2 days)

Long-term
Anxiety reduced and controlled, evidenced by avoidance of anxiety-producing situations and by positive responses to therapy (expected within 1 month)

NURSING INTERVENTIONS/INSTRUCTIONS

1. Assess mental and emotional status and effect of stressors on breathing and life-style; inner personal resources and ability to cope and respond to treatment; environment for excessive stimuli (first visit).
2. Provide an accepting environment for expression of fears and concerns (each visit).
3. Identify coping mechanisms used by client, and encourage client to use those that are effective (each visit).

4. Instruct client in relaxation techniques, music, guided imagery, and the use of autogenic technique during periods of dyspnea (first and second visits).

5. Instruct client to avoid stressful situations, excessive activity, and medications that are taken for anxiety that affect respiration (first visit).

6. Provide client with continuing information about status or condition, improvements, and treatments, and answer all questions (each visit).

7. Initiate referral to counseling or psychotherapy as indicated (any visit).

CLIENT AND FAMILY/CARETAKER INTERVENTIONS

1. Maintain calm, caring attitude during episodes of dyspnea; stay with client.
2. Attempt to prevent or discourage stressful situations.
3. Develop and use effective coping skills that decrease anxiety.
4. Ask questions about medications, equipment, or the disease when information is needed.
5. Adapt to chronic illness and long-term treatments.
6. Seek out assistance from psychotherapist to manage anxiety.
7. Consult physician if you are unable to control anxiety and respiration is affected.

Nursing diagnosis

Ineffective breathing pattern

Related factors: Anxiety; decreased energy and fatigue; decreased lung expansion; tracheobronchial obstruction

Defining characteristics: Dyspnea; tachypnea; cough with or without sputum; changes in rate and depth of respiration; use of accessory muscles; altered chest excursion; crackles, rhonchi; assumption of three-point position; prolonged expiratory phase; increased anteroposterior diameter of chest; abnormal arterial blood gas levels

OUTCOME CRITERIA

Short-term
Return to adequate breathing pattern and airway clearance, evidenced by satisfactory respiratory rate, ease, and depth at

baseline and by reduction in dyspneic episodes, hypoxia, stasis of secretions, and abnormal breath sounds (expected within 1 to 2 days)

Long-term
Maintenance of respiratory baselines, evidenced by breathing at optimal level within disease parameters (expected within 1 month)

NURSING INTERVENTIONS/INSTRUCTIONS

1. Assess respiratory status, including rate, depth, and ease; presence of dyspnea; use of accessory muscles, with lengthened expiratory phase; energy and fatigue level; ability to mobilize and remove secretions by coughing; breath sounds on auscultation for crackles or wheezes; hyperresonance on percussion; tactile fremitus (see Pulmonary System Assessment, p. 6, for guidelines) (each visit).

2. Provide postural drainage using gravity and percussion, avoiding any positions that may compromise the elderly client (first visit and as needed).

3. Instruct client to drink 2 to 3 liters (10 to 12 glasses) of fluids per day and to follow an activity regimen within tolerance level (first visit).

4. Demonstrate for and instruct client in deep breathing and coughing exercises, with pursed-lip breathing and abdominal breathing (first visit).

5. Inform client of positions for sleeping that will allow for ease in breathing and chest expansion (first visit).

6. Instruct client in administration of oral bronchodilators; use of small-volume nebulizer and hand-held measured-dose inhaler (carry at all times); and administration of cortiocosteriods orally and by hand-held measured-dose inhaler (first visit).

7. Instruct client in oxygen administration via nasal cannula from compressed cylinder, concentrator, or liquid oxygen system (first and second visits).

8. Encourage continued participation in pulmonary rehabilitation program at home (first visit).

9. Initiate referral to respiratory therapist and durable medical equipment agency (first visit).

10. Instruct client to cease smoking and to enter program for support if necessary.

11. Draw blood sample, or advise client to visit laboratory, for theophylline level check when ordered by physician.
12. Report to physician dyspnea not controlled by medication, inability to clear secretions from airway, confusion, or change in mentation.
13. Instruct client to wear Medic-Alert bracelet or carry card in purse or wallet stating condition and medications.
14. Instruct client to utilize American Lung Association for information and support services.

CLIENT AND FAMILY/CARETAKER INTERVENTIONS

1. Assess respiration for rate and ease twice daily.
2. Perform deep breathing exercises, four breaths 4 times per day.
3. Perform isometric exercises to strengthen diaphragm and intercostal muscles and lift 3-pound weights for upper-body strengthening daily as part of a pulmonary rehabilitation regimen, which should also include swimming, walking, or bicycling.
4. Maintain fluid intake of 8 to 10 glasses per day.
5. Use positioning and foam-rubber wedge or pillows for sleeping.
6. Administer medications correctly; avoid over-the-counter drugs unless advised by physician; report adverse effects to physician.
7. Administer oxygen correctly at 2 to 3 L/min (portable and stationary), and take safety precautions in presence of oxygen.
8. Avoid exposure to ouside and home pollutants such as sprays, fumes, smog or particulates in air, dog or cat hair, or other allergens.
9. Use humidification in home and change air conditioner and furnace filters monthly.

Nursing diagnosis

Activity intolerance

Related factors: Generalized weakness; sedentary life-style; imbalance between oxygen supply and demand

Defining characteristics: Tired, weak feeling; fatigue; exertional discomfort and dyspnea; awakening caused by dyspnea; hypoxia; increased pulse rate and blood pressure during activity

OUTCOME CRITERIA

Short-term
Increased endurance and ability to perform activities of daily living (ADL), evidenced by maintenance of respiration, pulse, and blood pressure while independently caring for self and performing routine tasks (expected within 1 week)

Long-term
Optimal activity level achieved and maintained within baseline respiratory and energy parameters (expected to be ongoing)

NURSING INTERVENTIONS/INSTRUCTIONS

1. Assess activity tolerance, pulse, and respirations before and after activity; assess for presence of dyspnea and increased work of breathing during activity; assess amount of sleep and rest (first visit).
2. Instruct client to rest after each activity and to pace activities around rest periods and use of bronchodilator (first visit).
3. Instruct client to use oxygen during activites if appropriate (first visit).
4. Instruct client in use of energy saving devices and aids (first and second visits).
5. Instruct client to build endurance by increasing activities every 2 to 3 days (each visit).
6. Arrange for home health aide (HHA) visits to assist with ADL.

CLIENT AND FAMILY/CARETAKER INTERVENTIONS

1. Exercise moderately and for short periods of time, as tolerated, and increase as energy and endurance increase.
2. Take pulse before and after activity; check for increases of 10 or more beats/min.
3. Rest every 3 hours and following activity such as bathing, walking, or using stairs.
4. Use stool to sit in shower, arm rests, aids for dressing, hand bars for support, aids for reaching and walking, wheelchair if necessary.

5. Use inhaler before activity; perform activity when systemic bronchodilator is at optimal effect.
6. Ask for assistance in ADL.
7. Use proper inspiration and expiration pattern when participating in an activity such as lifting during expiration.
8. Avoid continuing activity if you are dyspneic or fatigued.

Nursing diagnosis

High risk for infection

Related factors: Inadequate primary defenses; chronic disease

Defining characteristics: Stasis of secretions, inability to mobilize and remove secretions, loss of ciliary action, reduced pulmonary macrophages

OUTCOME CRITERIA

Short term
Prevention of pulmonary infection, evidenced by normal temperature and sputum that is clear and thin for easy removal (expected with daily assessment)

Long-term
Maintenance of pulmonary system free from acute infection (expected to be ongoing)

NURSING INTERVENTIONS/INSTRUCTIONS

1. Assess for temperature elevation, chest pain, change in color of sputum to yellow or green, and increased viscosity (each visit).
2. Instruct client in antibiotic and corticosteroid administration (first visit).
3. Inform client of precautions to take to avoid exposure to infection potential (first visit).

CLIENT AND FAMILY/CARETAKER INTERVENTIONS

1. Take temperature if you feel chilled and sputum changes color.
2. Avoid smoking and exposure to groups or to persons with upper respiratory infection.
3. Wash hands frequently, especially before treatments or eating and after using tissues for coughing and expectorating.

4. Cover nose and mouth when coughing. Dispose of tissues in bag that is waterproof; seal and discard.
5. Maintain environment that is humidified and well ventilated.
6. Secure pneumonia and flu immunizations.
7. Wash, rinse, and disinfect reusable equipment and supplies; air dry on clean toweling or hang over shower rail.
8. Discard disposable supplies in sealed waterproof bag.
9. Report temperature elevation, chills, yellow or green sputum, or chest pain to physician.
10. Take prescribed antibiotics at proper intervals and until all is used.

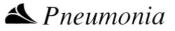

Pneumonia

Pneumonia is an inflammation of the lungs caused by bacteria, viruses, fungi, or protozoa. It may also be caused by aspiration of food, water, or gastric contents into the alveolar system. It is usually the result of an upper respiratory infection and may involve segments, a lobe, or an entire lung. The disease progresses from an initial filling of the alveoli and bronchioles with exudate to consolidation of the lung area as leukocytes attempt to destroy the organisms. The disease is especially life threatening in the elderly or chronically ill.

Home care is primarily concerned with teaching of medication regimen (antiinfectives based on identified causative pathogen) and prevention of complications.

Nursing diagnosis

Ineffective breathing pattern

Related factors: Chest pain; decreased energy and fatigue; inflammatory process; tracheobronchial obstruction

Defining characteristics: Dyspnea; tachypnea; respiratory depth changes; altered chest excursion; diminished breath sounds; cough with tenacious, purulent sputum; abnormal arterial blood gas values

OUTCOME CRITERIA

Short-term
Adequate oxygenation, as evidenced by respiratory rate, depth, and ease within normal baseline determinations, absence of dyspnea, cough less frequent, chest clear with normal breath sounds and air movement (expected within 7 to 10 days)

Long-term
Adequate respiratory functioning, as evidenced by breathing with optimal level of ease to maintain usual life-style (expected within 1 month)

NURSING INTERVENTIONS/INSTRUCTIONS

1. Assess physical status of respiratory system (see Pulmonary System Assessment, p. 6, for guidelines); note life-style, history, and trends (e.g., frequent upper respiratory infections, chronic respiratory disease, chronic illness, smoking, alcoholism, immunosuppressive therapy) to identify predisposing factors and to determine their implications for care and future teaching (first visit).
2. Monitor respirations for ease, rate, and depth; auscultate and percuss chest for diminished breath sounds and dullness (each visit). Instruct client to take respirations and record in log (first visit).
3. Assess skin color, constitutional symptoms, chills and fever, and pleuritic chest pain, and note sputum and its viscosity, amount, and change in color (each visit).
4. Assess fluid maintenance needs on the basis of age, weight and height, sex, general health, and insensible fluid losses. Instruct client to double maintenance needs, unless his or her status would be compromised (as with an elderly client or a client who has a cardiac or renal disorder) (first visit).
5. Note allergies to medications and instruct client in antiinfective therapy (penicillins, cephalosporins, oxacillin, nafcillin, tetracycline, erythromycin, lincomycin or clindamycin), including dose, frequency, food or drug interactions, and side effects (first visit).
6. Instruct client in splinting, deep breathing and coughing exercises, and how to expectorate; allow for return demonstration (each visit).

7. Monitor sputum culture results and x-ray results as available.
8. Refer client to respiratory therapy as indicated.
9. Instruct client to avoid indiscriminant or trivial use of antibiotics (last visit).
10. Suggest visit to physician for influenza and pneumonia immunizations, especially if client is elderly (last visit).

CLIENT AND FAMILY/CARETAKER INTERVENTIONS

1. Take respirations and record in log.
2. Monitor sputum (not saliva) and report changes in color, amount, or consistency to physician.
3. Administer antiinfective, antitussive, and expectorant as ordered, and take complete course of antiinfective prescription.
4. Drink predetermined amount of liquid at specified intervals over 24 hours.
5. Humidify environment; maintain optimal temperature and ventilation of environment.
6. Perform deep breathing and coughing exercises 3 to 4 times per day as tolerated.
7. Dispose of used tissues properly and wash hands when appropriate.

Nursing diagnosis

Hyperthermia

Related factors: Illness

Defining characteristics: Increase in body temperature above normal range; increased respiratory rate

OUTCOME CRITERIA

Short-term

Absence of temperature elevation, as evidenced by normal temperature and absence of chills, shaking, or diaphoresis (expected within 3 to 4 days)

Long-term

Afebrile; comfort at optimal level without recurrence of temperature elevation (expected within 1 week to 1 month)

NURSING INTERVENTIONS/INSTRUCTIONS

1. Monitor temperature for deviations from normal, and instruct client to take own temperature and record in log and to return demonstration (first visit).
2. Assess for presence of chills and diaphoresis with temperature elevation (each visit).
3. Supervise administration of antiinfectives (first visit; reinstruct on second visit).
4. Instruct client in administration of antipyretics on the basis of temperature elevation (first visit).
5. Instruct client in use of sponge bath and appropriate clothing and room temperature for comfort (first visit).
6. As temperature decreases, monitor white blood cell (WBC) count and sputum culture results if available.

CLIENT AND FAMILY/CARETAKER INTERVENTIONS

1. Take temperature twice daily, when you feel chilled or as needed, and record in log.
2. Take antipyretics correctly.
3. Maintain increased fluid intake.
4. Bathe by sponging or tub bath; maintain dry linens and room free of drafts at comfortable temperature and ventilation.

Nursing diagnosis

Pain

Related factors: Injuring agent of inflammatory process

Defining characteristics: Verbal expression of pain descriptors; holding chest to guard or protect it; changes in respiratory pattern

OUTCOME CRITERIA

Short-term
Control of pain, as evidenced by relaxed expression and posture, effortless respiration, and statements that pain has been relieved (expected within 2 to 7 days)

Long-term
Optimal comfort level, as evidenced by continued freedom from pain during respiration or activities of daily living (ADL) (expected within 1 week to 1 month)

NURSING INTERVENTIONS/INSTRUCTIONS

1. Assess pain location, frequency, severity, and characteristics and its relationship to condition and activity (each visit).
2. Instruct client in proper splinting (position, comfort, aids) before coughing and deep breathing exercises (first visit).
3. Instruct client in administration of mild analgesic before pulmonary exercises and before pain becomes severe (first visit).
4. Encourage rest periods and pacing of activities (first visit).

CLIENT AND FAMILY/CARETAKER INTERVENTIONS

1. Provide rest; assist with ADL.
2. Administer analgesic correctly; avoid use if it affects respiration.
3. Schedule activities around medication administration.
4. Notify physician if pain persists or symptoms escalate.
5. Take time to participate in activities; rest when needed, and resume activity if possible.

Nursing diagnosis

High risk for activity intolerance

Related factors: Presence of respiratory disease; deconditioned status; work of breathing (weakness, fatigue)

Defining characteristics: Weakness, fatigue, inability to perform ADL

OUTCOME CRITERIA

Short-term
Minimal fatigue expressed and increased activity tolerance as measured by increasing periods of wakefulness and progressive ability to perform ADL without fatigue (expected within 1 week)

Long-term
Independence in return to self-care, as evidenced by optimal level of care achieved and return to wellness (expected in 1 month)

NURSING INTERVENTIONS/INSTRUCTIONS

1. Obtain history, including ADL, levels of independence and endurance, family assistance and support (first visit).
2. Instruct client in performing personal hygiene and comfort measures; stress accessibility to personal items needed for care and to ask for assistance when needed (first visit).
3. Provide privacy, encourage rest, and instruct client to progressively increase activity at own pace (first and second visits).
4. Instruct client to exercise moderately for short periods of time as tolerated (first visit).

CLIENT AND FAMILY/CARETAKER INTERVENTIONS

1. Perform daily personal care with assistance or independently as able, without rushing and at tolerable pace.
2. Schedule periods of activity and rest on the basis of endurance and individual need.

Nursing diagnosis

Knowledge deficit

Related factors: Lack of information about disease, preventive measures, relapse or complications

Defining characteristics: Expression of need for information about disease process, causes, risk for reinfection or other complications

OUTCOME CRITERIA

Short-term
Adequate knowledge, as evidenced by statements of signs and symptoms of disease, transmission and causes of disease, complications of disease, and actions to take (expected within 3 to 7 days)

Long-term
Adequate knowledge, as evidenced by client's meeting requirements to achieve optimal level of health and functioning during progress to wellness (expected within 1 month)

NURSING INTERVENTIONS/INSTRUCTIONS

1. Assess life-style and ability to adapt, learning abilities and interests, family participation and support (first visit).
2. Instruct client to avoid exposure to upper respiratory infections, smoking, and changes in environmental temperature (first visit).
3. Instruct client in signs and symptoms and complications that may occur (e.g., chest pain, dyspnea, persistent temperature) and to report to physician (first visit).
4. Initiate referral to social services and support groups for educational materials and to stop smoking (first visit).
5. Suggest influenza and pneumonia immunization if appropriate (last visit).

CLIENT AND FAMILY/CARETAKER INTERVENTIONS

1. Avoid respiratory irritants, persons with infections, cigarette or cigar smoke.
2. Comply with suggested physician visits for follow-up evaluation and to report any complaints.
3. Contact and participate in community support groups focusing on respiratory health.
4. If elderly, secure influenza and pneumonia immunizations.

🔺 *Tracheostomy/Laryngectomy*

Laryngectomy is the partial or total surgical removal of the larynx, with or without a neck resection, to treat malignancy. A tracheostomy is a surgical opening in the neck through the skin and muscle and into the trachea; its purpose is to provide an airway in the presence of obstruction caused by tumor, foreign body, edema, or mucus or in conjunction with a laryngectomy or neck resection. The incision is made below the larynx, through the second or third tracheal ring, and a tracheostomy tube is inserted to maintain the opening and provide an airway. A shorter, wider laryngectomy tube is inserted during the laryngectomy procedure, which is followed by formation of a permanent stoma.

Home care is primarily concerned with respiratory care and patency of the tracheostomy following discharge from the hospital and with the teaching of tube changes and care, dressing and tie changes, and prevention of complications and emotional dysfunction associated with the presence of this artificial airway.

Nursing diagnosis

Ineffective airway clearance

Related factors: Tracheobronchial secretions, obstruction

Defining characteristics: Cough, effective or ineffective, with or without mucus removed via tube; thick and tenacious secretions obstructing tube patency; inability or refusal to remove and clean tube and protect from foreign materials

OUTCOME CRITERIA

Short term

Adequate oxygenation, as evidenced by satisfactory respiratory rate, depth, and ease; breath sounds within baseline levels; absence of obstruction of tube by secretions (expected within 2 to 3 days)

Long-term

Adequate respiratory function, as evidenced by client breathing through tracheostomy tube with optimal level of ease to maintain desired or limited life-style; adaptation to breathing through permanent healed stoma (expected within 1 to 3 months)

NURSING INTERVENTIONS/INSTRUCTIONS

1. Assess physical status of respiratory system; include vital signs, airway patency, breath sounds, skin integrity around tube and mucous membrane of stoma, sputum and characteristics (see Pulmonary System Assessment, p. 6, for guidelines) (each visit).
2. Instruct client to take and record own respirations and pulse (first visit).

3. Instruct client in use and cleaning of nightly humidifier if needed (first visit).
4. Ascertain that supplies are available for suctioning and portable suctioning machine, oxygen and supplies for administration if needed. Instruct in suctioning technique, using sterile or clean technique depending on wound healing (first and second visits).
5. Assess tracheal suctioning results and client's facility and comfort in performing procedure (each visit).
6. Instruct client to remove inner cannula and cleanse and reinsert if mucus has accumulated in tube (first visit; reinstruct on second visit).
7. Provide breathing exercises and instruct client to perform them independently (first visit; reinstruct on second visit).
8. Monitor results of laboratory tests and procedures, if available, and pulmonary function studies.

CLIENT AND FAMILY/CARETAKER INTERVENTIONS

1. Take and record pulse and respiratiory rate, depth, and ease.
2. Perform suctioning, with proper technique and cleanliness, when needed.
3. Maintain disinfection of reusable supplies and cleanliness of suctioning apparatus.
4. Change and cleanse inner cannula as needed.
5. Perform breathing exercises.
6. Note and report any change in skin at tracheostomy site (redness, pain, bleeding, drainage), change in color of sputum, or change in breathing.
7. Have emergency numbers available for immediate use by family or a recorded message to contact emergency assistance if client is left unattended.

Nursing diagnosis

Impaired verbal communication
Related factors: Physical barrier of tracheostomy
Defining characteristics: Inability to speak with tube in place

OUTCOME CRITERIA

Short-term
Ability to communicate, as evidenced by use of paper and pencil or magic slate or hand movements (expected within 2 to 5 days)

Long-term
Effective communication, as evidenced by use of and optimal adaptation to a communication method compatible with client's life-style, such as esophageal or electronic speech (expected within 1 to 3 months)

NURSING INTERVENTIONS/INSTRUCTIONS

1. Assess past communication styles and needs, life-style, interests, stamina, ability to participate in speech therapy, and family's interest and support of this alternative (first visit).
2. Use paper and pencil, slate, alphabet, or flash cards to communicate (each visit).
3. Exhibit patience with communication efforts; allow client to proceed at own pace and select own method for communicating (each visit).
4. Initiate referral to speech pathologist/therapist for esophageal or electronic speech (first visit).
5. Encourage interaction with other persons who have undergone laryngectomy (first visit).
6. Provide information about community agencies and support groups such as American Cancer Society, International Association of Laryngectomees, and speech clubs for assistance and support (first visit).

CLIENT AND FAMILY/CARETAKER INTERVENTIONS

1. Communicate effectively using preferred aids.
2. Participate in a program with a speech pathologist/therapist for esophageal or electronic speech.
3. Contact community reources for assistance and information.

Nursing diagnosis

Body image disturbance

Related factors: Biophysical factors

Defining characteristics: Presence of laryngectomy/tracheostomy tube, permanent stoma, change in structure and function of body part; dependence on alternative method of speech

OUTCOME CRITERIA

Short-term
Progress in adaptation to body function change and problems of image, as evidenced by communicating that comfort has increased as result of work with speech pathologist and use of alternative speech methods; increased interest in appearance and interaction with others (expected within 2 to 7 days)

Long-term
Improved self-concept and self-image, as evidenced by optimal level of health, full self-care in activities of daily living (ADL), and resumed social and work activities (expected within 1 to 3 months and ongoing)

NURSING INTERVENTIONS/INSTRUCTIONS

1. Assess client's ability to adapt, coping skills and mechanisms used, and family support (first visit).
2. Accept feelings of mutilation, grief, depression, and frustration with result of surgery (each visit).
3. Encourage family to communicate openly and display patience with speech efforts of client (each visit).
4. Promote independence in grooming and self-care (each visit).
5. Encourage progress in communication efforts and in speech therapy (each visit).
6. Assist client in life-style adaptations and clothing alternatives (each visit).
7. Initiate referral to counseling if appropriate (fourth or fifth visit).

CLIENT AND FAMILY/CARETAKER INTERVENTIONS

1. Treat client as a functioning member of the family.
2. Verbalize feelings and concerns; seek assistance if needed.
3. Participate in daily care and personal grooming.
4. Progress in therapy with speech pathologist.
5. Resume work or enter vocational rehabilitation program.
6. Resume social, recreational, and business activities.

Nursing diagnosis

High risk for impaired skin integrity

Related factors: External factors related to pressure of tracheostomy tube; secretions

Defining characteristics: Irritation, redness, or swelling of peristomal areas or tracheostomy site; crusting around tube or stoma; accumulation and drying of secretions at site

OUTCOME CRITERIA

Short-term
Reduced risk for skin impairment, as evidenced by the absence of any irritation or disruption in area of tracheostomy tube insertion site (expected within 3 days)

Long-term
Absence of any excoriation or impairment despite disruption of skin surface by stoma or tube site (expected within 1 week and ongoing)

NURSING INTERVENTIONS/INSTRUCTIONS

1. Assess skin at tracheostomy site for redness, excoriation, dried and crusting secretions (see Integumentary System Assessment, p. 31, for guidelines) (each visit).
2. Instruct client in cleansing around tube, application of antiseptic or antibiotic ointment, softening and removal of dried mucus, and application of clean dressing around tube; allow for return demonstrations (first visit).
3. Inform client of importance of cleaning area and changing dressing when soiled or wet or before secretions accumulate (first visit).

4. Inform client of importance of maintaining personal hygiene and avoidance of use of soiled or contaminated articles when caring for skin at site (first visit).

CLIENT AND FAMILY/CARETAKER INTERVENTIONS

1. Maintain clean, dry, tracheostomy site.
2. Avoid allowing secretions to accumulate or dry around peristomal area.
3. Cleanse, redress, and apply ointment to site as needed.
4. Replace tube if fit is not proper and manipulation irritates site.

Nursing diagnosis

Knowledge deficit

Related factors: Lack of information regarding self-care

Defining characteristics: Request for information on and instruction in care of laryngectomy/tracheostomy and prevention of pulmonary or surgical site infection; fear/avoidance/refusal to care for tube and site and perform treatments

OUTCOME CRITERIA

Short-term

Adequate knowledge, as evidenced by performance of tracheostomy tube removal, cleansing and reinsertion, suctioning, and tie and dressing changes; correct medication administration; and having a protocol for emergency contacts in place (expected within 1 week)

Long-term

Adequate knowledge, as evidenced by meeting requirements of altered life-style to achieve optimal level of health and functioning within established limits of artificial airway (expected within 1 to 3 months)

NURSING INTERVENTIONS/INSTRUCTIONS

1. Assess reaction to surgery, life-style, ability to adapt, performance of ADL, learning interest and abilities, and family participation and support (first visit).

2. Instruct client in removal, cleansing, and reinsertion of outer cannula and inner cannula; tie changes and how to tie knots; and dressing preparation and changes; instruct client in when to change or cleanse and technique to use in giving care and in tube changes; allow return demonstrations (first and second visits).

3. Instruct client in taking temperature, noting changes in sputum or skin around tube or stoma, changes in breathing, and what to report to physician (first visit).

4. Instruct client in handwashing technique and when to use it; cleansing and care of supplies and equipment; and disposal of used and contaminated disposable articles and supplies (first visit).

5. Instruct client to avoid exposure to respiratory infections, passive smoking, noxious odors and stimuli, and foreign materials or particles near the artificial airway (first visit).

6. Instruct client to wear loose clothing around stoma or to wear a cloth shield (first visit).

7. Instruct client to report excessive accumulation of mucus and inability to remove secretions or any difficulty in air flow through tube or stoma (first visit).

8. Instruct client to carry writing material at all times until a permanent method of communication has been established (first visit).

9. Instruct client to wear a medical alert bracelet, and help client to devise some emergency telephone communication if needed for assistance (first visit).

10. Instruct client to use inhalant therapy as ordered and humidification of the environment (first visit).

11. Instruct client in oral care, including frequency and type preferred (first visit).

12. Instruct client in medication administration, especially antiinfectives, including dose, times, food and drug interactions, and side effects; instruct client to complete the prescribed medication course (first and second visits).

13. Initiate referral to social services if indicated, and provide information about community agencies for information and support groups.

14. Refer home health aide (HHA) to assist with ADL as needed.

CLIENT AND FAMILY/CARETAKER INTERVENTIONS

1. Perform daily tracheostomy/laryngectomy care using proper technique and maintenance of airway patency.
2. Wash hands properly and at proper times, properly dispose of used articles, and properly disinfect and care for reusable articles and equipment.
3. Take temperature and assess for skin or breathing changes daily; report signs and symptoms indicating infection to physician.
4. Administer all prescribed medications correctly and report side effects or lack of improvement.
5. Avoid exposure to infectious agents, irritating or noxious stimuli, or foreign material near artificial airway.
6. Use protective cover over stoma.
7. Wear emergency information and carry emergency protocol for telephone assistance.
8. Maintain a supply of articles and equipment needed for care, and establish communication with a medical durable equipment company for 24-hour service and delivery of supplies.
9. Take advantage of community resources available to assist with information, support, and economic needs.

◣ *Tuberculosis*

Tuberculosis is an infectious disorder of the lungs but may affect other organs or systems, such as bones and joints, the central nervous system, the genitourinary tract, or the adrenal glands. It is caused by *Mycobacterium tuberculosis* and usually is contracted and transmitted by inhalation of air contaminated by droplets containing the organisms. This inflammatory pulmonary disorder forms tubercles that lead to formation of necrosis, caseation, fibrosis, and calcification in the affected areas of the lungs. The most susceptible groups include persons who are malnourished, persons who exhibit a low host resistance to the causative agent, and immunosuppressed individuals as in AIDS.

Home care concentrates on the teaching of daily personal hygiene, nutrition, rest, and a medication regimen.

Nursing diagnosis

Ineffective breathing pattern

Related factors: Decreased energy and fatigue; inflammatory process

Defining characteristics: Shortness of breath, fremitus, respiratory depth changes, diminished breath sounds, altered chest expansion, productive or nonproductive cough, blood-tinged sputum

OUTCOME CRITERIA

Short-term

Adequate oxygenation, as evidenced by respiratory rate, depth, and ease within preestablished baselines and by reduced frequency of productive coughing (expected within 1 to 2 weeks)

Long-term

Adequate respiratory functioning, as evidenced by client breathing with optimal level of ease to maintain desired or limited life-style, by x-ray study showing arrested or inactive stage of the disease, and by sputum culture conversion from positive to negative (expected within 2 to 5 months)

NURSING INTERVENTIONS/INSTRUCTIONS

1. Assess physical status of respiratory system (see Pulmonary System Assessment, p. 6, for guidelines) (first visit).
2. Monitor respirations for ease, rate, and depth; temperature for elevation; cough and mucus production for frequency, type, and characteristics; check for hemoptysis and dyspnea; also note dullness on percussion and crepitant crackles and rhonchi on auscultation. Instruct client in procedure for taking respirations and temperature and recording in a log (each visit).
3. Evaluate level of endurance when client is performing ADL; note onset of fatigue, cough or pain. Instruct client in measures to minimize or reduce energy expended and in establishing a rest schedule (first visit; reinstruct monthly).

4. Instruct client in effective cough procedure that does not cause stress to the chest wall and in how to collect an early-morning sputum specimen for laboratory analysis (first visit).
5. Suggest oral hygiene for frequent coughing and expectoration (first visit).
6. Monitor results of x-ray studies and sputum analysis as available, and incorporate information into clinical profile.
7. Refer client to self-help or support groups and local branches of organizations such as the American Lung Association and Smokenders (first visit).

CLIENT AND FAMILY/CARETAKER INTERVENTIONS

1. Take and record temperature and respiratory rate and depth as needed.
2. Adapt activities of daily living (ADL) to physical tolerance.
3. Perform oral hygiene 2 to 3 times daily or as needed.
4. Have laboratory tests done on sputum (collect and transport sputum specimen to laboratory as ordered).
5. Report acute dyspnea or hemoptysis to physician.

Nursing diagnosis

Altered nutrition: less than body requirements

Related factors: Inability to ingest nutrients because of biologic factors

Defining characteristics: Anorexia, lack of interest in food; weakness; fatigue; weight loss; inadequate nutritional intake

OUTCOME CRITERIA

Short-term
Adequate nutrition, as evidenced by stable weight, stable arm circumference, and energy level adequate to perform ADL (expected within 2 to 4 weeks)

Long-term
Optimal nutritional status maintained, as evidenced by normal weight for height and frame and compliance with prescribed diet, rest, and activity regimens (expected within 1 to 3 months)

NURSING INTERVENTIONS/INSTRUCTIONS

1. Assess nutritional status, food likes and dislikes, cultural and religious restrictions, caloric requirements and economic resources (first visit).
2. Take height and weight and compare with standardized charts; instruct client in taking weight (first visit).
3. Take arm measurements for baseline and later comparisons (first visit).
4. Instruct client to maintain a food diary for 1 week, including type and amount of food consumed and method of preparation (first and second visits).
5. Instruct client in food selections for a high-protein, high-carbohydrate diet. Incorporate assessment data and food diary into menu planning (first and second visits).
6. Provide information for vitamin supplements (first visit).
7. Suggest oral hygiene before each meal (first visit).
8. Suggest eating more frequent meals in smaller amounts if appetite is poor (first visit).
9. Refer home health aide (HHA) to assist with ADL and meal preparation.

CLIENT AND FAMILY/CARETAKER INTERVENTIONS

1. Weigh weekly using same scale, at same time of day, and wearing same amount of clothing, and record in a log.
2. Maintain a 7-day food diary listing types and amounts of all foods eaten.
3. Perform oral hygiene with mouth wash before meals, and brush teeth after meals.
4. Eat a high-protein, high-carbohydrate, high-calorie diet.
5. Use high-calorie supplements as needed.
6. Take daily vitamins.
7. Prepare foods that are preferred and related to cultural needs and that provide calorie requirements and social interaction.

Nursing diagnosis

Knowledge deficit

Related factors: Lack of information about measures to comply with medical regimen and about prevention of transmission of disease

Defining characteristics: Expression of need for information about the disease, how it is transmitted, long-term medication regimen, rest and activity requirements and limitations.

OUTCOME CRITERIA

Short-term
Adequate knowledge, as evidenced by client describing the causes, transmission, susceptibility, and progression of the disease; signs and symptoms of complications; and medication side effects; skin testing of contacts; compliance with medication regimen (expected within 1 to 2 weeks)

Long-term
Adequate knowledge, as evidenced by continued compliance with medication regimen and life-style adaptations and by x-ray films showing that the disease is in a dormant state; disease prophylaxis of contacts (expected within 2 to 5 months)

NURSING INTERVENTIONS/INSTRUCTIONS

1. Assess client's ability to perform ADL, life-style, ability and willingness to adapt and learn, and family support system. Integrate information with disease staging and progression (see Functional Assessment, p. 43, and Psychosocial Assessment, p. 41, for guidelines) (first visit).
2. Assess respiratory, renal, hepatic, hematopoietic, neurologic, visual, and auditory changes; note known allergies and ascertain pregnancy status (first visit and then monthly) (see respective assessments for guidelines).
3. Instruct client in causes, dormancy, and progression of disease, and relate them to plan for care (first visit).
4. Instruct client contacts (within last 3 months) to obtain skin testing and possible follow-up x-ray at local health department (first visit and reinstruct each visit).

5. Inform client contacts that medication is provided by the health department for both treatment and prophylaxis (first visit).

6. Instruct client to schedule rest and activity to avoid fatigue while maintaining endurance (first visit).

7. Instruct client in respiratory isolation procedures if necessary; suggest provision of a well-ventilated room supplied with disposable supplies and utensils and a waterproof bag for disposal (first visit).

8. Instruct client to cover nose and mouth when coughing or sneezing and in proper disposal of tissues and other used supplies (first visit).

9. Instruct client in proper hand washing technique and in when to perform procedure (first visit).

10. Instruct client in administration (including names, times, side effects, dosage, and food/drug/alcohol interactions) of isoniazid, ethambutol, rifampin, and streptomycin (and possibly capreomycin, pyrazinamide, ethionamide, clyceoserine, kanamycin, and amikacin); instruct client to avoid over-the-counter or nonprescribed drugs (first visit and reinstruct on second visit).

11. Instruct client contacts in administration and side effects of isoniazid (first visit).

12. Instruct client and family contacts to comply with scheduled appointments with private physician or public health department for follow-up testing and medication (each visit).

13. Inform client to report hypersensitivities (rash, urticaria), pruritis, difficulty in breathing, jaundice, urinary changes, peripheral neuritis, or changes in visual or hearing acuity (first visit).

14. Encourage client to be tested for HIV, since the incidence of TB is high among persons with HIV infection.

15. Initiate referral to public health agencies and social services and to self-help and support groups (first visit).

16. Refer HHA to assist when necessary.

CLIENT AND FAMILY/CARETAKER INTERVENTIONS

1. Administer prescribed medications correctly using check-off sheet, labeled tablet compartments, or another method as a reminder.

2. Secure medication in advance from public health services or home nurse to facilitate compliance.
3. Comply with diagnostic procedures (skin testing and x-ray, with return for test reading) and with prophylactic medication regimen as prescribed for family contacts.
4. Notify health care provider of pregnancy.
5. Perform ADL according to needs, resting before and after to avoid fatigue; secure physician permission to return to usual activities and work patterns.
6. Avoid alcohol, smoking, and any nonprescribed drugs.
7. Wash hands when needed, and dispose of used supplies and utensils in a sealed, waterproof bag.
8. Notify physician of untoward or toxic reactions to medications.
9. Utilize community resources.

Cardiovascular system

▲ Angina Pectoris/Coronary Artery Disease (CAD)

Coronary artery disease, also known as arteriosclerotic heart disease, is the narrowing or obstruction of the arteries of the heart by atherosclerotic plaque, causing a decrease in blood flow. It leads to a decrease in oxygen supply to the heart (ischemia), resulting in retrosternal or substernal chest pain or pressure that may extend to the left arm or jaw with varying degrees of severity and frequency. Typically, the pain is precipitated by exertion and relieved by a smooth-muscle relaxant or a vasodilator. Predisposing or risk factors include hypertension, elevated lipid panel, obesity, cigarette smoking, and diabetes mellitus.

Home care is primarily concerned with the teaching of medication regimens to prevent or control attacks and the control of risk factors by compliance with exercise and dietary regimens.

Nursing diagnosis

Pain

Related factors: Biologic injuring agents

Defining characteristics: Verbalization of pain descriptors (dull, crushing, tightness, choking, pressing feeling in chest); grimace; holding/guarding chest or arm; clenched fist over sternum; pain with activity and awakening from sleep; elevated pulse and blood pressure

OUTCOME CRITERIA

Short-term
Absence of pain, as evidenced by client's statement that pain is relieved or controlled by initiation of measures to prevent

discomfort; relaxed posture and expressions (expected within 1 to 7 days)

Long-term
Optimal comfort level and freedom from anginal pain, as evidenced by continued absence of pain and compliance with medication regimen related to anticipatory need and activity restrictions (expected within 1 month)

NURSING INTERVENTIONS/INSTRUCTIONS

1. Assess, and instruct client to assess, pain and characteristics, and precipitating and alleviating factors, with emphasis on early recognition of onset; have client maintain a diary with a record of each pain episode (first visit).
2. Monitor pain for type, location, intensity, and duration to establish individual anginal pattern, and instruct client to report any aberration in established pattern to physician (each visit).
3. Instruct client in administration of sublingual nitroglycerin for use at onset of pain (first visit):
   - Use at first sign of an attack (relate to pain diary).
   - Administer prescribed dose in tablet form under the tongue or in the buccal pouch and allow to dissolve; avoid swallowing the tablet.
   - Repeat dosage up to 3 times at 5-minute intervals if pain is not relieved.
   - Notify physician and call ambulance and go to emergency room if total of 3 tablets taken over 15 minutes does not relieve pain.
4. Instruct client in alternative form and route (inhalation amyl nitrite) if prescribed (first visit).
5. Instruct client to rest during acute episode and to maintain supine or semi-Fowler's position to reduce oxygen requirement (first visit).

CLIENT AND FAMILY/CARETAKER INTERVENTIONS

1. Maintain pain diary; identify trends and report to physician when necessary.
2. Administer and record medication to prevent or treat angina.
3. Use positions of comfort and take rest periods as needed.
4. Schedule medication regimen around activities.

5. Call physician and/or ambulance if 3 doses of nitroglycerin are ineffective.

Nursing diagnosis

Activity intolerance

Related factors: Imbalance between oxygen supply and demand

Defining characteristics: Abnormal response to activity (pulse, blood pressure, difficulty breathing, pain); ECG changes reflecting arrhythmias or ischemia; known presence of CAD

OUTCOME CRITERIA

Short-term
Increase in activity tolerance and endurance, as evidenced by client's statement that stressors have been avoided and pain episodes associated with activity have been decreased (expected within 1 to 7 days)

Long-term
Optimal activity and self-care achieved with adaptation to established limitations in functioning (expected within 2 weeks)

NURSING INTERVENTIONS/INSTRUCTIONS

1. Assess life-style, participation in activities of daily living (ADL) and effects of activity on angina (first visit).
2. Identify activities that increase oxygen consumption and cause pain (first visit).
3. Assist client to plan a progressive daily self-care schedule, and instruct him or her to refrain from any activity that precipitates symptoms, including exposure to cold, exertion after a meal, exertion from sexual intercourse (first visit).
4. Advise client that activity may be continued by modifying it in order that no symptoms of angina are elicited; that nitroglycerin may be prescribed prophylactically before activity is to be performed (first visit).
5. Initiate referral to physical and/or sex therapist as indicated (any visit).

CLIENT AND FAMILY/CARETAKER INTERVENTIONS

1. Maintain activity and rest schedule as planned.
2. Progress in ADL and endurance level without angina response.
3. Cease activity and rest when angina occurs.
4. Seek assistance to increase activity tolerance and sexual activity if needed.

Nursing diagnosis

Anxiety

Related factors: Threat of death; threat to or change in health status

Defining characteristics: Verbalization of fear of death from heart attack; increased tension and apprehension; feeling of uncertainty with life-style changes; fear of unspecific consequences

OUTCOME CRITERIA

Short-term
Decrease in anxiety, as evidenced by client's statement expressing reduction in and control of anxiety to manageable level (expected within 1 week)

Long-term
Continuing manageable level of anxiety with optimal pyschic and emotional functioning, as evidenced by resumption of daily living pattern with modifications to prevent angina episodes (expected within 2 weeks)

NURSING INTERVENTIONS/INSTRUCTIONS

1. Establish rapport and allow time and supportive environment for client to communicate concerns and fears (each visit).
2. Provide information about all tests and treatments to monitor and control condition (first visit).
3. Allow time for questions, and answer in understandable terms and with honesty (each visit).
4. Reaffirm positive life-style changes (each visit).
5. Refer client to counseling if anxiety becomes chronic (last visit).

6. Teach relaxation techniques if client is agreeable (first visit or when needed).

CLIENT AND FAMILY/CARETAKER INTERVENTIONS

1. Inquire about condition and methods to control anxiety.
2. Initiate necessary life-style changes.
3. Contact self-help groups or counseling.
4. Use relaxation techniques to control anxiety.

Nursing diagnosis

Knowledge deficit

Related factors: Lack of information about medical regimen

Defining characteristics: Request for information about medications, disease process, nutritional and activity restrictions, and health measures to prevent complications and decrease risks

OUTCOME CRITERIA

Short term

Adequate knowledge, as evidenced by client's ability to describe signs and symptoms and progression of the condition; compliance with exercise and dietary controls; and reduction in known stressors and smoking (expected within 1 week)

Long-term

Adequate knowledge of and compliance with medical regimen, as evidenced by client's meeting the requirements of a changed life-style to achieve optimal level of wellness and functioning (expected within 1 month and ongoing)

NURSING INTERVENTIONS/INSTRUCTIONS

1. Assess life-style and ability to adapt, dietary patterns, learning and coping abilities and interest, and family participation and support in the medical regimen (first visit).
2. Assess cardiovascular status (see Cardiovascular System Assessment, p. 9, for guidelines) and note blood pressure, pulse changes, angina pain patterns, history of chronic illness, use of caffeine, alcohol, and tobacco; assess for more distant heart sounds, fourth heart sound, more dif-

fuse apical pulse, presence of nausea, diaphoresis, cool extremities, and vertigo during acute episodes of angina (each visit).

3. Instruct client to maintain an activity diary and relate activities to angina episodes; teaching from the known to the unknown, allow client to verbalize signs and symptoms, precipitating factors, and first indication of onset (first visit and reinforce on second visit).

4. Instruct client to identify stressors, including heavy meals, exertion, exposure to cold, emotional upsets, or any combination of these (first visit).

5. Instruct client to closely follow prescribed health regimen for any chronic condition such as hypertension or diabetes mellitus (first visit).

6. Advise client to stop smoking, and refer client to support group if needed (first visit).

7. Instruct client to maintain a food diary; instruct client in lowering caloric intake for reducing weight if indicated, avoiding foods high in saturated fats and cholesterol, and limiting low-fat foods that contain monounsaturated and polyunsaturated fats; include low-sodium-intake instructions if recommended, and supply client with food lists and sample menus during teaching sessions (first visit and reinforce when needed).

8. Advise client to follow a paced, incremental walking program (first week).

9. Instruct client in administration of long-acting nitrites, beta-adrenergic blocking agents, calcium blockers, antilipidemics, and prophylactic antiplatelet agents, including dosage, route, frequency, side effects, and food/drug/alcohol interactions; instruct client to avoid skipping doses or abrupt discontinuation of medications and to avoid OTC drugs unless advised by physician (first visit).

10. Instruct client in administration of nitroglycerin before or during angina attack and to note vertigo, syncope, or headache with initial dose and tolerance to drug (first visit).

11. Advise client to carry medication at all times (away from body heat), to store it in a dark container, and to replace tablets every 3 months (first visit).

12. Instruct client to report any aberration in anginal pattern and pain that is not relieved by medication (first visit).

13. Instruct client to carry or wear identification information indicating condition and medications being taken (first visit and check for compliance on second visit).
14. Inform client of available social services, community agencies, resources, and groups for information and support (first visit).

CLIENT AND FAMILY/CARETAKER INTERVENTIONS

1. Administer medication appropriately and accurately.
2. Avoid identified stressors, and manage anginal episodes quickly and effectively.
3. Comply with dietary and exercise programs as instructed.
4. Limit alcohol intake, and reduce or cease cigarette smoking.
5. Notify physician of medication side effects, unrelieved pain, or changes in vital signs.
6. Utilize social services, nutritionist, or physical therapist as needed.

◢ Congestive Heart Failure (CHF)

Congestive heart failure (CHF) is a chronic, progressive syndrome characterized by the inability of the heart to act as a pump. The result is a cardiac output that is inadequate to meet the body's metabolic requirements. CHF results from myocardial infarction, coronary artery disease, inflammatory diseases of the heart, hypertension, valvular disorders, or any other condition that strains the heart over a long period of time. The compensatory mechanisms of increased heart rate and cardiac dilatation and hypertrophy are adaptive responses to diminished cardiac output. The cause determines whether hypertrophy occurs on the left or right side or involves both sides. Treatment is directed at management of specific etiologic and pathophysiologic factors, reversal of compensatory mechanisms, and elimination of contributing factors.

Home care is primarily concerned with assessment and with teaching the client about the disorder, the medical

regimen designed to prevent the occurrence of heart failure, and measures to treat this chronic condition.

Nursing diagnosis

Decreased cardiac output

Related factors: Mechanical factors causing alteration in preload and afterload; inotropic changes in the heart; structural factors

Defining characteristics: Alterations in hemodynamic readings (pulse, blood pressure); fatigue; dyspnea; rales; cyanosis; pallor; oliguria; left-sided heart failure with overlapping of symptoms of fluid excess as condition progresses

OUTCOME CRITERIA

Short-term
Adequate cardiac output, as evidenced by reduction in signs and symptoms of lowered cardiac output; compliance with medical regimen, resulting in return of vital signs to baseline ranges (expected within 2 to 7 days)

Long-term
Optimal cardiac status within disease limitations, as evidenced by ability to resume and maintain adapted life-style without distress or complications (expected within 2 to 4 weeks)

NURSING INTERVENTIONS/INSTRUCTIONS

1. Assess circulatory status, noting rate and rhythm of apical and peripheral pulses, blood pressure, presence of cough or dyspnea, activity intolerance levels, presence of S_3 or S_4 heart sounds, accentuated S_2, summative gallop (S_3 with S_1) (see Cardiovascular System Assessment, p. 9, for guidelines) (each visit).
2. Perform complete physical assessment, including renal, hepatic, and neurologic systems, and note any stressors that increase cardiac output, such as chronic inflammatory or infectious diseases, increased blood pressure, pulmonary emboli, arrythmias, anemia, or thyrotoxicosis (first visit).
3. Assess life-style and relate it to contributing factors as a basis for teaching, noting tobacco use, excessive alcohol, use, sodium and caffeine intake, stress, or overweight problems (first visit).

4. Instruct client to monitor and record apical and radial pulses; stress alterations that should be reported to physician rather than absolute values (first visit).
5. Instruct client to avoid fatigue by pacing activities and rest periods; instruct client to rest and sleep in semi-Fowler's position (first visit).
6. Instruct client in administration of vasodilators and advise client to note side effects, implication of decreased blood pressure on position, resultant headaches, and altered renal function; instruct client to avoid OTC drugs (first visit).
7. Instruct client in administration of cardiotonics; advise client to take pulse before administration and to withhold drug if pulse is lower than 60 beats/min; inform client of signs and symptoms of toxicity, including nausea, vomiting, anorexia, diarrhea, confusion, visual changes, and new or worsening pulse irregularities (first visit).
8. Instruct client to report deteriorating condition, including increasing fatigue with activity, dyspnea, pallor, diaphoresis, thready pulse or alteration in pulse baseline, persistent cough, feelings of suffocation, cyanosis, restlessness, anxiety, or panic (first visit).

CLIENT AND FAMILY/CARETAKER INTERVENTIONS

1. Monitor and record daily pulses, blood pressure, capillary refill, skin for any change in color.
2. Administer medications correctly, and state implications and expected results.
3. Avoid fatigue, stressors, and excessive activity.
4. List signs and symptoms of digitalis toxicity, and report if present.
5. Report changes in vital signs that indicate change in cardiac output.

Nursing diagnosis

Fluid volume excess

Related factors: Compromised regulatory mechanisms

Defining characteristics: Edema, unexplained weight gain, shortness of breath, orthopnea, change in respiratory pattern, oliguria, jugular vein distention, pulmonary effusion, congestion on x-ray, abnormal breath sounds (crackles), right-sided failure with overlapping symptoms of decreased cardiac output as condition progresses

OUTCOME CRITERIA

Short-term
Fluids in balance, as evidenced by intake and output returned to baselines, weight maintained, and edema reduced or absent (expected within 3 to 4 days)

Long-term
Fluid and electrolytes in balance, as evidenced by optimal weight and by achievement of optimal renal and pulmonary function for life-style requirements (expected within 1 month)

NURSING INTERVENTIONS/INSTRUCTIONS

1. Assess fluid requirements; calculate for age and weight (usually about 2L/day unless restricted) (first visit).
2. Measure height and abdominal girth, and instruct client to take daily weight at same time, on same scale, wearing same clothing, and to record and report weight gains (first visit).
3. Monitor for discrepancies between estimated intake and output and for pedal and ankle swelling, increasing fatigue, abdominal fullness, ascites, oliguria, and weight gain (each visit).
4. Assess chest sounds for crackles and changes in respiration (each visit).
5. Monitor and instruct client in diuretic therapy and potassium levels when they are available; encourage foods high in potassium, including citrus fruits, bananas, poultry, potatoes, and raisins, and/or administer potassium replacement if prescribed (first visit).
6. Monitor and instruct client in dietary sodium intake and for compliance with restrictions (first visit).
7. Instruct client to inform physician of edema, breathing changes or difficulties, or weight gain (first visit).

CLIENT AND FAMILY/CARETAKER INTERVENTIONS

1. Monitor weight and fluid intake and urinary output estimations.
2. Administer diuretics and electrolyte replacement properly.

3. Comply with sodium restriction.
4. Report weight gains, edema, or any other symptoms of fluid retention.

Nursing diagnosis

Fatigue

Related factors: Increased energy requirements, overwhelming physical and psychological demands

Defining characteristics: Verbalization of lack of energy, fatigue, inability to maintain usual routine; poor oxygenation of tissues; bed rest causing deconditioning

OUTCOME CRITERIA

Short-term
Decreasing fatigue, as evidenced by client's statement of increased energy and endurance and by participation in paced activities (expected within 1 week)

Long-term
Energy and endurance returned to baseline levels, as evidenced by achievement of self-care and mobility for optimal functioning within condition limitations (expected within 1 to 2 months)

NURSING INTERVENTIONS/INSTRUCTIONS

1. Assess life-style, ADL abilities, and limitations imposed by illness (first visit).
2. Identify activities that elicit symptoms and deplete energy reserves (first visit).
3. Assist client in progressive plan for daily care; instruct client to avoid any activity that precipitates symptoms, to pace activities, and to provide rest periods (first visit).
4. Employ energy-saving devices and techniques for ADL (each visit).
5. Inform client to avoid strenuous activity or exercise (first visit).
6. Refer HHA to assist with ADL.

CLIENT AND FAMILY/CARETAKER INTERVENTIONS

1. Identify physical and mental stressors, and avoid them when possible.
2. Progress in ADL within established limits.
3. Satisfy rest and sleep needs.

Nursing diagnosis

Ineffective individual coping

Related factors: Multiple life changes, inadequate coping methods

Defining characteristics: Verbalization of inability to cope or ask for help, inability to problem solve, chronic worry and anxiety; inappropriate use of defense mechanisms

OUTCOME CRITERIA

Short-term
Improved coping, as evidenced by client's statement of understanding of need for adaptations in life-style and positive coping strategies (expected within 1 week)

Long-term
Optimal coping, as evidenced by adaptations in life-style and by compliance with medical regimen to achieve health and optimal functioning (expected within 1 to 2 months)

NURSING INTERVENTIONS/INSTRUCTIONS

1. Assess mental and emotional status, coping abilities, use of defense mechanisms, and problem-solving skills (first visit).
2. Provide an accepting environment for expression of concerns (each visit).
3. Assist client to identify goals and positive coping mechanisms (each visit).
4. Allow client to participate in and plan care and to practice effective problem solving-skills (each visit).
5. Initiate referral to counseling or psychotherapist if indicated (any visit).

CLIENT AND FAMILY/CARETAKER INTERVENTIONS

1. Develop and use effective coping mechanisms.
2. Share concerns with family members, and request assistance and support when needed.
3. Plan care and solve problems that arise from inadequate care.
4. Manage care effectively and maintain a positive attitude.

Nursing diagnosis

Knowledge deficit

Related factors: Lack of information about condition

Defining characteristics: Request for information about disease and its effect; compliance with daily medical regimen

OUTCOME CRITERIA

Short-term
Adequate knowledge, as evidenced by client's description of disease process, signs and symptoms, complications, and effect of disease on body systems and general health (expected within 3 days)

Long term
Adequate knowledge, as evidenced by compliance with the medical regimen to meet requirements of a changed life-style for achievement of an optimal level of health and functioning (expected within 1 month)

NURSING INTERVENTIONS/INSTRUCTIONS

1. Assess life-style and ability to adapt, learning abilities and interest, and family participation and support (first visit).
2. Outline a program to teach disease process and preventive measures (first visit):
   • Medication administration, with complete information for accuracy and desired effects
   • Signs and symptoms of disease and of complications
   • Activity and rest program
   • Bowel hygiene and prevention of change in normal pattern
   • Diet for reduction, low in sodium, fats, and cholesterol

- Cessation of smoking; limitations of caffeine and alcohol
- Review of laboratory tests and changes needed
- Foods to avoid and include in dietary regimen

3. Instruct client to comply with physician and laboratory appointments and to check with physician for results and possible changes in therapy (first visit).
4. Instruct client to carry or wear medical identification information (first visit).
5. Refer client to agencies and support groups to assist in compliance with medical regimen if needed (any visit).

CLIENT AND FAMILY/CARETAKER INTERVENTIONS

1. Follow medical regimen as taught.
2. Report known signs and symptoms of complications if present.
3. Administer medications safely, with awareness of side effects or untoward effects to report.
4. Manage care with assistance of agency or group if needed.
5. Verbalize understanding that measures to maintain cardiac status are lifelong.

◣ *Coronary Bypass Surgery*

Coronary bypass is a surgical procedure that circumvents obstructed coronary arterial vessels through a process of myocardial revascularization. The resulting unobstructed blood flow oxygenates previously ischemic heart muscle. Autogenous blood vessels frequently used to bridge the occluded areas are the internal mammary arteries or the saphenous veins. The clinical profile would include a history of arteriosclerotic heart disease and coronary artery disease (CAD), notably unstable angina pectoris and localized rather than diffuse disease. Some controversy exists about the surgical procedure because, although it offers dramatic relief from pain and other syptoms, it may not necessarily positively affect the prognosis of the disease.

Home care is primarily concerned with postoperative teaching of the medical regimen to prevent complications

and with life-style changes that will promote wellness within limitations imposed by the procedure and the underlying heart condition.

Nursing diagnosis

Ineffective individual coping

Related factors: Multiple life changes, personal vulnerability

Defining characteristics: Verbalization of inability to cope, meet role expectations, problem solve; inappropriate use of defense mechanisms; alterations in societal participation; chronic worry and anxiety about outcome of surgery

OUTCOME CRITERIA
Short-term
Improved coping behaviors, as evidenced by statement of feeling more able to handle stressors and by use of appropriate and effective coping and defense mechanisms (expected within 1 to 2 weeks)

Long-term
Adequate and positive coping, as evidenced by progression from sick-role behaviors to relaxation and adaptive behaviors and by resumption of activities daily living (ADL) and other activities within limitations imposed by convalescence (expected within 1 to 2 months)

NURSING INTERVENTIONS/INSTRUCTIONS
1. Establish rapport and provide an accepting environment for expression of concerns and questions (each visit).
2. Assess mental status, ability to adapt, use of coping mechanisms, and internal resources, and explore with client the most effective coping mechanisms and selection of positive options (first visit).
3. Assess client's interest in and participation in activities and resumption of role and place in family (first visit).
4. Allow client to actively participate in plan of health care regimen (first visit).
5. Arrange for contact with support group.

CLIENT AND FAMILY/CARETAKER INTERVENTIONS

1. Express feelings and concerns.
2. Identify and use coping mechanisms that are the most effective, and develop coping skills as needed.
3. Participate in own health care planning.
4. Utilize support group for information and help.

Nursing diagnosis

Knowledge deficit

Related factors: Lack of information about postoperative care

Defining characteristics: Request for information regarding medications, cardiac rehabilitation, dietary restrictions, lifestyle changes, sexual function, and signs and symptoms to report to physician

OUTCOME CRITERIA

Short-term
Adequate knowledge of follow-up care, as evidenced by client's ability to describe the condition, risk factors, and required life-style adaptations and by compliance with medication, diet, and rehabilitation program (expected within 1 week)

Long-term
Adequate knowledge, as evidenced by client's complying with postoperative recommendations to achieve optimal level of health and functioning without complications (expected within 1 month and ongoing).

NURSING INTERVENTIONS/INSTRUCTIONS

1. Review physician's postoperative health regimen, amount and type of teaching done, and reinforcement needed in order that home care becomes a continuum of previous teaching (first visit).
2. Facilitate establishment of an environment that is conducive to learning and free of outside distractions, in which the client is free of pain and excessive anxiety, and teach care based on identified needs for information and demonstration (each visit).
3. Assess cardiovascular and respiratory status (see

Cardiovascular System Assessment, p. 9, and Pulmonary System Assessment, p. 6, for guidelines); note vital signs (compare to baselines), point of maximal intensity (PMI), and presence of irregularities or pain (each visit).

4. Instruct client to monitor and record pulse daily for 1 full minute after a 5-minute quiet period and to notify physician of changes or deviation from usual pulse rate and regularity (first visit).

5. Instruct client to take weekly weights at same time, with same clothing, and on same scale and to report unexplained gains or losses to physician (first visit).

6. Instruct client in need for rest, and plan to schedule activities around rest periods; suggest 8 hours of sleep per night; inform client of importance of following cardiac rehabilitation program without exception (first visit).

7. Inform client that activity progression will be determined by results of rehabilitation participation, and advise that sexual activity may begin 6 to 8 weeks after sugery based on physician recommendation (first visit).

8. Assess for incisional healing, discomfort at operative area, or change in wound, including redness, swelling, or drainage (each visit).

9. Assess for presence of chest pain, and differentiate between preoperative and postoperative pain (anginal or cardiac); instruct client in administration of analgesics (each visit).

10. Evaluate exercise tolerance, and advise against driving or sitting for long periods, abruptly changing positions from lying to sitting or sitting to standing, or lifting heavy objects (first visit).

11. Instruct client in administration and implications of antihypertensives, antiarrhymics, cardiotonics, diuretics, anti-coagulants, and analgesics (first visit and reinforce on second visit).

12. Instruct client to continue prescribed regimen for control of chronic conditions such as hypertension or diabetes mellitus (first visit).

13. Instruct client in low-calorie, low-cholesterol, low-fat, low-sodium diet; instruct client to avoid caffeine and alcohol except in small amounts (first visit and reinforce on second visit).

14. Instruct client to avoid Valsalva maneuver during bowel

elimination and to administer stool softeners to prevent constipation (first visit).

15. Remind client that smoking should be reduced and preferably eliminated, and suggest group support to assist in stopping (first visit).

16. Instruct client to report signs and symptoms of complications or regression to preoperative profile, including erratic pulse, chest pain, activity intolerance, fatigue, or unexplained anxiety and restlessness (first visit).

17. Instruct client to carry or wear identifying information about condition and medications (first visit).

18. Inform client of importance of compliance with medical regimen that includes cardiac rehabilitation and of follow-up appointments with physician and laboratory (first visit).

19. Monitor changes in medical orders and laboratory results when applicable (each visit).

20. Initiate referral to social worker, home health aide, and other support personnel and groups as appropriate (any visit).

CLIENT AND FAMILY/CARETAKER INTERVENTIONS

1. Monitor and record pulse daily and notify physician of changes.

2. Monitor weight weekly and report significant gains or losses.

3. Integrate rest periods with increasing activities; try to get 8 hours of sleep per night.

4. Participate in cardiac rehabilitation program, with a monitored walking program between sessions.

5. Resume sexual activity.

6. Manage incisional discomfort with medication; provide care for incisional site (handwashing, bathing, dressing).

7. Avoid sitting for extended periods of time, lifting heavy objects, or participating in strenuous exercises or sports.

8. Administer prescribed medications as instructed.

9. Continue medical regimens for treating chronic conditions.

10. Maintain diet that promotes ideal weight.

11. Prepare and eat diet with restrictions in sodium, cholesterol, and fat; limit caffeine and alcohol intake.

12. Maintain bowel elimination based on individual pattern.

13. Identify signs and symptoms of incisional infection, return

to preoperative heart abnormalities, or complications of surgical procedure, and report to physician.

14. Wear or carry medical identification at all times.

15. Comply with follow-up physician and laboratory appointments.

16. Participate in self-help or support groups, contact community agencies for information, and utilize nutritionist or sex therapist as needed.

◢ *Hypertension*

Hypertension can be defined as sustained arterial blood pressure of over 140 mm Hg systolic and 90 mm Hg diastolic. It causes arterial walls to become thickened, lose elasticity, and resist blood flow, which results in decreased blood supply to tissue and increased cardiac workload. The etiology of essential, or primary, hypertension is unknown. It can be treated and controlled, not cured. Secondary hypertension is associated with disorders of the kidney, adrenal glands, central nervous system, or great vessels or with the use of medications. In the absence of complications, essential hypertension is asymptomatic. Clinical manifestations are nonspecific and result from vascular changes in the heart, brain, or kidneys.

Home care is primarily concerned with the teaching of medication regimens to control the condition and preventive measures to control complications and risk factors.

Nursing diagnosis

Knowledge deficit

Related factors: Lack of information about medical regimen

Defining characteristics: Request for information about medications, dietary and exercise program, disease and its effects and complications

OUTCOME CRITERIA

Short-term
Adequate knowledge, as evidenced by client's ability to describe disease process and effects, signs and symptoms, risk factors, and life-style modification requirements; familiarity and compliance with medication regimen (3 to 7 days)

Long-term
Adequate knowledge, as evidenced by meeting requirements of modified life-style to control condition and achieve optimal health and functioning (expected within 2 weeks)

NURSING INTERVENTIONS/INSTRUCTIONS

1. Assess life-style, learning and adaptation abilities, interest level, and family participation and support (first visit).
2. Assess all systems for effect of long-term hypertension; note history for predisposing factors or disorders that relate to secondary hypertension (first visit).
3. Assess and instruct client in monitoring blood pressure and pulse (first visit).
4. Inform client of high-risk factors associated with condition, including smoking, obesity, high sodium, fat, and cholesterol intake, stress, and sedentary life-style, and include family members in teaching, since heredity plays a role in predisposition to increased blood pressure (first visit).
5. Advise client about life-style changes, methods of stress management, and dietary changes, and to have regular screening for blood pressure and circulatory and visual changes (first visit).
6. Instruct client to take blood pressure 3 times per week; emphasize sitting quietly for 5 minutes before taking pressure, using the right size of cuff, applying cuff smoothly and snugly and fastening securely, and positioning arm at heart level; instruct client to report repeated and unexplained elevations to physician (first visit and reinforce when needed).
7. Instruct client in administration of diuretics, antihypertensives, antilipidemics, potassium replacement, vasodilators, and sympathetic depressants, including doses, route, frequency, side effects, and food/drug/alcohol interactions; caution client not to alter doses or abruptly stop medication and to avoid OTC drugs unless recommended by physician (first visit and reinforce second visit).

8. Encourage client to participate in full range of previous activity as long as blood pressure is controlled; include an exercise program of walking, swimming, and biking, with 8 hours of sleep per night (first visit).

9. Advise client about weight reduction if needed; instruct client to maintain a food diary for 1 week, and offer a list of foods to avoid (ones that are high in cholesterol and saturated fats); encourage a more liberal intake of fruits and vegetables, whole grains, fish, and poultry (first and second visits).

10. Instruct client in sodium restriction (usually 2 g/day); advise client not to add salt to foods, and to avoid cured, processed, or convenience foods, and suggest use of herbs and spices for flavoring (first visit).

11. Inform client about foods that are high in potassium with diuretic therapy, including a list of those to include and avoid, especially if potassium supplement not given (first visit).

12. Suggest that client reduce or stop smoking and limit or avoid alcohol intake and hot baths or hot tub (first visit).

13. Instruct client to rise slowly from lying position to avoid orthostatic hypotension (first visit).

14. Instruct client to carry or wear identification information about condition and medications (first visit).

15. Emphasize importance of keeping appointments with physician for monitoring condition and therapy changes if needed, as well as for laboratory testing (first visit).

16. Initiate referral to community agencies and groups for information and support or counseling, including American Heart Association and smoking and weight control groups.

CLIENT AND FAMILY/CARETAKER INTERVENTIONS

1. Monitor blood pressure as instructed and recommended, and record in log to review with physician.

2. Administer medications correctly and record any side effects.

3. Participate in an exercise program that is ongoing and progressive as appropriate.

4. Avoid alcohol and tobacco in excess; reduce frequency.

5. Comply with dietary restriction of sodium, fat, and cholesterol.

6. Monitor weight weekly if on reduction diet, and adjust caloric intake accordingly.
7. Wear or carry identification information.
8. Maintain laboratory and physician appointment schedule.
9. Utilize support groups and couseling services if needed.

Nursing diagnosis

High risk for injury

Related factors: Internal factor of complication of hypertension

Defining characteristics: Failure to comply with medical regimen; sustained elevated blood pressure; cardiovascular and central nervous system symptomatology (hypertensive crisis, heart attack, cerebrovascular accident)

OUTCOME CRITERIA

Short-term
Absence of signs and symptoms of complication, as evidenced by compliance with medication regimen (expected within 1 week)

Long-term
Optimal cardiovascular, neurologic, and renal system function, as evidenced by life-style modification and ongoing compliance with medical regimen to achieve health and wellness without complications (expected within 1 month and ongoing).

NURSING INTERVENTIONS/INSTRUCTIONS

1. Assess for behaviors that indicate resistance to or inability to comply with prescribed treatment regimen (first visit).
2. Reinforce instruction in diet, exercise, and medication programs and limitations in stress, alcohol, tobacco, and weight gain (first visit).
3. Assess for markedly elevated blood pressure, headache, visual disturbance, nausea, vomiting, palipitations, restlessness, confusion, tachycardia, dysrhymthmias, chest pain, or dyspnea, and instruct client in noting and reporting such signs and symptoms (each visit).
4. Encourage client to participate in plan and take control of care (each visit).
5. Assist client with compliance by writing out plan and expectations (first visit).

6. Encourage client to ask questions, seek information, and participate in discussions about condition; praise compliance and accomplishments (each visit).
7. Inform client of importance of life-style changes that maintain blood pressure status and prevent complications (each visit).

CLIENT AND FAMILY/CARETAKER INTERVENTIONS

1. Comply with life-style changes and medical regimen.
2. Report signs and symptoms of complications immediately to physician.
3. Support all attempts at management of care and prevention of complications.
4. Secure and read information about condition and consequences of poor control of hypertension.

Nursing diagnosis

Ineffective management of therapeutic regimen (individual)

Related factors: Complexity of therapeutic regimen

Defining characteristics: Inappropriate choices of daily living for meeting the goals of a treatment or prevention program; failure to achieve weight loss and lower cholesterol level; inaccurate medication administration; observed smoking; reduction in exercise program; verbalization that action not taken to reduce risk factors for prevention of complications

OUTCOME CRITERIA

Short-term
Verbalization of and specific plans and behaviors for therapeutic regimen, as evidenced by intention of following recommended dietary, exercise, and medication regimens with commitment (expected within 1 week)

Long-term
Compliance with management of therapeutic regimen, as evidenced by active particpation in therapy and by demonstration of behaviors consistent with goals of therapy to achieve optimal health and prevent complications (expected within 1 month and ongoing)

NURSING INTERVENTIONS/INSTRUCTIONS

1. Assess reasons for client's disregarding therapeutic regimen and which aspects are difficult to comply with (first visit).
2. Provide client with detailed written instructions and a plan for specific behaviors, such as medications regimen via oral route, and include a simplified method if several medications are taken per day; regimen should be tailored to client life-style in peak action and scheduling where possible (first and second visits).
3. Inform client of consequences of smoking, and assist him or her to develop a plan to quit smoking, cope with withdrawal symptoms, deal with the possibility of a relapse, and use available resources and community programs (first visit).
4. Assist client to plan realistic dietary modifications; inform client of the benefits of the diet and the effects of noncompliance (first and second visits).
5. Inform client that behavior changes take time, and suggest methods to reinforce behavior changes and environmental changes to accomodate daily routines (first visit).
6. Instruct client in monitoring behavior(s) regularly, recording for analysis, and the need for alternative behaviors or strengthening of existing behaviors (first and second visits).

CLIENT AND FAMILY/CARETAKER INTERVENTIONS

1. Demonstrate accurate performance of specific health behavior(s) consistent with goals of therapeutic regimen.
2. Verbalize and adhere to a plan to follow diet, quit smoking, follow exercise program, and take medications as prescribed.
3. Establish a system to administer medications accurately and to manage the medication regimen for optimal effects in accordance with life-style.
4. Use resources and support groups to assist with compliance.
5. Modify life-style to fit management of therapeutic regimen and changes when needed.

◣ *Myocardial Infarction (MI)*

A myocardial infarction results from a partial or complete occlusion of a coronary artery. It is caused by atherosclerotic buildup in the artery, resulting in narrowing of the artery, a thrombus in the artery, or arterial spasm, leading to ischemia and necrosis of the heart tissue. The location of the infarct may vary, but most occur in the area of the left ventricle. Management is directed at preventing further damage, preventing recurrence or complications, and control of symptomatology.

Home care is primarily concerned with assessment and with the teaching of a medication regimen, control of risk factors to prevent recurrence, and measures to allow the heart to heal.

Nursing diagnosis

Pain

Related factors: Biologic injuring agents

Defining characteristics: Verbalization of pain descriptors (deep, crushing, squeezing chest pain in varying degrees of intensity); chest pain radiating to left arm, jaw, or neck (substernal or visceral); changes in vital signs; arrthymias; holding chest; dyspnea; nausea; vomiting; sense of impending doom; diaphoresis; restlessness

OUTCOME CRITERIA

Short-term
Reduced pain, as evidenced by client's statement that pain has been relieved; relaxed facial expressions and posturing; and participation in activities of daily living (ADL) without pain (expected within 1 week)

Long-term
Absence of pain, as evidenced by progression to optimal level of health and performance of ADL without pain recurring (expected within 2 weeks)

NURSING INTERVENTIONS/INSTRUCTIONS

1. Assess pain location, severity, and type; precipitating factors; effect of medication on pain (each visit).
2. Instruct client in medication administration to relieve pain (nitrites) (first visit).
3. Instruct client to notify physician if pain returns or is not controlled and have emergency numbers available (first visit).
4. Instruct client to stay calm and to rest in semi-Fowler's position or with head elevated until emergency assistance arrives (first visit).

CLIENT AND FAMILY/CARETAKER INTERVENTIONS

1. Administer medications correctly and effectively.
2. Report complaints of pain to physician.
3. Maintain calm environment and reduce stressors when pain occurs.
4. Call on emergency services if pain and associated symptoms occur indicating heart attack.

Nursing diagnosis

Activity intolerance

Related factors: Imbalance between oxygen supply and demand

Defining characteristics: Verbal report of fatigue or weakness; abnormal heart rate or blood pressure or dyspnea in response to activity; reduced energy and endurance level

OUTCOME CRITERIA

Short-term

Increased activity and endurance, as evidenced by performance of ADL and other activities and by progressive moderate exercising and ambulation (expected within 2 to 3 weeks)

Long-term

Participation and independence in ADL and mobility to achieve optimal level of health and functioning with progressive increase in endurance (expected within 1 to 2 months)

NURSING INTERVENTIONS/INSTRUCTIONS

1. Review results of discharge treadmill exercise test if done (first visit).
2. Assess for and encourage participation in ADL and diversional activities (each visit).
3. Encourage gradual increase in an individualized daily exercise/walking program based on absence of symptoms, results of treadmill exercise test, and physician recommendation; relate activities to age, general condition, cardiac status, interests, and life-style (each visit).
4. Instruct client to rest before and after exercise program; to avoid heavy lifting, stress, large meals, extremes in temperature, and stimulants (caffeine) or any combination of these; and to avoid isometric exercises (first visit and reinforce on second visit).
5. Instruct client to cease activity and notify physician if activity intolerance occurs, including unwarranted fatigue, shortness of breath, diaphoresis, weakness, pulse not reverting to baseline within 5 minutes after rest, change in pulse trends, or chest pain (first visit).
6. Encourage client to enroll and participate in formal cardiac rehabilitation program with prescription from physician (first visit).
7. Refer home health aide to assist in ADL.

CLIENT AND FAMILY/CARETAKER INTERVENTIONS

1. Participate in planned activities with progressive increases.
2. Schedule rest periods with activities, and plan diversional activities.
3. Refrain from cardiac stressors and extreme exertion or activities.
4. Adjust work to activity tolerance.
5. Report new or recurrent symptoms of activity intolerance.

Nursing diagnosis

Decreased cardiac output

Related factors: Electrical factor of alteration in rate, rhythm, and conduction

Defining characteristics: Changes in hemodynamic readings; arrhythmias; ECG changes

OUTCOME CRITERIA

Short-term
Adequate cardiac output, as evidenced by vital signs returning to baseline determinations (expected within 2 to 3 days)

Long-term
Cardiac output maintained, as evidenced by vital signs and cardiac status returning to level to achieve optimal functioning without complications (expected within 2 weeks).

NURSING INTERVENTIONS/INSTRUCTIONS

1. Assess circulatory status, noting blood pressure, point of maximal impulse (PMI), pulse rate and rhythm, capillary refill time, skin color and temperature, presence of pain or edema, fatigue, weakness, nausea, vomiting, or unexplained restlessness or anxiety (see Cardiovascular System Assessment, p. 9, for guidelines) (first visit and ongoing).
2. Instruct client to monitor vital signs and record in a log, noting any changes to report to or ask physician about (first visit).
3. Instruct client in administration of and assessment of response to medications (vasodilators, beta blockers, calcium channel blockers, antihypertensives, diuretics, inotropic agents, low-dose aspirin), including dose, route, frequency, side effects, food/drug/alcohol interactions, and implications for self care; emphasize compliance with regimen and avoidance of OTC drugs, and caution against altering, omitting, or abruptly stopping any of the prescribed medications (first visit and reinforce on each visit).

CLIENT AND FAMILY/CARETAKER INTERVENTIONS

1. Administer all prescribed medications correctly, and monitor for desired effects.
2. Monitor vital signs daily as instructed, in different positions and at different times, and record; identify changes to report.
3. Report signs and symptoms of reduced cardiac output.

Nursing diagnosis

Sexual dysfunction

Related factors: Altered body function caused by disease process

Defining characteristics: Verbalization of the problem; actual or perceived limitations imposed by disease; fear of heart attack and death

OUTCOME CRITERIA

Short-term
Improved sexual adequacy, as evidenced by client's statement of awareness that sexual activity is allowed and that options with intimacies are being explored (expected within 1 week)

Long term
Optimal sexual relationship with significant partner achieved with required adaptations (expected within 2 months)

NURSING INTERVENTIONS/INSTRUCTIONS

1. Assess sexual history, concerns, beliefs and attitude about sexual activity after MI; activity tolerance and results of treadmill exercise test and 2-flight stair-climb test; review drug profile and relate to persistent problems with decreased libido or impotence (first visit).
2. Provide written information about sexual activity after MI to client and partner (first visit).
3. Encourage expression of concerns and questions after initial assessment, and include partner in all discussions (each visit).
4. Encourage nonsexual activities that promote intimacy, including participating in activities together and talking together (first visit).
5. Advise client about sexual options that minimize cardiac workload (first visit):
   - Rest before sexual activity, or engage in activity after a night's rest.
   - Take prophylactic nitrite, if prescribed, before activity.
   - Use side-to-side or less taxing positions.

- Avoid activity after eating a large meal or drinking alcoholic beverages.
- Avoid extremes of temperature, stress, and fatigue.
- Avoid anal intercourse.
6. Instruct client to cease activity and to notify physician if intolerance to sexual activity occurs, including persistent increase in pulse and respirations after activity, chest pain at any time, or extreme protracted fatigue following activity (first visit).
7. Refer client to sex therapist if appropriate (any visit).

CLIENT AND FAMILY/CARETAKER INTERVENTIONS

1. Verbalize concerns, and inquire about sexual activity.
2. Communicate concerns with partner.
3. Promote intimacy through nonsexual as well as sexual approaches.
4. Structure sexual activity to minimize stressors and distractors.
5. Verbalize effect of fear and certain medications on sexual activity, desire, or performance.
6. See therapist with partner if needed.

Nursing diagnosis

Knowledge deficit

Related factors: Lack of information about post–myocardial infarction medical regimen

Defining characteristics: Request for information about medications, dietary and fluid needs, need for life-style changes, and follow-up requirements; denial of condition

OUTCOME CRITERIA

Short-term
Adequate knowledge, as evidenced by client's ability to describe signs and symptoms of condition, management of risk factors, and compliance with medical regimen (expected within 1 week)

Long-term
Adequate knowledge, as evidenced by client's meeting requirements of adapted life-style to achieve optimal health

and functioning without complications (expected within 1 month)

NURSING INTERVENTIONS/INSTRUCTIONS

1. Assess life-style, ability to adapt, coping and learning abilities, and family participation and support (first visit).

2. Assess for precipitating or risk factors associated with the condition, including family history, previous MI, hypertension, diabetes mellitus, obesity, sedentary life-style, hyperlipidemia, and personality response to stress; adapt teaching to data (first visit).

3. Instruct client in circulatory assessment, to monitor resting pulse for 1 full minute daily, and to withold inotropic agent if pulse is less than 60; inform client of signs and symptoms of cardiac complications to report, including changes in pulse or blood pressure, chest pain, edema, skin color change, fatigue, weakness, nausea, vomiting, or restlessness (first visit).

4. Instruct client in administration of medications (vasodilators, beta blocker, calcium channel blockers, antihypertensive, diuretics, anticoagulants, antilipidemics, inotropic agents, low-dose aspirin), and prepare a written schedule with administration instructions for client (first visit).

5. Instruct client to weigh weekly on same scale, at same time of day, and wearing same clothing (first visit).

6. Assess nutritional status and caloric requirements, and instruct client in reduction diet to maintain ideal weight and in low-cholesterol, low-fat, sodium restricted diet as prescribed (first visit and reinforce on second visit).

7. Instruct client to avoid smoking, stress, alcohol, and stimulating beverages (first visit).

8. Inform client of importance of compliance with exercise and cardiac rehabilitation program (each visit).

9. Instruct client in bowel program and to avoid straining at defecation (first visit).

10. Assist client in identifying stressors, and teach relaxation techniques and stress management (each visit).

11. Offer food list and sample menus of food and fluid inclusions and restrictions (first visit).

12. Instruct client to maintain fluid intake, to monitor intake and output for balance, and to compare with weight gains or losses and presence of edema (first visit).

13. Instruct client to avoid high altitudes; inform client of possible limitation of air travel (first visit).

14. Instruct client to notify physician of deteriorating condition or complications, including erratic pulse, dyspnea, unexplained anxiety, feelings of confusion or impending doom, persistent or recurrent chest pain, or fever (first visit).

15. Encourage client to comply with physician and laboratory appointments (first visit).

16. Advise client to carry or wear identification and information regarding health status (first visit).

17. Initiate referral to counseling, community agencies and groups for smoking cessation and weight loss, and the American Heart Association for literature and support (first visit).

CLIENT AND FAMILY/CARETAKER INTERVENTIONS

1. Administer all medications safely as instructed.
2. Monitor vital signs and report changes.
3. Balance work, rest, exercise, and diversional activities.
4. Avoid smoking, stressful situations, and alcohol.
5. Maintain ideal weight.
6. Prepare and consume special diet of calculated calories, low in sodium, cholesterol, and fat.
7. Maintain bowel pattern of soft, formed stool.
8. Report symptoms of condition change, or inquire if unsure about changes to physician.
9. Comply with physician and laboratory appointments.
10. Wear medical identification at all times.
11. Contact support or self-help groups as needed.

▲ *Pacemaker Implantation*

A permanent pacemaker is an electric device, inserted in the chest wall, that maintains a normal rhythm of myocardial contractions by delivering an electrical stimulus to the myocardium. A pacemaker may stimulate the heart at a constant and fixed rate (asynchronous, competitive), or it may deliver a stimulus on demand (synchronous, noncompetitive) when the heart does not contract at a set rate. A transvenous approach is frequently done, in which the electrode (lead) is inserted percutaneously through the right cephalic, jugular, or subclavian vein and positioned in the right ventricle. The distal end of the electrode is attached to the pulse generator (pacemaker), which is placed in a subcutaneous pocket in the upper chest. The pacemaker contains circuitry and battery programs for a heart rate generally between 50 and 100 beats/min. The pacemaker regulates the heart rate, which results in an adequate cardiac output. Permanent pacemakers are inserted in clients with heart block, dysrhythmias, or conduction defects.

Home care is primarily concerned with the teaching of the medical regimen that is followed and the monitoring of pacemaker functioning and heart rate to prevent complications.

Nursing diagnosis

High risk for infection
Related factors: Invasive procedure of pacemaker insertion

Defining characteristics: Redness, swelling, pain, fluid collection at the site of insertion; temperature elevation

OUTCOME CRITERIA
Short-term
Absence of infection, as evidenced by clean and dry insertion site, with healing in progress and edges of incision well approximated (expected within 3 days)

Long-term
Skin integrity maintained at incisional site, as evidenced by completely healed incision without irritation, discomfort, or disruption of skin (expected within 4 to 6 weeks)

NURSING INTERVENTIONS/INSTRUCTIONS
1. Assess, and instruct client to assess, vascular (cutdown) access and pacemaker insertion sites for local heat, erythema, edema, tenderness or pain, drainage, or disruption of suture edges (each visit).
2. Instruct client in hand-washing technique and clean wound and skin care (first visit and reinforce on second visit).

3. Monitor temperature and instruct client in taking temperature and noting chilling or flushing and reporting these changes and elevations over 100° F to physician (first visit).
4. Instruct client in antibiotic prophylactic therapy if prescribed (first visit).

CLIENT AND FAMILY/CARETAKER INTERVENTIONS

1. Monitor temperature and condition of sites.
2. Verbalize signs and symptoms to report.
3. Provide clean wound care; perform hand washing before giving any care to wounds.
4. Administer antibiotic therapy.
5. Utilize positions that prevent pressure on sites and promote comfort.

Nursing diagnosis

Anxiety

Related factors: Change in health status; fear of death

Defining characteristics: Verbalization of fear of pacemaker malfunction and consequences; feeling of helplessness caused by dependence on pacemaker; increased apprehension and uncertainty

OUTCOME CRITERIA

Short-term
Reduction in anxiety, as evidenced by client's statement that anxiety has decreased, that muscles and posturing have relaxed, and that pacemaker function and limitation imposed on life-style are understood (expected within 2 to 3 days).

Long-term
Anxiety controlled and managed, as evidenced by life-style changes made to achieve level of health commensurate with pacemaker and medical regimen (expected within 2 weeks)

NURSING INTERVENTIONS/INSTRUCTIONS

1. Assess mental and emotional status and effect of stress on pacemaker function (see Psychosocial Assessment, p. 41, for guidelines) (first visit).

2. Assess for inner personal resources, ability to cope, and responses to presence of pacemaker (first visit).
3. Provide an accepting environment, and allow for expression of fears and concerns regarding pacemaker function (each visit).
4. Instruct client in relaxation techniques, and help client to identify and avoid stressful situations (first and second visits).
5. Provide continuing information about condition, improvements, tests, and treatments, and answer all queries honestly and in understandable language (each visit).
6. Initiate referral for counseling for stress and anxiety reduction as indicated (any visit).

CLIENT AND FAMILY/CARETAKER INTERVENTIONS

1. Verbalize and vent concerns regarding pacemaker, restrictions, and knowledge needed to prevent complications.
2. Inquire about pacemaker and its function and about changes in life-style expected.
3. Use relaxation and diversional techniques to decrease anxiety.
4. Consult physician if you are unable to control anxiety and if it affects daily activities.

Nursing diagnosis

Knowledge deficit

Related factors: Lack of knowledge about pacemaker

Defining characteristics: Request for information about pacemaker function, pacemaker monitoring, malfunction of pacemaker battery, failure to capture or sense, or malpositioning or malfunctioning of pacing catheter

OUTCOME CRITERIA

Short-term

Adequate knowledge of pacemaker, as evidenced by client's ability to describe type of pacemaker, why it is needed, how it functions, and symptoms and signs of pacemaker failure or complications and consequences; pulse maintained at set rate and regularity (expected within 3 days)

Long-term
Adequate knowledge of safe, appropriate pacemaker functioning, as evidenced by meeting requirements of pacemaker monitoring and functioning and associated medical regimen to
achieve optimal level of cardiac function and general health
(expected within 2 to 4 weeks)

NURSING INTERVENTIONS/INSTRUCTIONS

1. Assess life-style, ADL abilities, ability to learn and adapt,
   interest in learning pacemaker functioning, and family
   participation and support (first visit).
2. Assess cardiovascular status; note blood pressure, pulse
   rate, and rhythm of apical and peripheral pulses (see
   Cardiovascular System Assessment, p. 9, for guidelines)
   (each visit).
3. Review pacemaker instruction manual and note implications for client teaching (first visit).
4. Instruct client in administration of medications for underlying conditions and cardiac medications prescribed (first
   visit).
5. Instruct client to take and record radial pulse daily; stress
   resting 5 minutes before taking pulse and monitoring
   pulse for 1 full minute; instruct client to report to physician any significant deviation from pacer setting or any
   change that reflects pre-pacemaker condition (first visit
   and reinforce on second visit).
6. Instruct client in normal function of the heart and how the
   pacemaker performs to maintain heart rate (first visit).
7. Monitor client for signs and symptoms of decreased cardiac output, including fatigue, vertigo, decreased blood
   pressure, slow or erratic pulse, shortness of breath, diminished peripheral pulses, altered mental status, or chest
   pain, and instruct client to notify physician if any occur
   (first visit).
8. Inform client of range of activities allowed or when they
   may be resumed, such as sexual activity, according to
   physician recommendations; instruct client to avoid contact sports, constrictive clothing around pacemaker, jerky
   or exaggerated movements on pacemaker side, or toying
   with insertion sites (first visit).
9. Inform client of sources of electromagnetic interference
   and implications for pacemaker (first visit).

- Ground all home appliances (electric and battery operated) and maintain them in good working order.
- Client may use light switches, radios, television, and most household convenience appliances as long as none are held over the insertion site.
- Avoid proximity to microwave ovens (stay at least 6 feet away if in use); avoid large electrical generators.
- Move away from any field that interferes with pacemaker function, and normal function will resume.
- Always inform other professionals (dentist, technician, physician) about presence of pacemaker before having any procedure or testing done.
- When travelling by air, inform security personnel before passing through metal detector, since pacemaker will trigger alarm.

10. Instruct client in telephone pacemaker check (done every 3 months) and to keep physician appointments for monitoring pacemaker and evaluation at least twice a year (first visit).
11. Inform client of need for battery change and unit replacement, and instruct client to schedule evaluation before and near "expiration date" (first visit).
12. Instruct client in range-of-motion exercises on side of pacemaker if needed (first visit).
13. Instruct client to carry pacemaker history at all times with information that includes type, manufacturer, model and serial number, programmed rate, location of pulse generator, implant date, medications being taken, and name and number of attending physician (first visit and reinforce on second visit).
14. Instruct client to have emergency number at hand at all times (first visit).
15. Provide list of agencies and groups that can assist with information and support (first visit).

CLIENT AND FAMILY/CARETAKER INTERVENTIONS

1. Monitor pulse daily as instructed.
2. Administer medications safely and effectively.
3. Report signs and symptoms of pacemaker malfunction to physician.

4. Report signs and symptoms indicating change in cardiac output as a result of malfunction to physician.
5. Engage in full range of activities, with adaptations to minimize injury or electromagnetic interference.
6. Monitor pacemaker function periodically by telephone or by clinic or hospital visit.
7. Carry pacemaker information at all times.
8. Comply with instruction to avoid complication of pacemaker dysfunction.
9. Comply with appointments and schedules for evaluation and battery change.
10. Utilize community resources for information and support.

◣ *Peripheral Vascular Disease (PVD)*

Peripheral vascular disease refers to a condition characterized by interference with blood flow to or from the extremities; the condition may involve either arteries or veins of the extremities. It may be caused by atherosclerosis or arteriosclerosis resulting in narrowing of the arteries, inflammation (as in thrombosis or thromboangiitis obliterans), or vasospasms (as in Raynaud's disease or varicose veins). Whether PVD is caused by inefficient cardiac pump actions or obstructed, damaged, inflamed, or infected vessels, the defining characteristic is a decreased peripheral blood flow resulting in ischemia.

Home care is primarily concerned with the teaching of a medical regimen that enhances circulatory status in the extremities and prevents complications associated with impaired peripheral circulation.

Nursing diagnosis

Altered peripheral tissue perfusion

Related factors: Interruption of arterial flow or venous congestion

Defining characteristics: Arterial flow—intermittent claudication, absent or weak peripheral pulses, decreased capillary filling time, cold feet, pallor on elevation, rubor when dependent, delayed healing, atrophy of skin, hair loss. Venous flow— aching; heavy sensation; Homan's sign; deep muscle tenderness and cramping pain; swelling, warmth, and increased pigmentation of area; prominent superficial veins; stasis ulcer

OUTCOME CRITERIA

Short-term
Improved circulation to extremities, as evidenced by return to baseline lower-extremity color, temperature, size, and peripheral pulse; absence of discomfort in extremities (expected within 1 week)

Long-term
Adequate perfusion of extremities, as evidenced by return of circulation to baselines with optimal use and functional ability of extremities (expected within 1 to 2 months)

NURSING INTERVENTIONS/INSTRUCTIONS

1. Assess circulatory status and effect on extremities (see Cardiovascular System Assessment, p. 9, for guidelines) (first visit).
2. Review history for age at onset of circulatory problem, cardiac status, number of pregnancies, chronic disease, familial tendency toward circulatory problems, trauma, infections, use of tobacco and alcohol, or weight problem (first visit).
3. Differentiate between arterial and venous deficiency or dysfunction (first visit).
4. Assess peripheral pulses, capillary refill time, skin color and integrity, temperature, pain in extremities, paresthesia, degree of motion and sensation, and calf measurement (each visit).
5. Instruct client to protect extremities against chilling; to avoid use of constrictive hose or clothing and accessories; to avoid prolonged standing or leg crossing; and to avoid use of heating pad or hot water bottle (first visit).
6. Instruct client in a walking program and elevation of legs above heart level when sitting to reduce venous congestion (first visit and reinforce on second visit).
7. Instruct client in measures to increase arterial flow, including elevating head using a foam rubber wedge, resting with legs below heart level, performing postural exercises, and

walking as prescribed (first visit and reinforce on second visit).

CLIENT AND FAMILY/CARETAKER INTERVENTIONS

1. Protect extremities from temperature extremes or burns or trauma.
2. Avoid application of heat, constriction of circulation to extremities, and prolonged sitting or standing.
3. Rest and exercise daily as prescribed to promote circulation and prevent pain.
4. Perform ROM, Buerger-Allen, and walking exercises as prescribed.

Nursing diagnosis

High risk for impaired skin integrity

Related factors: Internal factor of altered circulation

Defining characteristics: Skin discoloration, thickening, scarring; dermatitis; altered sensation; ischemic lesion; stasis ulcer

OUTCOME CRITERIA

Short-term
Absence of skin breakdown, as evidenced by intact skin and absence of irritation, excoriation, and trauma (expected within 2 days)

Long-term
Skin integrity maintained, as evidenced by skin intact and circulation inproved, allowing for optimal health and use of extremities (expected within 1 month)

NURSING INTERVENTIONS/INSTRUCTIONS

1. Assess skin for breakdown areas and deviations from baseline condition (see Integumentary System Assessment, p. 31, for guidelines) (first visit).
2. Instruct client to monitor skin on extremities for trauma or any disruptions and to notify physician of changes (first visit).
3. Instruct client to avoid injury (first visit).
   - Avoid scratching or rubbing extremities.
   - Wear sturdy, well-fitting shoes with clean, loose-fitting white cotton hose.

- Bathe in tepid water with a neutral soap and dry thoroughly.
- Trim nails straight across.
- Apply cream to skin on extremities.
4. Instruct client in application of antiembolic hose or elastic bandages (first visit and reinforce on second visit).
5. Inform client that bed cradle may be used to keep linens off extremities (first visit).
6. Apply Unna boot or dressings on leg ulcer as ordered (any visit).
7. Refer to podiatrist or perform routine foot care to treat ingrown nails, corns, callouses (first visit).

CLIENT AND FAMILY/CARETAKER INTERVENTIONS

1. Monitor skin daily and report abnormalities to physician.
2. Avoid conditions or trauma that injures skin on extremities.
3. Wear support hose and proper shoes and socks.
4. Maintain skin integrity in presence of circulatory disorder.
5. Utilize podiatrist for foot care if needed.
6. Provide daily foot and skin care on both extremities.

Nursing diagnosis

Knowledge deficit

Related factors: Lack of information about circulatory disorder

Defining characteristics: Request for information about disease and its effects, measures to prevent symptoms and complications of disorder, and mobility requirements and restrictions

OUTCOME CRITERIA
Short-term
Adequate knowledge, as evidenced by client's statement of signs and symptoms of circulatory deficiency and escalating condition, compliance with medical regimen, and adaptive life-style behaviors (expected within 4 to 7 days)

Long-term
Adequate knowledge, as evidenced by client's meeting requirements to achieve optimal level of health and functioning within limitations imposed by chronic circulatory condition; absence of complications (expected within 1 to 2 months)

NURSING INTERVENTIONS/INSTRUCTIONS

1. Assess life-style, adapting abilities, learning interest and abilities, and family participation and support (first visit).
2. Assess mobility status, including ability to walk without pain or discomfort, claudication, or aching extremities with increased ambulation, and instruct client to rest when pain occurs (first visit).
3. Instruct client to cease or reduce smoking and give rationale (first visit).
4. Instruct client to reduce weight or to maintain desired body weight, and assist client to plan low-fat, low-cholesterol diet (first visit).
5. Instruct client in medication administration, including vasodilators, adrenergic blocking agents, and analgesics, and instruct client to avoid OTC drugs without physician advice (first visit and reinforce on second visit).
6. Assess client's knowledge of condition and its signs and symptoms, and instruct client to notify physician of deteriorating condition or worsening symptoms indicating complications, including severe pain with or without activity, decrease in or loss of sensory or motor function, and changes in skin appearance or temperature (first visit).
7. Instruct client to obtain adequate rest, including 8 hours sleep per night, to maintain proper positioning of extremities based on arterial or venous insufficiency, to follow only the prescribed activity and exercise regimen, and to stop activity when pain occurs (first visit).
8. Instruct client in stress management techniques, or inform client of availability of assistance from counseling (any visit).
9. Refer client to support group for weight reduction or to stop smoking (first visit).

CLIENT AND FAMILY/CARETAKER INTERVENTIONS

1. Administer medications safely and monitor effects.
2. Notify physician if signs and symptoms of circulatory compromise are present.
3. Participate in programs to reduce weight and stop smoking.
4. Maintain reduction diet and restrict intake of fat and cholesterol.

5. Maintain rest and exercise programs.
6. Avoid stressful situations; practice stress-reducing exercises.
7. Reconcile pain with activity needs.

◣ *Thrombophlebitis*

Thrombophlebitis refers to a venous thrombus accompanied by venous inflammation, usually occurring in the lower extremity. Symptoms may vary; they depend in part on location and which vessels are affected. The causes of thrombophlebitis include venous stasis, venous trauma, and increased blood coagulation. The condition may be complicated by vessel obstruction by the clot or movement of the clot into the circulation (embolus).

Home care is primarily concerned with the control of factors that contribute to thrombus formation and the prevention of chronic venous insufficiency or pulmonary emboli by teaching the client the medical regimen and the importance of compliance with instruction.

Nursing diagnosis

Pain

Related factors: Biologic injuring agents

Defining characteristics: Verbalization of pain descriptors; pain, warmth, redness, edema of calf; Homan's sign; protective behavior of affected leg

OUTCOME CRITERIA

Short-term

Decreased pain, as evidenced by client's statement of pain reduction; relaxed posture and absence of guarding behavior; decrease in inflammation of calf; and resumption of physical activity (expected within 1 week)

Long-term
Absence of pain, as evidenced by independence in ADL and by activity to achieve optimal level of health and functioning without discomfort (expected within 2 to 4 weeks)

NURSING INTERVENTIONS/INSTRUCTIONS

1. Assess pain, including type, location, severity, and influence of position and activity (each visit).
2. Encourage periods of rest with leg elevated and supported; perform ROM exercises as prescribed (active or passive) (each visit).
3. Instruct client to avoid any constriction of popliteal space on affected leg (first visit).
4. Apply warm soaks or compresses to affected leg, and teach client to perform procedure (first visit).
5. Encourage client to perform as many of ADL as possible, and instruct client in ambulation as allowed (first visit).
6. Instruct client in application of anti-embolic hose if prescribed (first visit).
7. Instruct client in administration of analgesics, and especially note any interactions with anticoagulant therapy (first visit).
8. Refer HHA to assist with ADL.

CLIENT AND FAMILY/CARETAKER INTERVENTIONS

1. Provide activity and rest with progressive increases daily.
2. Administer medications and heat treatments as instructed.
3. Use aids in ambulation as needed.
4. Participate in ADL, and progress until independence is achieved.
5. Report return of pain to physician.
6. Utilize physical therapist if appropriate.

Nursing diagnosis

Knowledge deficit

Related factors: Lack of information about medical regimen and preventive measures

Defining characteristics: Request for information about risk factors for recurrence or complication of condition, activity and weight restrictions, and normal peripheral perfusion

OUTCOME CRITERIA

Short-term
Adequate knowledge, as evidenced by client's statement of effects of activity and weight on condition; compliance with medication regimen; and adequate perfusion of extremity (expected within 2 to 3 days)

Long-term
Adequate knowledge, as evidenced by client's meeting requirements to achieve optimal functioning of extremity without complications or recurrence of condition (expected within 1 month)

NURSING INTERVENTIONS/INSTRUCTIONS

1. Assess for knowledge of disease and history or life-style that includes risk factors for the condition, including use of contraceptives, past surgeries and injuries, use of tobacco, tendency toward overweight, and blood pressure problems (first visit).
2. Assess extremies for integrity, color, warmth, size (take calf measurements bilaterally), motion, pain, presence of peripheral pulses, capillary refill time, and paresthesias (each visit).
3. Instruct client in calf assessment and to report asymmetry caused by edema (first visit).
4. Instruct client in weight reduction, including reducing calories in diet and following exercise program when appropriate (first visit and reinforce on second visit).
5. Instruct client in leg exercises, ROM exercises, and a progressive walking program with or without aids (each visit).
6. Suggest reduction in or cessation of smoking; refer client to support group for assistance (first visit).
7. Instruct client to avoid constricting clothing, prolonged sitting or standing, or crossing legs while sitting or resting; to elevate the legs above heart level when sitting; and

to position the legs to avoid popliteal compression by use
of pillows under the knees (first visit).

8. Measure and apply elastic anti-embolic hose from toes to
knees or to groin area smoothly; instruct client in application and how to avoid bunching or rolling down of hose
and to remove for sleep (first visit).

9. Suggest use of bed cradle or other device to keep covers
off leg (first visit).

10. Instruct client to avoid rubbing or massaging extremity
(first visit).

11. Instruct client in administration of anticoagulants, including dose, frequency, side effects, and food/drug/alcohol
interactions; to avoid OTC drugs that contain aspirin or
other drugs (nonsteroidal anti-inflammatories) that inter-
fere with platelet function; and to comply with laboratory
testing for prothrombin time as prescribed (first visit and
reinforce on second visit).

12. Instruct client in signs and symptoms of effects of anticoagulant therapy, including bleeding of gums, ecchymoses,
epistaxis, and blood in urine or stool or sputum, and to
report such incidents to physician (first visit).

13. Instruct client to report any change in skin integrity of
extremity, such as stasis dermatitis or ulceration, and to
report any signs and symptoms of pulmonary emboli,
including anxiety, restlessness, breathlessness, syncope,
increased pulse and respirations, cough, or pleuritic pain
(first visit).

14. Instruct client to carry or wear identification indicating
medications being taken (first visit).

15. Refer client to podiatrist if appropriate (any visit).

CLIENT AND FAMILY/CARETAKER INTERVENTIONS

1. Monitor extremities, including skin of extremities, daily
for signs and symptoms to report.

2. Comply with leg exercise, activity program, and dietary
program as instructed.

3. Avoid circulatory compromise in clothing, positioning,
movement, pressure, or massage.

4. Reduce smoking and alcohol and caffeine intake.

5. Engage in weight-reduction program if needed.

6. Wear anti-embolic hose properly; remove every 8 hours for skin and leg assessment.
7. Administer anticoagulant therapy correctly, based on periodic prothrombin time testing.
8. Avoid trauma, medications, or straining that increases the risk of bleeding, and report bleeding from any orifice, skin, or mucous membrane; report the presence of blood in any excretions or secretions.
9. Comply with laboratory testing and physician appointments.
10. Wear identifying information.
11. Utilize podiatrist for foot care.

Neurologic system

◣ Alzheimer's Disease

Alzheimer's disease is a degenerative disease of the brain. It is a progressive dementia type of disease characterized by a large loss of cells from the cerebral cortex and other areas. It results in behavior changes, memory loss, and impaired intellectual functioning. The brain changes include atrophy with wide sulci, senile plaques, and neurofibrillary tangles. The exact cause is unknown, but the disease is believed to be associated with genetic, viral, autoimmune disease, and choline acetyl-transferase deficiency etiologies. The degree of severity of the dementia is a clinical judgment; diagnosis of Alzheimer's disease is made after years of evaluation of the presenting signs and symptoms.

Home care is primarily concerned with the teaching of safety and the medical regimen and with preservation of cognitive, social, physical, and psychological function.

Nursing diagnosis

Altered thought processes

Related factors: Physiologic changes

Defining characteristics: Cognitive dissonance; memory deficit or problems; impaired ability to make decisions, grasp ideas, problem solve, reason, and conceptualize; altered attention span; disorientation to time, place, person, circumstances, and events; hallucinations; inappropriate or non-reality-based thinking

OUTCOME CRITERIA

Short-term

Preservation of cognitive and intellectual function, as evidenced by an ability to maintain reality within disease limitations (expected within 2 weeks, depending on stage of illness)

Long-term
Optimal cognitive and intellectual functioning within parameters established for the stage of the disease (expected ongoing)

NURSING INTERVENTIONS/INSTRUCTIONS

1. Assess short-term memory deficits; orientation to time, place, and person; effect of medications on cognitive function; reactions to stimulation; aggressive, abusive behavior (each visit).
2. Instruct family or caretaker to provide orientation-based stimulation, including clocks, calendars, and familiar objects within reach, and to repeat or correct misunderstood or confusing interactions (first visit).
3. Instruct family to approach client calmly and quietly, in a nonthreatening manner, to treat client with dignity and respect, and to avoid hostility and criticisms when behavior is unacceptable (first visit).
4. Instruct family to allow client time for accomplishing tasks, to set up a schedule for care and events, and to allow for time to respond to client's questions (first visit).
5. Instruct family to limit stimulation to what client can manage without confusion and agitation and to reduce environmental stimulation such as noise and excessive lighting (first visit).

CLIENT AND FAMILY/CARETAKER INTERVENTIONS

1. Orient client to time, place, and person, and help client maintain a realistic thought process when appropriate.
2. Modify environment to enhance cognitive ability. Permit hoarding, pictures of past life, and use of a telephone.
3. Maintain a supportive, nonjudgmental environment.
4. Allow client time to accomplish tasks, to communicate, and to process thinking in order to reduce frustration and agitation.
5. Avoid actions that cause overstimulation or sensory overload.

Nursing diagnosis

High risk for injury

Related factors: Internal biochemical regulatory function of brain

Defining characteristics: Integrative dysfunction; sensory dysfunction; wandering; unsafe environment; restlessness; balance and coordination problems; lack of awareness; disorientation; forgetfullness

OUTCOME CRITERIA

Short-term
Reduction in risk for physical trauma, as evidenced by absence of environmental hazards and accidental injury (expected within 1 week)

Long-term
Absence of injury, as evidenced by adjustment of environment and provision of assistance necessary for safe ambulation and ADL practices (expected within 1 to 2 weeks and ongoing)

NURSING INTERVENTIONS/INSTRUCTIONS

1. Assess gait for instability, muscle weakness, and sensory-perceptual dysfunction; assess environment for hazards to be corrected (first visit).
2. Instruct family or caretaker in environmental changes to be made: clear pathways; remove or move furniture; remove small rugs; make slippery floors safe; remove matches from accessibility and remain with client when he or she is smoking; other adjustments, such as hand bars, assistive aids for walking (first visit).
3. Instruct family to secure and install a signalling device that will sound an alarm when client wanders past a certain point (first visit).
4. Provide assistance, and incorporate appropriate amount of assistance and appropriate frequency of ambulation into daily activity plan (first visit and reinforce on second visit).
5. Instruct family to reorient client to environment when necessary, to orient client to anything new in the immediate surroundings, to place articles for frequent use within reach, and to maintain same placement of articles and furniture (first visit).
6. Instruct family to avoid application of hot articles to the skin, offering food that is hot, or hot water for bathing (first visit).
7. Instruct family to store medications in a safe, locked cabinet (first visit).
8. Inform family that low-heeled, nonskid shoes should be

used by client for walking; instruct client to use a wide base when standing or ambulating (first visit).

CLIENT AND FAMILY/CARETAKER INTERVENTIONS

1. Identify and eliminate or control hazards in the environment.
2. Prevent falls or other injuries or trauma.
3. Provide identification bracelet or alarm device to prevent wandering away and reduce risk for injury.
4. Assist and supervise activities on the basis of client's cognitive and mentation status.
5. Incorporate ambulation and diversional activities into client's daily schedule.

Nursing diagnosis

Self-care deficit (bathing/hygiene, dressing/grooming, feeding, toileting)

Related factors: Perceptual or cognitive impairment; motor deficits

Defining characteristics: Inability to perform ADL; inability to recognize need for daily personal care; inability to use articles or utensils; inability to distinguish what is appropriate from what is inappropriate in dressing, grooming and toileting

OUTCOME CRITERIA

Short-term
Self-care maintained within limitations imposed by disease, as evidenced by personal appearance and care being adequate and appropriate (expected within 1 to 2 weeks)

Long-term
Appropriate pattern of ADL achieved, as evidenced by cleanliness and adequate hygiene, grooming, dressing, eating, and toileting with or without assistance or assistive aids (expected within 1 month and ongoing)

NURSING INTERVENTIONS/INSTRUCTIONS

1. Assess areas of self-care deficits and causes for them, need for assistance or supervision, and need for assistive aids

(see Functional Assessment, p. 43, for guidelines) (each visit).

2. Instruct family or caretaker to verbally remind or use cues for client to perform specific activity and to give only the assistance that is needed while avoiding expectations of task performance that may be frustrating (each visit).

3. Provide and instruct client and family in use of assistive aids and devices for eating, including large or padded handles on utensils, plate guard, placing food within view, and removing items not needed for meal (first visit).

4. Provide and instruct client and family in use of aids for toileting, including raised toilet seat, commode, hand bar for holding, and undergarmets that are easy to remove and replace, offering toileting opportunity or remind to use toilet (first visit).

5. Provide and instruct client and family in use of aids for bathing, dressing, and grooming, including Velcro closures, zippers, large neck openings, elastic waists, articles within reach; suggest possibility of purchasing several articles of clothing that are the same if client likes to wear the same things every day; lay out clothing daily in order of application and demonstrate use of articles if needed (each visit).

6. Provide and instruct client in use of a stool in the shower or hand bars to get in and out of the tub; supervise client in regulating the water temperature (first visit).

7. Refer HHA to assist in ADL as needed.

8. Initiate referral to physical and/or occupational therapy (any visit).

CLIENT AND FAMILY/CARETAKER INTERVENTIONS

1. Assist in ADL as needed.

2. Supervise self-care activities without impinging on independence and causing frustration; avoid rushing client to complete a task.

3. Provide assistive aids to enhance self-care in ADL.

4. Recognize client's capabilities, and assist in areas of self-care deficits.

5. Maintain adequate personal care, grooming, hygiene, and appearance.

Nursing diagnosis

High risk for violence directed at others

Related factors: Brain pathology

Defining characteristics: Restlessness; irritability; combative behavior; fear, bewilderment; agitation; outbursts when unable to complete tasks; lack of rest and sleep; frustration

OUTCOME CRITERIA

Short-term

Minimal violence directed at others, as evidenced by reduction in agitation, frustration, and combative behavior (expected within 1 to 2 weeks)

Long-term

Absence of other-directed violence, as evidenced by lack of agitation, frustration, and combative behavior (expected ongoing)

NURSING INTERVENTIONS/INSTRUCTIONS

1. Assess possible sensory overload, reactions to events and precipitating factors, depression, coping mechanisms used, misinterpretation of environment, and sleep and rest patterns (each visit).
2. Note behaviors indicating suspiciousness, fear, irritability, agitation, or combativeness (each visit).
3. Provide for verbalization of feelings to avoid suppressed feelings that lead to frustrations; instruct family or caretakers to avoid assigning tasks or having expectations that cause frustrations (each visit).
4. Promote a calm environment, and instruct family or caretaker to reduce stimuli, to avoid distressing client, and to provide diversion to diffuse a situation that does distress client (first visit).
5. Instruct family or caretaker to approach slowly and in a calm manner, to use slow gestures, and to keep hands where client can see them (first visit).
6. Instruct and reinforce regularly to avoid giving care or bothering client when agitated; limit foods and beverages containing caffeine (chocolate, coffee); face client when

present during upsets or combative periods and protect self from possible injury from client (each visit).
7. Instruct family to avoid allowing client excessive napping and to offer daily activities; remind client when bedtime approaches, and fulfill rituals before sleep; if client is awakened during night, reassure him or her with a quiet, calm voice that it is night and time for sleep (first visit).

CLIENT AND FAMILY/CARETAKER INTERVENTIONS

1. Identify cause of agitation and combative behavior, and take measures to prevent violence and frustration.
2. Respond to client's emotions, and provide a calm, reassuring environment.
3. Allow for open expression of anxiety, frustrations, and feelings with an accepting attitude.
4. Allow client as much control over environment as possible.
5. Provide for rest and sleep needs as determined by previous patterns.
6. Eliminate or minimize stimuli or expectations that agitate client.

Nursing diagnosis

Altered family processes

Related factors: Situational crisis of progressive degeneration of brain function of family member

Defining characteristics: Family system unable to meet physical and emotional needs of family and ill family member; family unable to express or accept feelings and security needs of members; family unable to accept change or deal with traumatic experience of caring for ill member

OUTCOME CRITERIA

Short-term

Progressive adaptation to care of family member, as evidenced by family's statement of decreased anxiety and fatigue and by effective use of coping mechanisms (expected within 1 to 2 weeks)

Long-term
Optimal adjustment and adaptation to care of ill member, as evidenced by satisfactory physical, social, and psychological health of family members (expected within 1 month and ongoing)

NURSING INTERVENTIONS/INSTRUCTIONS

1. Assess family interventions, dynamics, supportive behaviors, past patterns of social and diversional activities, past roles, and overall health status of caregiver(s) (see Family Assessment, p. 46, for guidelines) (first visit).
2. Inform family that disorder is progressive, that no cures are available, and that care is supportive (first visit).
3. Include all family members or significant persons in all teaching and planning of care, with scheduling and incorporation into daily routines (each visit).
4. Discuss possible hired help or respite care to assist in care and supervision of client, day care program, or other useful programs to relieve family from constant attendance to client needs (any visit).
5. Inform and instruct family in relaxation and coping techniques and in strategies to manage own behavior caused by unrelieved responsibilities (first and second visits).
6. Instruct family or caretakers to monitor their own health needs, and help them to identify problem areas for referral and evaluation if needed; emphasize the need to maintain their physical and emotional health (first and second visit).
7. Inform family of the importance of continuing or maintaining social and diversional activities and of the availability of social supports to participate in care (first visit).
8. Discuss anxiety produced by role reversal and feeling of powerlessness in caring for parent (any visit).
9. Instruct family in, and encourage them to discuss, methods to deal with client behavior and reactions (first visit).
10. Refer family to social services for assistance with finances or consultation with legal advisor if needed for client who has changes in cognitive ability and competence (any visit).
11. Refer family or caretaker to family counseling or individual counseling as appropriate (any visit).

12. Suggest and discuss local and national resources, such as
    Alzheimer's Disease and Related Disorders Association
    and Children of Aging Parents, for information and sup-
    port (first visit).
13. Discuss the need for long-term placement in the future as
    disease progresses or if family resources become
    exhausted (any visit).

CLIENT AND FAMILY/CARETAKER INTERVENTIONS

1. Verbalize feelings and concerns.
2. Identify problems in family and how family solves them
   together.
3. Resolve life-style changes together.
4. Seek out and participate in support group activity.
5. Utilize respite day care assistance.
6. Maintain family health: physical, emotional, and social.
7. Consult with social worker, financial counselor, and legal
   advisor for assistance.
8. Consider and begin to adapt to future long-term custodial
   care.

Nursing diagnosis

Caregiver role strain

Related factors: Unpredictable illness course or instability in
care receiver's health; psychological or cognitive problems in
care receiver; lack of respite for caregiver

Defining characteristics: Report of not having enough
resources to provide care (emotional and physical strength,
help from others); worry about the receiver's health and emotional state or about having to place care receiver in an institution; feeling that caregiving interferes with other roles

OUTCOME CRITERIA
Short-term
Caregiver role strain identified, as evidenced by verbalization
of difficulties encountered in performing care and concern
about ability and conflicts in giving care and adapting to role
(expected within 1 week)

Long-term
Adaptation to, and reduction of strain in, caregiver role, as evidenced by continued safe and appropriate care provided without compromise to caregiver's own physical and emotional needs (expected within 1 month and ongoing).

NURSING INTERVENTIONS/INSTRUCTIONS

1. Assess demands and care needs of receiver and ability and desire of caregiver to perform role; participation of family members in care (first visit).
2. Assess relationship between care receiver and caregiver before illness and stressors placed on the relationship by the progressive nature of the disorder (first visit).
3. Assist caregiver to monitor his or her continued ability to perform care and treatments and provide for day-to-day needs and how care receiver's behavior and needs change this ability; maintenance of routines; need for additional resources (aides, homemaker, respite care, friends, family) (each visit).
4. Discuss role performance and whether expectations are realistic; flexibility of role and decision-making process (first visit).
5. Initiate referral to HHA, social services, or psychological counseling, and suggest other community resources to contact for assistance with economic, mental health, or physical health needs (any visit).

CLIENT AND FAMILY/CARETAKER INTERVENTIONS

1. Develop coping strategies for the caregiving role and flexibility in day-to-day functioning.
2. Explore financial, legal, and physical assistance sources and consider referral to these services.
3. Maintain own health and well-being in caregiver role.
4. Utilize respite care and assistance from others for relief from stress of constant caregiving.
5. Maintain ongoing caregiving and treatment regimen.

Nursing diagnosis

Knowledge deficit

Related factors: Lack of information about disease and care

Defining characteristics: Expressed need for information about medication administration, measures to prevent acute or chronic illness, prognosis, and progression of disease

OUTCOME CRITERIA

Short-term
Adequate knowledge, as evidenced by family or caregiver's statement of correct medication scheduling and administration and methods to identify health problems (expected within 1 week)

Long-term
Adequate knowledge, as evidenced by optimal health and function within disease limitations (expected ongoing)

NURSING INTERVENTIONS/INSTRUCTIONS

1. Instruct family or caregiver in assessment for presence of urinary tract infection, upper respiratory infection, or other physical manifestations that might arise when client is unable to communicate symptoms; instruct family in taking temperature and recognizing changes in vital signs or urine or stool characteristics or expressions (nonverbal) of pain in any area and to report them to the physician (each visit).
2. Instruct family in administration of tranquilizers, antidepressants, and sedatives, including dose, action, frequency, side effects to report, when to discontinue the drug, and food and drug interactions (first visit and reinforce second visit).
3. Inform family that it is important to prevent exposure to infections and that health maintenance measures are important to prevent hospitalization, which would be traumatic for the client and might hasten progression of the disease (first visit).
4. Instruct family in daily nutritional, fluid, and elimination needs, and provide written lists of high-calorie foods that can be managed successfully, even if finger foods; a daily intake of 8 glasses of fluid per day if appropriate; use of

stool softeners or suppository to prevent constipation and fecal impaction; regularity in elimination pattern for urination and defecation (first visit).

CLIENT AND FAMILY/CARETAKER INTERVENTIONS

1. Manage daily elimination needs; provide for basic nutritional and fluid needs.
2. Take preventive measures to ensure health of client.
3. Correctly administer medications and report untoward effects.
4. Assess and report changes in physical health status.

▲ Amyotrophic Lateral Sclerosis (ALS)

Amyotrophic lateral sclerosis is a motor neuron disease with the presenting symptoms associated with the part of the nervous system most affected. It is characterized by progressive degeneration of the corticospinal tracts and the anterior horn cells or bulbar efferent neurons. This degeneration causes muscle weakness and atrophy, beginning in the hands and spreading to the forearms and legs, and may eventually become generalized. In some cases, chewing, talking, and swallowing are affected. Muscle fasciculations are also commonly apparent. The exact cause is unknown, and treatment is based on symptomatic relief.

Home care is primarily concerned with the maintenance and teaching aspects of preservation of muscle function and independence in and control of therapy and care.

Nursing diagnosis

Impaired physical mobility

Related factors: Neuromuscular impairment
Defining characteristics: Inability to purposefully move with-

in physical environment, including bed mobility, transfer, and ambulation; decreased muscle strength, control, or mass

OUTCOME CRITERIA

Short-term
Preservation of physical mobility, as evidenced by ambulation and participation in activities of daily living (ADL) within limitations imposed by disease (expected within 1 week and ongoing)

Long-term
Optimal continued ability to perform gross and fine motor activities to achieve and maintain functioning (expected ongoing)

NURSING INTERVENTIONS/INSTRUCTIONS

1. Assess degree of mobility, range of motion, weakness of upper extremities, muscle wasting, and fasciculations (see Musculoskeletal System Assessment, p. 25, for guidelines) (each visit).
2. Assess ability to wash body parts, put on or take off clothing, get to and use toilet, bring food from receptacle to mouth, and difficulty in chewing and swallowing (first visit).
3. Instruct client in strengthening exercises to maintain function for as long as possible (first and second visits).
4. Instruct client in use of assistive devices for ambulation and ADL, and help client to obtain necessary equipment to maintain independence, such as lift, hospital bed, wheelchair, and spring seats (first visit).
5. Instruct client in positioning, transfer, and turning techniques (first visit and reinforce as needed).
6. Initiate referral to physical and occupational therapists, if appropriate, to address above interventions (any visit).
7. Refer home health aide to assist in ADL.

CLIENT AND FAMILY/CARETAKER INTERVENTIONS

1. As long as possible, perform ADL and walking activities with or without use of assistive aids, as disease progression allows.
2. Use techniques to assist in turning, positioning, and transfer.

3. Maintain function within disease limitations as long as possible, with as much independence as possible.
4. Comply with physical and occupational therapy schedule and practice activities as instructed.

Nursing diagnosis

Ineffective individual coping

Related factors: Personal vulnerability; multiple life changes; consequences of fatal chronic illness

Defining characteristics: Verbalization of inability to cope or ask for help; chronic worry and anxiety; chronic fatigue; chronic depression; emotional tension; inability to meet basic needs and role expectations

OUTCOME CRITERIA

Short-term
Adequate coping, as evidenced by client's statement of need for life-style changes, expectations of disease and prognosis, need for improved coping mechanisms (expected within 1 week)

Long-term
Adequate coping, as evidenced by progressive grieving throughout illness, with reduction in anxiety and worry about prognosis and debilitation (expected within 3 months and ongoing)

NURSING INTERVENTIONS/INSTRUCTIONS

1. Establish rapport; provide an accepting environment for expression of concerns and questions (each visit).
2. Assess mental status, ability to adapt, use of coping mechanisms, and internal resources, and explore with client the most effective coping mechanisms and selection of positive options (first visit).
3. Help client to identify goals and positive coping mechanisms (each visit).
4. Allow client to participate in and plan care and practice effective problem-solving skills (each visit).
5. Instruct client to avoid events that produce stress or prevent

use of constructive coping mechanisms or behavior (first visit).

6. Instruct client in coping, communication, and problem-solving skills (first and second visits).

7. Instruct client in relaxation techniques, and in diversional techniques such as music, muscle relaxation, and reading (first visit).

CLIENT AND FAMILY/CARETAKER INTERVENTIONS

1. Develop effective use of coping mechanisms.
2. Avoid stress-provoking events.
3. Engage in relaxation and diversional activities.
4. Request assistance when needed.
5. Reduce and/or control anxiety level; express feelings and concerns.
6. Adapt to change in life-style to comply with medical regimen.

Nursing diagnosis

Altered nutrition: less than body requirements

Related factors: Inability to ingest food

Defining characteristics: Dysphagia; decreased gag reflex; weight loss; muscle wasting; inability to chew food

OUTCOME CRITERIA

Short-term
Adequate nutrition, as evidenced by intake of nutrients via mouth, nasogastric tube, or total parenteral nutrition (expected within 1 week)

Long-term
Adequate nutritional intake by appropriate method and route to maintain sustenance for as long as disease permits (expected ongoing)

NURSING INTERVENTIONS/INSTRUCTIONS

1. Assess nutritional status, caloric and vitamin/mineral needs, ability to chew and swallow, presence of choking episodes, weight loss, and ideal weight (see Gastrointestinal System Assessment, p. 17, for guidelines) (each visit).

2. Instruct client to weigh weekly at same time, on same scale, wearing the same clothing, and compare with ideal weight (first visit).

3. Assess for feeding method, presence of nasogastric tube, gastrostomy, esophagostomy, right atrial catheter and feeding provided (first and second visits).

4. Instruct caregiver to offer soft foods, as in casseroles, that can be easily managed for oral feeding; client should avoid liquids after chewing food (first visit).

5. Instruct caregiver to offer foods that are hot or cold to stimulate mouth receptors; avoid semisolid foods and milk (first visit).

6. Instruct client to position himself or herself upright with neck flexed during feedings or meals (first visit).

CLIENT AND FAMILY/CARETAKER INTERVENTIONS

1. Maintain nutritional status via oral, intravenous, or gastrostomy route.

2. Maintain actual weight, or as close to it as possible with consideration of muscle wasting; weigh weekly.

3. Calculate caloric intake and compare with weight loss.

4. Minimize the risk of choking and aspiration of food.

5. Prepare and ingest foods that are easy to chew and swallow.

Nursing diagnosis

Knowledge deficit

Related factors: Lack of information about disease

Defining characteristics: Expressed need for information about medical regimen, safety precautions to prevent trauma, and measures to maintain function

OUTCOME CRITERIA

Short-term

Adequate knowledge, as evidenced by client's ability to describe progressive characteristics of the disease, the medical regimen, and precautions to be taken to maintain function for as long as possible (expected within 1 week)

Long-term
Adequate knowledge, as evidenced by compliance with treatments for optimal preservation of abilities for functioning (expected ongoing based on disease progression)

NURSING INTERVENTIONS/INSTRUCTIONS

1. Assess life-style, ability to adapt, extent of disease and its effects, learning ability and interest, and family participation and support (first visit).
2. Inform client of disease process, prognosis, reason for loss of neuromuscular function, and the primary symptoms of the disease (first visit).
3. Inform client of and stress need for continuing activity and socialization; offer suggestions for diversional activities to support cognitive abilities; emphasis continuing need for self-care and independence for as long as possible (each visit).
4. Suggest use of a companion, ways to change life-style, and methods of stress and anxiety management (first visit).
5. Assist client with compliance with medical regimen by writing out plan of care and activities and realistic expectations (first visit and reinforce or revise on second visit).
6. Instruct client in medication adminstration, including dose, time, frequency, action of drug, side effects, and food and drug interactions (first visit).
7. Instruct client in skin care, massage and protective padding of bony areas, and importance of changing positions every 2 to 4 hours; report any breakdown or skin changes that do not disappear (first visit).
8. Refer client to speech pathologist if he or she is still able to speak, or if client is having a problem with swallowing; suggest a microphone for amplification or electrolarynx for phonation; if client is unable to speak, use environmental control system activated by pictures or slight movements (eye opening or closing) (first visit).
9. Instruct client that risk for infection is high, especially respiratory infection, and to avoid people with upper respiratory infections or other illnesses; dispose of tissues properly; instruct caregiver to use proper hand-washing technique before giving care; report any respiratory changes to the physician (first visit).

10. Inform client of, and instruct in and provide, mechanical ventilator assistance if client is at end stage and remaining at home and family or caretaker is able to manage this care (each visit).
11. Refer client and family to community agencies or social worker for assistance and support (any visit).

CLIENT AND FAMILY/CARETAKER INTERVENTIONS

1. Support all care and treatments, and prevent complications.
2. Adapt to and comply with the medical regimen.
3. Manage life-style changes and support independence in functional activities.
4. Maintain cognitive abilities and provide stimulation.
5. Report complications when appropriate.
6. Secure assistance with physical, economic, or psychological referral as needed.

◣ *Cerebrovascular Accident (CVA)*

Cerebrovascular accident is the cerebral inefficiency or hemorrhage resulting from blood flow disturbance caused by infarction or rupture of a blood vessel. The blood flow interruption may be caused by a thrombosis or an embolism, and the hemorrhage may be caused by a congenital aneurysm, trauma, or hypertension. Transient ischemic attacks (TIA) are temporary disturbances that may precede a CVA. Both types of CVA may have abrupt onsets, with the hemorrhagic type having the most acute and destructive onset. The extent of neurologic deficits and their permanence depend on the person's age and health status and on the site and size of the lesion.

The nature of the home care required depends on the severity and extent of the neurologic deficit; home care is primarily concerned with teaching the medical regimen that is used to treat the underlying condition and with rehabilitation and aftercare to maximize the health and wellness potential of the client.

Nursing diagnosis

Impaired physical mobility

Related factors: Neuromuscular impairment

Defining characteristics: Hemiplegia; hemiparesis; inability to purposely move within physical environment, including bed mobility, transfer, and ambulation; immobility

OUTCOME CRITERIA

Short-term
Progressive return of physical mobility, as evidenced by ambulation within limitations imposed by condition (expected within 1 week)

Long-term
Optimal continued return of mobility, as evidenced by maximal level of ability to ambulate, transfer, and perform other activities (expected ongoing)

NURSING INTERVENTIONS/INSTRUCTIONS

1. Assess degree and type of mobility impairment, range of motion (ROM), ability to transfer and change positions, muscle flaccidity, spasticity, and reflexes (see Musculoskeletal System Assessment, p. 25, for guidelines) (each visit).
2. Perform and instruct client in passive ROM exercises, with progress to active ROM exercises as appropriate in affected extremities (each visit).
3. Instruct client to position affected extremities using pillows, trochanter roll (hip), or other aids (footboard); place affected side with joint at higher level than joint proximal to it (first visit).
4. Instruct client to support limbs when repositioning (first visit).
5. Instruct client to elevate head of bed 15 degrees when in supine position and to use hard devices to support hand and soft devices to support leg (first visit).
6. Instruct client to limit turning to and lying on affected side for 1 hour and to avoid allowing the affected arm to rest on chest when in side-lying position (first visit).

7. Instruct client in exercises and movements, such as sitting up in bed or at side of bed, using head and body supports to prevent falling out of bed, moving to sitting position from lying position, moving from bed to chair, and moving from sitting position to standing position (first visit and reinforce each visit).

8. Initiate referral to physical and/or occupational therapy, and inform client of importance of compliance with exercises taught and use of aids to maximize self-mobility (first visit).

CLIENT AND FAMILY/CARETAKER INTERVENTIONS

1. Perform exercises and ambulation with or without aids.
2. Use techniques to assist in turning, positioning, and transfer.
3. Maintain ambulation within limitations.
4. Prevent contractures, maintain circulation, and maintain tone of muscles.
5. Comply with physical rehabilitation schedule, and practice activities as instructed.

Nursing diagnosis

Self-care deficit (bathing/hygiene, dressing/grooming, feeding, toileting)

Related factors: Perceptual impairment; paralysis; urinary/bowel incontinence

Defining characteristics: Inability to wash body parts, put on or take off clothes, get to and use toilet or be aware of urge to eliminate, bring food from receptacle to mouth; inadequate nutritional intake; inability to swallow

OUTCOME CRITERIA

Short-term
Progressive return to self-care, as evidenced by participation in feeding, toileting, bathing, personal hygiene, dressing, and grooming (expected within 1 week)

Long-term
Optimal return of functional abilities, as evidenced by maximal level of ability to perform activities of daily living (ADL)

with or without assistance or assistive aids (expected within 2 to 3 months and ongoing)

NURSING INTERVENTIONS/INSTRUCTIONS

1. Assess client's ability to perform self-care; ability to swallow and eat; ability to get on and off bedpan or use commode; ability to use one hand if hemiplegic; neurologic impairment (tactile, visual, auditory, kinesthetic) and response to stimuli (see Functional Assessment, p. 43, for guidelines) (each visit).
2. Instruct family or caregiver to provide assistance or supervision as needed for performance of ADL (first visit).
3. Provide and instruct client in use of assistive aids and devices for eating, including large, swivel, or padded handles on utensils; plate guard; placing food within view; and removing items not needed for meal (first visit).
4. Provide and instruct client in use of aids for toileting, including raised toilet seat, commode, hand bar, and undergarments that are easy to remove and replace (first visit).
5. Provide and instruct client in use of aids for bathing, dressing, and grooming, including Velcro closures, zippers, large neck openings, elastic waists, and articles that may be placed in a holder or stuck to wall or counter (first visit).
6. Initiate referral to occupational therapy for instruction and practice in ADL and suggestions for other assistive aids or performance of above interventions as appropriate (any visit).
7. Refer home health aide for assistance in ADL (first visit).

CLIENT AND FAMILY/CARETAKER INTERVENTIONS

1. Assist with ADL while encouraging independence.
2. Use assistive aids and devices in performance of ADL.
3. Maintain functional abilities in daily activities.
4. Comply with occupational rehabilitation schedule and practice activities as instructed.

Nursing diagnosis

Impaired verbal communication

Related factors: Physical barrier of decreased circulation in brain

Defining characteristics: Inability to speak (aphasia); dysarthria

OUTCOME CRITERIA

Short-term
Adequate communication, as evidenced by ability to communicate needs effectively (expected within 1 week)

Long-term
Return to communication patterns, as evidenced by optimal speech or development of an effective method of communication (expected within 2 to 3 months and ongoing)

NURSING INTERVENTIONS/INSTRUCTIONS

1. Determine communication deficits and remaining strengths or positive features (first visit).
2. Instruct family or caregiver to speak to client in short simple statements, to ask questions that need a yes or no answer, to speak slowly and in a normal tone, and to allow time for a response (first visit).
3. Instruct client to use gestures, paper and pencil, slate board, pictures, or cards and to reinforce established communication techniques if appropriate (first visit).
4. Instruct client in oral and facial exercises to improve muscular integrity (first and second visits).
5. Initiate referral to speech pathologist for therapy (any visit).

CLIENT AND FAMILY/CARETAKER INTERVENTIONS

1. Speak to client slowly and clearly and in a normal tone.
2. Avoid interruptions, forcing client to communicate, or criticism of his or her speech.
3. Use facial expressions or pantomine to communicate.
4. Use pencil and paper, slate board, pictures, cards, or any other effective method to communicate.
5. Maintain a quiet environment, position speaker in front of client, and decrease distractions.
6. Anticipate needs if client is unable to express them.
7. Comply with speech pathologist's schedules and instructions.

Nursing diagnosis

High risk for trauma

Related factors: Weakness; balancing difficulties; reduced temperature and/or tactile sensation; neurologic deficit

Defining characteristics: Hemiparesis; hemiplegia; loss of muscle tone; visual-spatial misperception; inability to orient self and movement in the environment; unsteady gait; lack of safety precautions in the environment; neurosensory impairment (tactile)

OUTCOME CRITERIA

Short-term
Minimal possibility of trauma, as evidenced by absence of falls or injury, and by client's statement of safety precautions to take (expected within 1 week and ongoing)

Long-term
Absence of trauma, as evidenced by safe environment maintained to accomodate neurologic deficits (expected within 1 month and ongoing)

NURSING INTERVENTIONS/INSTRUCTIONS

1. Assess sensory perception to hot/cold, sharp/dull; awareness of body parts; visual or auditory deficits; presence and degree of paralysis and ability for ambulation and movement; disorientation or change in mentation (each visit).
2. Instruct client and family to adjust environment to reduce possibility of falls and trauma by arranging furniture for holding, providing clear pathways, removing a door to accomodate a wheelchair, removing small rugs, and providing proper lighting and to use assistive aids when walking or refer to occupational therapy for this assistance (first visit).
3. Provide, and instruct family or caregiver to provide, a consistent approach when assisting with ambulation and ADL (first visit).
4. Instruct client to turn head and scan environment; instruct caregiver to approach on affected side and to place objects on affected side if visual field impairment is present (first visit).

5. Instruct client to protect affected limbs from extremes of hot or cold or from hot or cold applications to limbs if tactile perception is affected (first visit).
6. Instruct family or caregiver to supervise all activities if judgment of position, distance, or rate of movement is impaired (first visit).
7. Instruct family or caregiver in skin care if tactile perception is affected, ·including assessment and protection and massage of pressure points, frequent changes of position (every 2 hours), cleansing, and application of an emollient to the skin (first and second visits).

CLIENT AND FAMILY/CARETAKER INTERVENTIONS

1. Allow as much independence as possible.
2. Protect client from falls and from trauma to skin and affected limbs.
3. Promote visual field enhancement.
4. Adapt environment to deficits and for safe mobility.

Nursing diagnosis

Knowledge deficit

Related factors: Lack of information about disease and treatments

Defining characteristics: Expressed need for information about medication, medical regimen, and rehabilitation program

OUTCOME CRITERIA

Short-term
Adequate knowledge, as evidenced by client's statement of nutritional, fluid, elimination, and medication regimen and rehabilitation needs (expected within 3 days)

Long-term
Adequate knowledge, as evidenced by compliance with medical regimen and achievement of optimal health and functioning (expected within 1 to 3 months)

NURSING INTERVENTIONS/INSTRUCTIONS

1. Assess life-style, learning and adaptation abilities, interest level, and family participation and support (first visit).

2. Assess all systems for effect of long-term hypertension; note history for predisposing factors or disorders that relate to secondary hypertension (first visit).

3. Assess and instruct client in monitoring blood pressure and pulse (first visit).

4. Advise client about life-style changes, methods of stress management, and dietary changes; to have regular screening for blood pressure, circulatory, and visual changes; and to have laboratory testing if Coumadin therapy is prescribed (first visit).

5. Instruct client in administration of antihypertensives, anticoagulants, diuretics, stool softeners, and vitamin/mineral supplements, including dose, route, frequency, side effects, and food and drug interactions (first visit).

6. Instruct client in constipation program to include increased fluid intake (8 to 10 glasses/day), increased bulk in diet, and daily activity and exercise program (first visit).

7. Instruct client in dietary inclusion of foods or preference that are textured for easy swallowing; use of thickeners; placing foods on unaffected side of mouth and allowing plenty of time for meals; avoiding milk and foods that are too thin and smooth (first visit).

8. Instruct client in urinary bladder rehabilitation by offering elimination opportunity every 2 hours; scheduling voiding at certain times with fluid intake and temporary measures such as pads or waterproof undergarments (first and second visits).

9. Inform client of importance of compliance with physical, occupational, and speech therapy regimens (first visit).

10. Instruct client to report changes such as headache, vertigo, changes in mentation, or visual disturbances to the physician (first visit).

11. Inform client that emotional lability is not uncommon and of the possibility of becoming depressed and the need for counseling services if appropriate (any visit).

12. Inform client of agencies such as American Heart Association to contact for information, assistive devices, and support services (first visit).

CLIENT AND FAMILY/CARETAKER INTERVENTIONS

1. Adapt to life-style changes to accomodate medical regimen.
2. Verbalize nutritional, fluid, and elimination measures to ensure optimal function.
3. Comply with medication and rehabilitation schedules, and carry out safe interventions as instructed.
4. Verbalize signs and symptoms to report indicating possible recurrence of stroke.
5. Utilize community agencies for assistance and support.

Nursing diagnosis

Ineffective family coping: compromised

Related factors: Prolonged disease or disability that exhausts the supportive capacity of significant people

Defining characteristics: Expression of concern or complaint about client's health problem; lack of information about residual damage from stroke

OUTCOME CRITERIA

Short-term
Improved coping, as evidenced by acknowledgement of disabling effects of disease and required life-style changes and by cooperation and participation in treatment regimen (expected within 1 week)

Long-term
Optimal level of participation and support by family members to facilitate changes in client's life-style and improvement in health status (expected within 1 to 2 months)

NURSING INTERVENTIONS/INSTRUCTIONS

1. Assess family interactions and coping abilities, strengths of individual members, level of participation and support, and resources available and utilized by family (see Family Assessment, p. 46 for guidelines) (first visit).
2. Provide accurate information to family about treatment regimen and deficits that cannot be changed; allow time for questions or clarifications (each visit).
3. Encourage family to discuss strengths and options for

change and to identify coping mechanisms used (each visit).

4. Include family members in teaching and realistic planning of care (each visit).
5. Inform client and family that full or partial recovery may take a long time (first visit).
6. Inform client and family of government and community agencies available for support and assistance (first visit).
7. Initiate referral to social services, and encourage family to contact counselor if appropraite (any visit).

CLIENT AND FAMILY/CARETAKER INTERVENTIONS

1. Verbalize concerns and feelings about burden of care of family member with chronic disorder.
2. Seek assistance if needed.
3. Participate in planning and implementing care.
4. Adapt to limitations of client, and integrate them into family activity.
5. Cope with client's response to the losses.
6. Continue family activities and open communication.

◣ *Head Injury*

Head injury is penetration of the skull or traumatic impact to the skull that damages the brain tissue at the point of impact. The injury may be a concussion, cerebral contusion, laceration, or brainstem trauma and may result in edema, hemorrhage causing increased intracranial pressure, amnesia, hemiplegia, impaired consciousness, breathing impairment, or coma. Head injury is usually the result of an accident.

Home care depends on the extent and severity of the injury and is primarily concerned with teaching of the medical regimen and treatment of the residual effects to facilitate restoration of normal function.

Nursing diagnosis

High risk for injury

Related factors: Internal regulatory function; physical function; psychological function

Defining characteristics: Inability to purposefully move about; unsteady gait; sensory/perceptual deficits; disorientation; change in consciousness; visual disturbances; seizure activity

OUTCOME CRITERIA

Short-term

Improved function within limitations imposed by condition, as evidenced by mental alertness; return of thought processes; orientation to time, place, and person; and resumption of mobility and activities of daily living (ADL) without injury (expected within 1 week or as practical)

Long-term

Progressive return to optimal health and functioning without injury, with awareness of residual deficits (expected within 3 to 6 months)

NURSING INTERVENTIONS/INSTRUCTIONS

1. Assess for presence of reflexes, mentation changes, changes in motor or sensory function, paralysis, visual impairment, and cognitive ability (each visit).
2. Inform client of possible changes in judgment, emotional control, and social restraint in association with this condition (first visit).
3. Instruct family or caregiver to adjust environment to prevent trauma from falls or other injury, to reorient client as needed, to provide supervision and/or assist with ambulation and ADL as needed, and to provide assistive aids as needed (each visit).
4. Instruct family or caregiver in measures to protect client from injury during seizure activity, including staying with client, turning client on side, avoiding restraining client, and placing pillow under head (first visit).
5. Refer home health aide to assist with ADL as needed.
6. Consult with home care rehabilitation specialist (any visit).

CLIENT AND FAMILY/CARETAKER INTERVENTIONS

1. Provide assistance with ambulation and ADL with or without aids.
2. Maintain safe environment with clear pathways and lighted rooms; make sure client has proper shoes and glasses.
3. Prevent injury during seizure activity with protective measures.
4. Note and report changes in mentation or behavior.

Nursing diagnosis

Knowledge deficit

Related factors: Lack of knowledge about consequences of injury

Defining characteristics: Expressed need for information about injury, effects, prognosis, and medication and rehabilitative regimens

OUTCOME CRITERIA

Short-term
Adequate knowledge, as evidenced by client's ability to describe cause and effects of the injury and the medication and rehabilitative regimens (expected within 1 week)

Long-term
Adequate knowledge, as evidenced by compliance with medical regimen to achieve optimal health and functioning and progressive recovery (expected within 1 to 6 months)

NURSING INTERVENTIONS/INSTRUCTIONS

1. Assess life-style, ability to adapt, learning ability and interest, cognitive deficits, and family participation and support (first visit).
2. Inform family that time and patience are needed to deal with the deficits or problems and that the appearance of client may not be an indication of level of recovery if any (first visit).
3. Instruct family or caregiver in medication administration, usually anticonvulsants, anticoagulants, and muscle relaxants, including dose, action, frequency, side effects, and

food and drug interactions, and not to skip doses or discontinue without advice of physician (first visit).
4. Instruct family or caregiver in doing neurologic checks and assessment of mentation and changes in consciousness to report (each visit).
5. Inform client that recovery may take 6 months, including rehabilitation to treat specific residual deficits of posttraumatic stage (first visit).
6. Instruct family in appropriate interaction patterns to avoid family dysfunction and that client should avoid alcohol, driving, use of hazardous equipment, and unsupervised smoking (first visit).
7. Inform family of importance of keeping appointments with rehabilitation team and with agencies that assist with economic, psychological, and physical support (any visit).

CLIENT AND FAMILY/CARETAKER INTERVENTIONS

1. Adapt to change in life-style to include rehabilitation.
2. Participate in and support client's recovery from chronic problems and mental and emotional sequelae.
3. Administer medications correctly, and report side effects or ineffective response from medciations.
4. Provide a safe environment, including avoidance of alcohol, smoking alone, use of guns and hazardous machinery or appliances, driving a car, and use of OTC drugs.
5. Maintain rehabilitation schedule as prescribed.

⬥ *Multiple Sclerosis (MS)*

Multiple sclerosis is a chronic slowly progressive central nervous system disease causing demyelination in the brain and spinal cord. It is associated with an immunologic abnormality causing an inflammatory process that is responsible for the loss of the myelin sheath from the axon cylinders of the nerves, primarily in the white matter. The disease is characterized by remissions and exacerbations of symptoms, which include transient weakness, stiffness and fatigue of a limb, gait disturbances, vertigo, loss of bladder and bowel control, visual disturbances, emotional lability, and lack of judgment.

Home care is primarily concerned with the teaching of safety and the medical regimen and with the preservation of physical and mental function.

Nursing diagnosis

Self-esteem disturbance

Related factors: Biophysical, psychosocial factors

Defining characteristics: Verbal responses to change in body function; self-negating verbalizations; expression of shame (incontinence); inability to deal with illness; hestitancy to change life-style; inability to perform activities of daily living (ADL); depression

OUTCOME CRITERIA

Short-term
Improved self-esteem, as evidenced by client's statement of ability to cope with long-term debilitation and changes in life-style associated with dysfunction (expected within 1 week).

Long-term
Progressively more positive attitude about prolonged illness, with participation in treatment regimen to achieve optimal health and functioning within limitations of disease (expected within 2 to 3 months and ongoing)

NURSING INTERVENTIONS/INSTRUCTIONS

1. Assess client for behavioral changes and emotional status, including anxiety and depression, feelings of powerlessness, and use and effectiveness of coping mechanisms (each visit).
2. Focus on remaining abilities, and instruct family to maintain a positive attitude and support (each visit).
3. Discuss effect of illness on self-concept (any visit).
4. Encourage client to participate in treatments and ADL; instruct family to assist when needed but to allow for independence when possible (first visit).
5. Allow for expression of feelings and concerns about neurologic functioning and effect on life-style (each visit).
6. Refer client to counseling and social services if appropriate.

CLIENT AND FAMILY/CARETAKER INTERVENTIONS

1. Set goals and participate in treatments.
2. Identify and use coping mechanisms that are effective.
3. Use a planned program for entire day to deal with boredom and anxiety.
4. Maintain independence, and use measures to reduce embarrassment caused by changes in function.
5. Ventilate feelings during nurse's visits.
6. Improve self-concept with adaptation to prolonged dysfunction.
7. Accept and participate in counseling services if needed.

Nursing diagnosis

Altered patterns of urinary elimination

Related factors: Sensorimotor impairment

Defining characteristics: Urgency, frequency, dribbling, incontinence, retention, or spastic or flaccid bladder, depending on site of lesion

OUTCOME CRITERIA

Short-term
Progressive absence of urinary elimination impairment, as evidenced by reduction in incontinence episodes and retention with residual less than 150 ml (expected within 1 to 2 weeks)

Long-term
Urinary continence and absence of retention, as evidenced by establishment of urinary elimination pattern for optimal functioning (expected within 2 to 3 months and ongoing)

NURSING INTERVENTIONS/INSTRUCTIONS

1. Assess for presence of spastic bladder (incontinence), flaccid bladder (retention), suprapubic distention, or cloudy, foul-smelling urine (first visit).
2. Instruct client and family in administration of cholinergic or anticholinergic medications to relieve bladder symptoms, including action, dosage, frequency, side effects, precautions, and food and drug interactions (first visit).
3. Instruct client and family in fluid needs (8 to 10 glasses per

day), and assess for possible urinary bladder infection if residual is present (first visit).

4. Perform Credé maneuver or relex stimulation manually, and instruct in use of these methods if retention is present (first and second visits).
5. Instruct client or family to perform catheterization on intermittent basis if ordered to treat retention (any visit).
6. Instruct client in protection methods to prevent embarrassment from incontinence.
7. Refer client to bladder training program if appropriate (any visit).

CLIENT AND FAMILY/CARETAKER INTERVENTIONS

1. Maintain fluid intake of 3000 ml/day.
2. Participate in methods to stimulate or control urinary elimination.
3. Administer medications correctly to relieve bladder symptoms.
4. Monitor intake and output; assess for presence of urinary tract infection.
5. Utilize garment protectors and waterproof underwear.
6. Participate in bladder training program.

Nursing diagnosis

Impaired physical mobility

Related factors: Neuromuscular impairment

Defining characteristics: Inability to purposefully move within physical environment, including bed mobility, transfer, and ambulation; weakness; pain and spasms of muscles; unsteady gait; limb stiffness; vertigo; paresthesias; inability to perform ADL

OUTCOME CRITERIA

Short-term

Adequate mobility and activity performance, as evidenced by preservation of ability to ambulate and participate in ADL within limitations imposed by disease (expected within 1 to 2 weeks)

Long-term

Optimal ability to perform gross and fine motor activities to achieve and maintain present functioning (expected within 1 to 2 months and ongoing)

NURSING INTERVENTIONS/INSTRUCTIONS

1. Assess mobility status; presence and duration of muscle spasms; risk for injury related to altered mobility, paralysis, or paresthesia; need for wheelchair (see Musculoskeletal System Assessment, p. 25, for guidelines) (each visit).
2. Instruct client and family in administration of antispasmodics to decrease spasticity, including dose, time, frequency, precautions, and side effects (first and second visits).
3. Emphasize and instruct client in daily exercises, including stretching and stride increasing by walking with feet farther apart (for gait training) (first visit).
4. Instruct client to apply ice to spastic muscle (or use warm bath) before exercising and to rest between exercises (first visit).
5. Instruct client in use of assistive devices for self-care, instruct family to assist while encouraging independence (each visit).
6. For a safe environment, and especially to prevent falls, instruct family to clear pathways, remove small rugs, and provide rails or assistive aids for ambulation (first visit).
7. Initiate referral to physical and occupational therapists as needed.
8. Refer client to home health aide (HHA) and homemaker services as needed.

CLIENT AND FAMILY/CARETAKER INTERVENTIONS

1. Administer medications correctly and report side effects; avoid driving and hazardous activities, use of alcohol, and abrupt discontinuation of medications.
2. Meet needs for ADL with or without assistance and use of aids.
3. Relieve muscle spasticity, increase coordination, and use nonaffected muscles for impaired ones if possible.
4. Participate in physical therapy with water exercises, massage, and occupational therapy as needed.
5. Provide safe environment for functioning.

6. Utilize HHA and homemaker services to assist with ADL, meal preparation, and shopping; utilize any other services that are needed.

Nursing diagnosis

Knowledge deficit

Related factors: Lack of information about disease and manifestations

Defining characteristics: Expressed need for information about changes in life-style to promote functional maintenance and to maintain general health

OUTCOME CRITERIA

Short-term
Adequate knowledge, as evidenced by client's statement of precautions and treatments to implement and methods to ensure health and functioning (expected within 1 week)

Long-term
Adequate knowledge, as evidenced by maintenance of general health and functioning and by compliance with medical regimen and instructions (expected within 1 to 2 months)

NURSING INTERVENTIONS/INSTRUCTIONS

1. Assess life-style, ability to adapt, learning ability and interest, and family participation and support (first visit).
2. Inform client and family of cause of disease and reason for neurosensory and neuromuscular dysfunction (first visit).
3. Inform client and family of, and stress need for, long-term physical therapy and maintenance of mobility and independent functioning (first visit).
4. Instruct client to avoid fatigue, extremes of heat and cold, and any exposure to people with illness or infections; instruct client to balance rest and activity (first visit).
5. Instruct client to avoid constipation by increasing fiber and fluids in dietary intake, including items from the basic four food groups, and eating well-balanced, nutritious meals (first and second visits).
6. Inform client that tinnitus or decreased auditory acuity, and visual changes such as blurred vision or patches of

blindness, are caused by CNS involvement; suggest large print and other aids available for visual or auditory deficits (first visit).

7. Instruct client and family in skin care if client is confined to wheelchair or bed.

8. Review and instruct client in administration of all medications, and instruct client to avoid OTC drugs unless advised by physician (first and second visits).

9. Inform client of eventual possible sexual dysfunction, impotence in males, decreased libido, and decreased vaginal lubrication in women and suggest resources (any visit).

10. Instruct client and family in grieving process and reason for behaviors that are normal and perhaps predictable as function is lost (each visit).

11. Inform client and family that signs and symptoms of disease and changes in behavior (anger, depression) may be initiated by fatigue, infection, or physical or emotional stress or trauma (any visit).

12. Refer client and family to National Multiple Sclerosis Society and local agencies for information and support (any visit).

CLIENT AND FAMILY/CARETAKER INTERVENTIONS

1. Describe health measures to prevent complications and maintain function.

2. Avoid stress, fatigue, formation of contractures, and skin breakdown by compliance with physical therapy protocol.

3. Participate in goal setting and decisions regarding care schedule.

4. Maintain nutritional status needed for health and functioning; include vitamins, fiber, and fluid intake of 3000 ml/day.

5. Avoid exposure to or involvement in activities that predispose to infections.

6. Seek out assistance for sexual dysfunction and alternate sexual expression.

7. Adapt to and comply with complete medical regimen safely and appropriately.

8. Contact and utilize social services and community agencies for information and support.

◢ *Parkinson's Disease*

Parkinson's disease is a chronic, progressive central nervous system disorder characterized by muscular rigidity, a slow decrease in movement, and tremors. It involves the degeneration of the brain centers that control movement and is associated with low concentrations of dopamine, which account for the symptoms of the disease. The incapacitation that occurs from this disease may take years to develop.

Home care is primarily concerned with the teaching of medication administration and self-care activities to ensure basic needs, depending on symptomatic effects of the disease.

Nursing diagnosis

Impaired physical mobility

Related factors: Neuromuscular impairment; decreased strength and endurance

Defining characteristics: Inability to purposefully move within physical environment, including ambulation, bradykinesic tremor, contractures, deformities, unsteady gait, muscle rigidity

OUTCOME CRITERIA
Short-term
Preservation of physical mobility, as evidenced by ambulation and participation in activities of daily living (ADL) within limitations imposed by disease (expected within 1 week and ongoing)

Long-term
Continued optimal ability to perform gross and fine motor activities to achieve or maintain present functioning throughout illness (expected ongoing)

NURSING INTERVENTIONS/INSTRUCTIONS
1. Assess degree of mobility, range of motion (ROM), presence of contractures, bradykinesia, ability to stand from sitting position, need for assistive aids (see Musculoskeletal System Assessment, p. 25, for guidelines) (first visit).

2. Assess client's ability to wash body parts, put on or take off clothing or fasten clothing, bring food to mouth to feed self, and perform personal hygiene and grooming activities (see Functional Assessment, p. 43, for guidelines) (first visit).
3. Instruct client in daily ambulation and active or passive ROM and other exercises in all extremities, head, and neck; include stretching, stride increasing, and facial exercises (first and second visits).
4. Instruct client to use straight chair for sitting and how to get up using arm rests, to carry object in hand or place hand in pocket to reduce tremors, to change positions to avoid resting tremor, to lift toes when stepping and step over imaginary or real lines, and to step backward once and forward with two steps to correct akinesia or freezing (first visit and when needed).
5. Instruct client in application of hot packs and use of massage to reduce muscle rigidity (first visit).
6. Encourage and instruct client in use of assistive aids for ADLs, and provide assistance by home health aide referral when needed (any visit).
7. Initiate referral to physical and occupational therapists as appropriate (first visit).

CLIENT AND FAMILY/CARETAKER INTERVENTIONS

1. Perform ambulation and exercises, ADL, and other activities within limitations imposed by disease.
2. Make use of measures to facilitate mobility, reduce tremor, and change positions.
3. Use aids to facilitate ADL and maintain independence.
4. Participate in physical and occupational therapy.
5. Make use of measures to reduce muscle rigidity.

Nursing diagnosis

Ineffective individual coping

Related factors: Personal vulnerability, multiple life changes

Defining characteristics: Verbalization of inability to cope, inability to meet basic needs, alteration in societal participation, change in usual communication patterns, chronic anxiety, depression, loss of control

OUTCOME CRITERIA

Short-term
Adequate coping, as evidenced by progressive participation in treatment program and use of coping and problem solving skills (expected within 1 week)

Long-term
Adequate coping, as evidenced by attitude and life-style changes indicating achievement of optimal physical and emotional functioning (expected within 3 months and ongoing)

NURSING INTERVENTIONS/INSTRUCTIONS

1. Assess for verbalization of behavioral changes indicating anxiety, lability, depression, social isolation, or body image disturbance; assess use and effectiveness of coping mechanisms (see Psychosocial Assessment, p. 41, for guidelines) (each visit).
2. Discuss self-concept, including appearance and loss of neurologic and musculoskeletal functioning (drooling, tremor, slurred speech); discuss adjustment to and acceptance of the disease (each visit).
3. Instruct client to use typewriter, slate, or paper and pencil to assist in communication (first visit).
4. Inform client and family of need for socialization and of agencies and groups in the community that perform services and provide information and support (first visit).
5. Assist client to establish realistic goals for functioning, and instruct client in coping and problem-solving skills to achieve these goals (first and second visits).
6. Initiate couseling as appropriate (any visit).

CLIENT AND FAMILY/CARETAKER INTERVENTIONS

1. Use a planned program for entire day to deal with anxiety and depression.
2. Identify and use coping skills that are effective.
3. Set realistic goals and participate in treatments.
4. Maintain independence and use measures to reduce embarrassment from changes in functioning.
5. Ventilate feelings and concerns; accept counseling if needed.

6. Improve self-concept with adjustment to the disease and its problems.

Nursing diagnosis

Knowledge deficit

Related factors: Lack of information about disease

Defining characteristics: Expressed need for information about disease's cause, effects, and prognosis; medication administration; fluid/nutritional/activity regimen; preservation of abilities; prevention of injury

OUTCOME CRITERIA

Short-term

Adequate knowledge, as evidenced by client's description of disease's cause and progressive nature, medical regimen, and precautions for preventing complications (expected within 1 week)

Long-term

Adequate knowledge, as evidenced by compliance with medical regimen for optimal preservation of functional abilities (expected within 1 month and ongoing)

NURSING INTERVENTIONS/INSTRUCTIONS

1. Inform client of disease process and cause and of reason for loss of neurologic and musculoskeletal functioning (first visit).
2. Inform client of and stress need for continuing activity and socialization, and need for self-care and independence in ADL to maintain functioning (first visit).
3. Instruct client to take frequent rest periods throughout the day (first visit).
4. Instruct client and family in nutritional needs, including small, frequent meals of high-calorie, protein food choices and a selection of high-fiber foods and fluid intake of up to 3000 ml/day to maintain nutrition and prevent constipation; inform client and family that accidents involving food and drinks are common and need to be ignored and treated with kindness; suggest eating slowly and chewing foods thoroughly (first and second visits).

5. Instruct client and family in administration of medications, including dose, action, frequency, side effects, precautions, and signs and symptoms to report to physician as a result of medication; discuss stool softeners, antiparkinsonian drugs (dopaminergic, anticholinergic, antihistamine), and antidepressants, and instruct client to avoid OTC drugs unless advised by physician (first visit and any visit as needed).
6. Instruct client and family in safety measures, including removal of small rugs and furniture from pathways and use of elevated chair and toilet seat (first visit).
7. Inform client that exercises to strengthen muscles used for speaking, chewing, and swallowing should be included in daily physical therapy and refer to speech pathologist if appropriate (first visit).
8. Inform of and direct client and family to community resources, including American Parkinson Disease Association, for information and support (first visit).

CLIENT AND FAMILY/CARETAKER INTERVENTIONS

1. Adapt and comply with medical regimen.
2. Administer medications correctly as prescribed, and report untoward effects.
3. Participate in activity, rest, and fluid and nutritional program within limitations or restrictions imposed by disease.
4. Establish and maintain adequate bowel elimination, weight, and nutritional status.
5. Institute measures to prevent falls and encourage independence.
6. Contact and utilize community agencies for information and support.

◢ *Seizure Disorders*

Seizures are recurrent paroxysmal disorders of cerebral function that are characterized by altered consciousness, sensory phenomena, motor activity, or changes in behavior. Any seizure pattern that is recurrent is known as epilepsy. Seizures are classified as partial or generalized and may be caused by cerebral or systemic disorders, such as acute infections (including central nervous system infections), cerebral hypoxia, cerebral fracture, brain lesions/tumors, toxic agents, congenital brain defects, cerebral edema, cerebral trauma, cerebral hemorrhage, cerebral infarct, and anaphylaxis. Seizure activity resulting from any cause may be transient and not recur after the disorder is corrected or ends.

Home care is primarily concerned with the teaching of medication administration to control seizures and with prevention of physical and psychological trauma that may result from seizure activity.

Nursing diagnosis

High risk for injury

Related factors: Internal regulatory function (sensory, integrative dysfunction)

Defining characteristics: Musculoskeletal trauma from falls; oral tissue trauma from biting; soft-tissue bruising; lack of safety precautions; uncontrolled movements

OUTCOME CRITERIA

Short-term
Minimal injury or absence of injury, as evidenced by mouth, tongue, bone, or soft-tissue damage being controlled or absent during and following seizure activity (expected within time frame of seizure)

Long-term
Absence of injury, as evidenced by no breaks in skin or mucous membranes or bones as seizures are controlled (expected ongoing)

NURSING INTERVENTIONS/INSTRUCTIONS

1. Assess type and frequency of seizure activity, loss of consciousness, loss of muscle tone, tongue biting, falling to the floor, weakness or paralysis, presence of aura (first visit).
2. Instruct caregiver to allow client to slide to floor; place client in side-lying position; avoid restricting any movement, jerking, or stiffening; loosen constricting clothing (first visit and reinforce on second visit).

3. Instruct caregiver to remain with client during entire seizure and to place small pillow under head or place head in lap (first visit).
4. Instruct client and family to remove harmful objects from the immediate environment (first visit).
5. Instruct client and caregiver to note if aura is present, how seizure began, and how it progressed and lasted; presence of cyanosis, excessive saliva, incontinence, and sleep period to report (first visit).
6. Instruct client to prevent seizure activity by avoiding emotional and physical stress or stimulation that triggers seizure (noise, lights, drugs) (first visit).

CLIENT AND FAMILY/CARETAKER INTERVENTIONS

1. Perform measures to prevent trauma during seizure activity.
2. Provide safe environment during seizure activity.
3. Assess aspects of seizure activity and report to physician for evaluation.
4. Remain and support client during seizure activity.
5. Avoid actions and stimuli that cause seizure activity.

Nursing diagnosis

Anxiety

Related factors: Threat to self-concept; threat of change in health status

Defining characteristics: Verbalized apprehension and uncertainty about unpredictable seizure activity; social withdrawal; feelings of inadequacy; stigma attached to presence of disorder

OUTCOME CRITERIA

Short-term
Reduced anxiety, as evidenced by client's statement that anxiety is at manageable level, embarrassment controlled, and social and family interactions improved (expected within 1 to 2 weeks)

Long-term
Anxiety level at optimal level for achievement of health and functioning, with self-concept enhanced (expected within 2 to 3 months)

NURSING INTERVENTIONS/INSTRUCTIONS

1. Assess anxiety level; social interactions and how condition impacts life-style and self-esteem; perception of how others view disease (first visit and as needed).
2. Allow client to express feelings about diagnosis of epilepsy (each visit).
3. Assist client to develop coping strategies to reduce anxiety, and instruct client in relaxation techniques, including reading, music, imagery, and relaxation exercises (first and second visits).
4. Inform client of importance of maintaining social relationships and recreation and occupational activities (each visit).
5. Initiate referral to counseling if appropriate (any visit).

CLIENT AND FAMILY/CARETAKER INTERVENTIONS

1. Discuss feelings, anger, and anxiety regarding condition.
2. Develop coping skills to reduce anxiety.
3. Utilize relaxation techniques to reduce anxiety.
4. Maintain relationships and activities for optimal functioning.
5. Adapt to life-style that includes stigma or misconception of the disease by others.
6. Participate in counseling services if needed.

Nursing diagnosis

Knowledge deficit

Related factors: Lack of information about disorder

Defining characteristics: Expressed need for information about medication administration and compliance and about cause, treatment, and prognosis of disorder

OUTCOME CRITERIA

Short-term
Adequate knowledge, as evidenced by client's ability to discuss cause, treatment, prognosis, and medication regimen (expected within 1 week)

Long-term
Adequate knowledge, as evidenced by compliance with medical regimen to achieve optimal health and functioning (expected within 1 month)

NURSING INTERVENTIONS/INSTRUCTIONS

1. Assess life-style, ability to adapt, learning ability and interest, and family participation and support (first visit).

2. Inform client of cause of seizure activity and of the importance of compliance with follow-up visits for laboratory testing and physician evaluation (first visit).

3. Instruct client in administration of anticonvulsant therapy, including dosage, route, action, and side effects to assess and report (gingival hypertrophy, visual disturbances, rashes, confusion); food and drug interactions; not to discontinue medication without physician advice; and to avoid OTC drugs without physician advice (first and second visits).

4. Instruct client to have dental checkups every 6 months; instruct client in teeth care, including brushing and use of dental floss to prevent oral infection (first visit).

5. Instruct client to report fever, sore throat, fatigue, or weakness, which may indicate agranulocytosis, and inform client of need to have complete blood count done every 6 months if ordered (first visit).

6. Instruct client to avoid late-night television, alcohol, fatigue, and stimulants known to cause seizure activity (first visit).

7. Inform client of immediate actions to take at onset of seizure and when to notify emergency service (first visit).

8. Suggest wearing an identification bracelet or carrying a card in a purse or wallet indicating condition, medication, physician, and physician's telephone number (first visit).

9. Inform client of antidiscrimination laws affecting work and other activities (first visit).

10. Inform client of National Epilepsy League and other agencies available for support and of groups for people with the disorder (any visit).

CLIENT AND FAMILY/CARETAKER INTERVENTIONS

1. Promote independence and avoid overprotection.

2. Comply with medication administration as instructed, and maintain regimen unless advised to change by physician; keep follow-up appointments

3. Manage life-style changes, and adapt to changes brought

about by disorder; utilize resources available for information and support.
4. Report complications of condition when appropriate.
5. Carry identification information.

◢ *Spinal Cord Injury*

Spinal cord injury is the contusion, compression, hemorrhage, laceration, or transection of the spinal cord, causing loss of neurologic function. The injury may be acute, in which all sensation and reflex activity below the injury level are lost, or partial, in which some motor and sensory loss occurs, depending on the tracts affected. The injury is usually the result of car or sports accidents, falls, wounds from guns or implements of war, or diseases of the spinal cord.

Home care depends on the extent of the injury and is primarily concerned with teaching of the medical regimen and with rehabilitation and aftercare to maximize health and function.

Nursing diagnosis

Impaired physical mobility

Related factors: Neuromuscular impairment, perceptual impairment

Defining characteristics: Paraplegia, quadriplegia; immobility; inability to purposefully move within physical environment, including bed mobility, transfer, and ambulation; spasticity; muscle weakness

OUTCOME CRITERIA

Short-term
Enhanced mobility, as evidenced by improved activity and movement, ability to transfer and change positions, and absence of contractures and muscle atrophy (expected within 1 to 2 weeks)

Long-term
Achievement of optimal mobility, movement, and activity for health and functioning within injury limitations (expected ongoing)

NURSING INTERVENTIONS/INSTRUCTIONS

1. Assess degree and type of injury and impairment; muscle strength; presence of spasticity, muscle wasting, and sensorimotor deficits (see Musculoskeletal System Assessment, p. 25, for guidelines) (each visit).
2. Perform and instruct client in passive, assistive, or active range-of-motion (ROM) exercises, to be done every 2 to 4 hours or as prescribed by physical therapist (first and second visits).
3. Instruct client in positioning and position changes and to provide any assistance needed; suggest prone position to relieve pressure on susceptible areas and use of fracture board under mattress to prevent sagging of mattress (first and second visits).
4. Instruct client in removal and application of hand or foot splints (or, for feet, to use tennis shoes with the toe cut out) to prevent contractures; avoid use of footboard, which may promote development of plantar flexion (first visit).
5. Instruct client, and support physical therapy instructions, in methods to move and turn in bed, and to transfer to chair, wheelchair, car, or elsewhere (any visit).
6. Instruct client to schedule rest periods to alternate with ROM and muscle strengthening exercises and activities.
7. Inform client of comfort resulting from warm baths and massage and their role in preventing spasticity (first visit).
8. Initiate referral to physical and/or occupational therapist for rehabilitation to maximize function remaining and to obtain special equipment for ambulation and other activities.
9. Provide information for securing bed with trapeze, Hoyer lift, transfer board, and other aids and protective devices (first visit).

CLIENT AND FAMILY/CARETAKER INTERVENTIONS

1. Perform exercises alternating with rest periods daily.
2. Progress in transfer techniques, movement, and activities, and improve in use of assistive aids and devices.

3. Maintain optimal independence in mobility and activities within injury limitations.
4. Secure necessary equipment and supplies for optimal movement.
5. Encourage and praise all attempts and accomplishments of client and goal achievement.
6. Comply with rehabilitation regimen initiated by the physical therapist.
7. Perform follow-up muscle and joint preservation measures.

Nursing diagnosis

High risk for impaired skin integrity

Related factors: External factors of pressure, physical immobilization, excretions from urine and bowel incontinence; internal factors of altered sensation and nutrition

Defining characteristics: Disruption of skin surface, redness at bony prominences, inability to change position

OUTCOME CRITERIA

Short-term
Reduction in risk for breaks in skin integrity, as evidenced by intact skin and absence of reddened areas (expected within 1 week)

Long-term
Skin integrity maintained, as evidenced by absence of actual skin breakdown or injury or signs and symptoms of beginning breakdown (expected ongoing)

NURSING INTERVENTIONS/INSTRUCTIONS

1. Assess skin at pressure areas for redness and perineal area for irritation or excoriation if client is incontinent of urine and/or feces (see Integumentary System Assessment, p. 31, for guidelines) (each visit).
2. Instruct client in proper positioning and position changes to relieve pressure and shearing forces on skin (first visit).
3. Instruct client in massage technique using lotion for hands, feets, and bony prominences in particular (first visit).
4. Instruct client in perineal care following elimination or incontinence, including washing with mild soap, rinsing

with warm water, patting dry, and applying skin protector (first visit).

5. Instruct client to eliminate any crumbs or debris in bed, chair, or other area that comes in contact with skin (first visit).

6. To prevent burns to areas deprived of sensation, instruct client to avoid use of hot water for bathing or application of heat or spilling hot foods (first visit).

7. Perform decubitus care if break in skin is noted, and instruct client to assess, to perform treatment appropriate for stage of decubitus, and to report poor response to treatment (any visit).

CLIENT AND FAMILY/CARETAKER INTERVENTIONS

1. Assess skin condition daily and perform measures to prevent breakdown.

2. Use aids to prevent skin pressure.

3. Avoid excessive heat or cold in contact with paralyzed area.

4. Eliminate pressure and shearing or mechanical forces that injure skin.

5. Perform movements and transfers without skin trauma, with or without assistance.

Nursing diagnosis

Self-care deficit (bathing/hygiene, dressing/grooming, feeding, toileting)

Related factors: Neuromuscular impairment, impaired mobility status

Defining characteristics: Inability to wash body parts, put on or take off clothes, get to and use toilet or be aware of urge to eliminate, bring food from receptable to mouth; paralysis

OUTCOME CRITERIA

Short-term

Ability to perform activities of daily living (ADL), as evidenced by beginning participation in feeding, toileting, bathing, personal hygiene, dressing and grooming, within limitations imposed by injury (expected within 1 to 2 weeks)

Long-term
Optimal participation in self-care for ADL with or without asssitve aids or devices to achieve independence (expected within 2 to 3 months and ongoing)

NURSING INTERVENTIONS/INSTRUCTIONS

1. Assess client's ability to perform self-care (paraplegic, quadriplegic), including ability to feed self; use bedpan, urinal, or commode; and bathe, groom, and clothe self (see Functional Assessment, p. 43, for guidelines) (each visit).
2. Provide assistance or supervision as needed for performance of ADL, and instruct client to ask for assistance when needed (each visit).
3. Instruct client in and suggest use of assistive aids and devices for eating, dressing, grooming, personal hygiene, and toileting, and inform client of clothing and utensils to purchase to enhance self-care (first visit).
4. Instruct client to allow time to perform activities without rushing, for best results (first visit).
5. Initiate referral to occupational therapist for instruction and support in ADL and for suggestions for other aids (any visit).
6. Refer home health aide (HHA) to assist with ADL as needed.

CLIENT AND FAMILY/CARETAKER INTERVENTIONS

1. Participate in ADL with progressive results, with or without the use of assistive aids or devices.
2. Perform self-care independently with maximal rehabilitative potential.
3. Assist client to maintain functional abilities in daily activities.
4. Comply with occupational rehabilitation schedule, and practice activities as instructed.

Nursing diagnosis

Ineffective individual coping

Related factors: Multiple life changes; inadequate coping method

Defining characteristics: Inability to cope, meet role expectations, meet basic needs; chronic anxiety; poor self-esteem; fear and feelings of grief; negative feelings about body; change in sexual function; feelings of dependence, helplessness

OUTCOME CRITERIA

Short-term
Improved individual coping, as evidenced by client's statement of realization of life-style changes that need to be made and willingness to adapt and learn effective coping mechanisms (expected within 1 to 2 weeks)

Long-term
Effective coping and adaptation to changed self-concept, as evidenced by achievement of requirements for optimal health and functioning within injury limitations, returning to employment, and retraining in sexual function and other life changes (expected within 3 months and ongoing)

NURSING INTERVENTIONS/INSTRUCTIONS

1. Assess for anxiety; depression; feelings about appearance and loss of neurologic functioning and effect on self-concept and body image; use and effectiveness of coping mechanisms; and behavioral and emotional changes and reasons for them (each visit).
2. Instruct client in development of new coping skills while maintaining current skills that are successful; assist client with problem-solving skills (first and second visits).
3. Include client in setting realistic goals for functioning and in developing the treatment plan and methods to evaluate progress (each visit).
4. Instruct client to avoid emotional and physical stress (first visit).
5. Show care, concern, and willingness to assist in coping with life-style changes (each visit).
6. Allow for expressions of feelings, concerns, and fears about the future, and inform client that this is acceptable behavior (each visit).
7. Refrain from using words such as "quad" or "cripple"; use words such as "disabled" or "handicapped" (each visit).
8. Initiate referral to social services, psychotherapy, sex counseling, occupational retraining, and rehabilitation as needed (any visit).

CLIENT AND FAMILY/CARETAKER INTERVENTIONS

1. Use planned program during the entire day to meet goals and prevent depression, boredom, and fatigue.
2. Ventilate feelings and grief as needed.
3. Identify and use coping mechanisms that work; try alternative methods to cope.
4. Seek counseling from appropriate referrals and rehabilitation resources; join groups whose members have had similar experiences.

Nursing diagnosis

Bowel incontinence

Related factors: Neuromuscular involvement

Defining characteristics: Involuntary passage of stool, constipation, loss of voluntary function and urge to defecate

OUTCOME CRITERIA

Short-term
Adequate elimination, as evidenced by reestablishment of regular, soft, formed stool pattern (expected within 1 to 2 weeks)

Long-term
Establishment of bowel elimination pattern without incontinence of stool or constipation (expected ongoing)

NURSING INTERVENTIONS/INSTRUCTIONS

1. Instruct client to have bowel evacuation at same time each day; instruct client to use gentle pressure on abdomen, gentle digital anal stimulation, and Valsalva maneuver to promote bowel movement (first and second visits).
2. Instruct client to drink 8 to 10 glasses of fluid per day and prune juice at bedtime (first visit).
3. Instruct client to add fiber to daily diet and suggest foods to include (first visit).
4. Instruct client to administer suppository 30 minutes before scheduled elimination during training for stool continence (first visit and reinforce on second visit).
5. Review and reinforce a total bowel regimen that includes

fluids, diet, scheduling, stool softener, suppository, and digital stimulation (each visit).

CLIENT AND FAMILY/CARETAKER INTERVENTIONS

1. Maintain daily or every-other-day bowel evacuation regimen.
2. Prepare and ingest high-fiber diet, and maintain fluid intake as instructed.
3. Administer medication as appropriate to enhance elimination at scheduled times.

Nursing diagnosis

Reflex incontinence

Related factors: Neurologic impairment (spinal cord injury)

Defining characteristics: No awareness of bladder filling or fullness; no urge to void; uninhibited bladder contraction/spasm; neurogenic bladder; bladder distention; frequent voiding in small amounts; constant dribbling

OUTCOME CRITERIA

Short-term
Improved bladder function, as evidenced by reduction in incontinence episodes with use of catheter or training program (expected within 1 to 2 weeks)

Long-term
Ability to maintain bladder function, with absence of infection, to achieve optimal urinary continence (expected ongoing)

NURSING INTERVENTIONS/INSTRUCTIONS

1. Instruct client in noting and reporting cloudy, foul-smelling urine (first visit).
2. Instruct client to increase fluid intake to 10 glasses per day, and suggest acid-ash juices such as cranberry juice (first visit).
3. Instruct client in use of indwelling catheter, if present, noting patency and using sterile technique in catheter and meatal care (first and second visits).
4. Instruct client in application and care of condom catheter if used (first visit).

5. Instruct client or family member in intermittent catheterization using sterile technique and care of catheters if procedure is appropriate (first and second visits).

6. Inform client of training program and instruct client in scheduling voiding and in performing Credé technique if bladder is not distended, or refer client to a rehabilitation program if rehabilitation is possible (first visit).

7. Initiate referral to enterostomal therapist, if appropriate (any visit).

CLIENT AND FAMILY/CARETAKER INTERVENTIONS

1. Perform assessment for urinary bladder infection whether catheter is used or not.

2. Perform intermittent catheterization using sterile or clean technique as appropriate.

3. Maintain catheter patency and catheter care or condom catheter procedures.

4. Participate in urinary control rehabilitation program if appropriate.

Nursing diagnosis

Knowledge deficit

Related factors: Lack of information about disability

Defining characteristics: Expressed need for information about medical and rehabilitative regimen and prevention of trauma or injury

OUTCOME CRITERIA

Short-term
Adequate knowledge, as evidenced by client's statement of treatment regimen and potential for injury or complications (expected within 1 week)

Long-term
Adequate knowledge, as evidenced by achievement of requirements for optimal health and functioning within limitations imposed by injury (expected within 1 to 2 months and ongoing)

NURSING INTERVENTIONS/INSTRUCTIONS

1. Assess life-style and ability to adapt, learning abilities and interest, and family participation and support (first visit)
2. Include all family members and care providers in instructions (each visit).
3. Assist client to write plan incorporating medical regimen and rehabilitation schedules and instruction, and revise daily as needed (each visit).
4. Instruct client to modify environment to prevent falls, to provide space needed for use of assistive aids such as a wheelchair, and to secure supplies and equipment that will ensure a safe home environment for ADL and other activities (first visit).
5. Instruct client to protect affected areas from excessively hot or cold applications or from trauma resulting from decreased sensory perception and motor deficits (first visit).
6. Instruct client in need to maintain fluid intake of up to 3 liters per day and a diet high in calories, protein, and carbohydrates, and offer food lists and sample menus to assist in planning meals (first visit).
7. Instruct client in signs and symptoms of respiratory infection and to report change in respiration, yellow or other color change in sputum, or temperature elevation (first visit).
8. Inform client of possible autonomic dysreflexia and actions to take to prevent this condition (first and second visits).
9. Inform client of importance of compliance with physical, occupational, psychological, and other therapy if applicable and to comply with scheduled visits to physican (first visit).
10. Inform client of stages of grieving and behavioral changes that can be expected to achieve stage of adjustment (each visit).

CLIENT AND FAMILY/CARETAKER INTERVENTIONS

1. Identify hazards and eliminate or modify them.
2. Use assistive and supplemental aids.
3. Maintain open communication during grieving process.

4. Assess for and report complications.
5. Maintain scheduled appointments for rehabilitative therapy.
6. Utilize agencies for assistance in transportation, information, support, food services, housekeeping services, and others.
7. Comply with fluid, nutritional, rest, activity, and other regimens included in medical regimen with as much independence as possible.

Nursing diagnosis

High risk for caregiver role strain

Related factors: Inexperience with caregiving; complexity/amount of caregiving tasks; duration of caregiving required; inadequate physical environment for providing care (housing, transportation, equipment, accessibility)

Defining characteristics: Report of not having enough resources to provide care (emotional and physical strength, help from others); difficulty in performing specific caregiving activities (bathing, cleaning up after urinary or bowel incontinence, moving and transferring, catheterization, managing discomforts and total care needs)

OUTCOME CRITERIA

Short-term
Identification of potential for caregiver role strain, as evidenced by caregiver's verbalization of difficulties encountered in performing care and concern about ability and conflicts in giving care (expected within 1 week)

Long-term
Prevention of caregiver role strain, as evidenced by caregiver's providing of continued, progressive, and safe care without compromise to own physical and emotional needs (expected within 1 month and ongoing)

NURSING INTERVENTIONS/INSTRUCTIONS

1. Assess severity of disability and care needs of the receiver of care and ability of caregiver to perform role (first visit).
2. Assess relationship between care receiver and caregiver before the illness and stressors placed on the relationship

by the complexity of needs caused by the illness (first visit).

3. Assist caregiver to monitor continued ability to perform care and treatments, day-to-day needs that may need to be changed or learned, changes in stressors and strains, maintenance of routines, and need for additional resources (aides, friends, family) (first visit).

4. Discuss role performance, whether expectations are realistic, and flexibility of role and decision-making process (first visit).

5. Initiate referral to HHA, social services, or psychological counseling to assist with economic or mental or physical health needs (any visit).

CLIENT AND FAMILY/CARETAKER INTERVENTIONS

1. Develop ability to cope with caregiver role; incorporate flexibility into day-to-day functioning.

2. Explore financial, legal, and physical assistance sources, and consider a referral to these services.

3. Maintain own health and well-being in caregiver role.

4. Maintain ongoing care and treatment regimen for care receiver.

Gastrointestinal system

◣ Cirrhosis of Liver

Cirrhosis of the liver is a chronic disease characterized by structural and degenerative changes causing liver dysfunction and possible liver failure. Changes include the destruction of the liver parenchyma with the development of fibrous tissue that surrounds the hepatocytes and separates the lobules and, finally, the formation of nodules as the liver attempts to regenerate itself. Cirrhosis may be caused by chronic alcoholism, long-standing right-sided heart failure, alterations in the immune system, stasis of bile in the liver, or hepatic or other infections.

Home care is primarily concerned with ongoing assessment of the chronic symptomatology of the disease, elimination of the underlying cause if possible, and the teaching involved in promoting maintenance of health status and prevention of further liver damage and complications.

Nursing diagnosis

Altered nutrition: less than body requirements

Related factors: Inability to ingest food because of biologic factors; inability to digest foods because of biologic factors

Defining characteristics: Anorexia; nausea; vomiting; inability to metabolize fats, proteins, and carbohydrates and store nutrients; diarrhea or constipation; excessive fluid losses; weight loss; abdominal pain

OUTCOME CRITERIA

Short-term
Adequate nutritional intake, as evidenced by compliance with a diet that facilitates appropriate weight maintenance for size, age, and frame; client's verbalization of foods to be included

in a high-carbohydrate, moderately high-protein diet; abstinence from alcohol (expected within 3 days)

Long-term

Adequate nutrition, as evidenced by food consumption and weight within expected requirements; continued abstinence from alcohol; achievement of optimal health and functioning within limitations imposed by disease (expected within 1 to 3 months and ongoing)

NURSING INTERVENTIONS/INSTRUCTIONS

1. Assess nutritional status and dietary inclusions and restrictions needed in presence of disease and in accordance with stage and symptoms of the disease (see Gastrointestinal System Assessment, p. 17, for guidelines) (first visit).
2. Instruct client to maintain a log of types and amounts of food eaten; review intake and use data as a basis for teaching diet; coordinate with dietitian (first, second, and third visits).
3. Assess alcohol intake and provide client with the rationale for avoiding all alcoholic beverages (each visit).
4. Assess for presence of anorexia, nausea, vomiting, malaise, fatigue, muscle wasting; suggest a period of rest before meals (first visit).
5. Measure height and weight and calculate weight requirements (first visit).
6. Measure abdominal girth (each visit).
7. Assist client in planning and selecting foods for high-carbohydrate and moderate protein diet totaling about 2000 to 3000 calories per day; suggest supplemental feedings if needed (first visit and reinforce on second visit).
8. Instruct client to restrict fluids in presence of edema or ascites (any visit).
9. Instruct client to avoid salty and convenience foods and to restrict sodium intake to 200 to 500 mg/day in presence of edema or ascites; instruct client in how to read labels on foods to determine sodium content (first visit).
10. Instruct client in administration of vitamins and minerals, antiemetics, and other prescribed drugs; instruct client to avoid OTC drugs unless advised by physician (first visit).
11. Instruct client to eat smaller, more frequent meals rather than three large meals (first visit).

12. Advise client to perform oral hygiene after meals and to use hard candy or sips of carbonated beverages or dry foods for nausea (first visit).
13. Initiate referral to nutritionist.
14. Refer home health aide (HHA) to assist with activities of daily living (ADL) and food preparation.

CLIENT AND FAMILY/CARETAKER INTERVENTIONS

1. Adhere to prescribed diet as instructed; maintain food diary.
2. Limit sodium, fluids, or protein if indicated.
3. Avoid alcohol.
4. Weight daily and report any significant gains or losses.
5. Administer medications and vitamin supplement.
6. Eat six times per day in small amounts; adjust intake if nausea or vomiting is present.
7. Provide pleasant environment for meals.
8. Maintain oral hygiene.
9. Consult with nutritionist if needed.

Nursing diagnosis

High risk for infection

Related factors: Inadequate secondary defenses; malnutrition

Defining characteristics: Leukopenia; chronic inadequate nutritional intake and metabolism; elevated temperature; changes in breathing, urine characteristics, or any part of body

OUTCOME CRITERIA
Short-term
Reduced risk for infection development, as evidenced by temperature and white blood count within normal ranges, lung fields clear, and skin intact (expected within 3 days)

Long-term
Absence of signs and symptoms of infection in any organ system (expected within 2 weeks)

NURSING INTERVENTIONS/INSTRUCTIONS

1. Assess skin for jaundice, pruritis, and evidence of scratches or excoriation (first visit).

2. Instruct client in relief measures for pruritis, including cool compresses, emollient baths, patting instead of rubbing skin dry, and use of mild soap and soft towel (first visit).

3. Instruct client to avoid scratching itchy areas and to keep fingernails short and clean and well filed for smoothness (first visit).

4. Assess lungs for decreased breath sounds, cough, adventitious sounds, or change in respiratory rate, depth, or ease (first visit).

5. Instruct client to take temperature and notify physician of elevations or of changes in respiratory pattern or airway clearance (first visit).

6. Instruct client to avoid exposure to persons with infections (first visit).

7. Instruct client in antibiotic administration as prescribed (first visit).

8. Refer HHA when necessary to assist.

CLIENT AND FAMILY/CARETAKER INTERVENTIONS

1. Maintain personal hygiene; adjust bathing, grooming, and dressing to enhance body image and protect jaundiced skin.

2. Administer medications as instructed.

3. Report signs and symptoms of infection to physician if present.

4. Monitor temperature if symptoms appear.

5. Maintain absence of infection of skin, lungs, or any other organ.

Nursing diagnosis

Altered protection

Related factors: Abnormal blood profile

Defining characteristics: Inability of liver to convert ammonia to urea, to produce coagulation factors, and to absorb vitamin K; leukopenia; ecchymoses; petechiae; bleeding from gums, mucous membranes

OUTCOME CRITERIA

Short-term
Control of bleeding tendency, as evidenced by absence of bleeding from any site (expected within 3 days)

Long-term
Maintenance of blood profile within normal ranges within limitations imposed by severity of disease (expected within 2 to 4 weeks)

NURSING INTERVENTIONS/INSTRUCTIONS

1. Assess for bleeding, including petechiae, ecchymoses, oozing or frank bleeding from any orifice or skin site; check hemoglobin and hematocrit levels if available; instruct client to report any bleeding to physician (each visit).
2. Instruct client to avoid trauma and constrictive clothing and to protect vulnerable areas from injury (first visit).
3. Instruct client in administration of vitamin K if appropriate (first visit).
4. Instruct caregiver/HHA to avoid toothbrushing and rectal temperatures.

CLIENT AND FAMILY/CARETAKER INTERVENTIONS

1. Identify and report signs and symptoms of bleeding.
2. Administer prescribed medications.

Nursing diagnosis

Altered thought processes

Related factors: Physiologic changes

Defining characteristics: Confusion, memory deficit, disorientation, lethargy

OUTCOME CRITERIA

Short-term
Improvement in neurologic function and mentation, as evidenced by stability in orientation and mental functioning (expected within 1 week)

Long-term
Appropriate level of mental function within limitations
imposed by disease status (expected within 2 to 4 weeks)

NURSING INTERVENTIONS/INSTRUCTIONS

1. Assess mentation, including confusion, lethargy, irritability, depression, personality and behavioral changes, slurred speech, and psychotic ideations, and instruct client to report any of these conditions to physician (each visit).
2. Encourage client to participate in interactions with others and to use clock, calendar, newspaper, radio, and other stimulation that may be preferred (first visit).
3. Inform client of reason for mental changes if they occur (first visit).
4. Refer client to psychological counseling if appropriate (any visit).
5. Refer HHA to assist with ADL.

CLIENT AND FAMILY/CARETAKER INTERVENTIONS

1. Identify and report mental and emotional changes.
2. Provide stimulation and reality reinforcement.
3. Administer medications if prescribed.

Nursing diagnosis

Body image disturbance

Related factors: Biophysical factors caused by disease process

Defining characteristics: Jaundice; pruritis; skin irritation from scratching; chronic fatigue; estrogen-androgen imbalance; ascites; edema

OUTCOME CRITERIA

Short-term
Improvement in self-image, as evidenced by participation in care and interest in appearance and by some resumption of outside activities or interactions (expected within 3 to 7 days)

Long-term
Adaptation to temporary and permanent changes in body image, as evidenced by resumption of self-care activities and

social and work activities to achieve optimal level of function within disease limitations (expected within 1 to 3 months)

NURSING INTERVENTIONS/INSTRUCTIONS

1. Assess ability of client and family to cope and adapt (first visit).
2. Allow time for and acceptance of expressions of concern and negative comments about appearance (each visit).
3. Assess behavioral and emotional trends and changes, and integrate them into clinical profile for disease progression and encephalopathy (each visit).
4. Assess and discuss appearance and measures to minimize the effects of edema, jaundice, weight changes, loss of hair, menstrual irregularities, impotence, and changes in sex characteristics (first visit and reinforce as needed).
5. Initiate referral to counseling or support group.

CLIENT AND FAMILY/CARETAKER INTERVENTIONS

1. Express concerns and feelings about changes.
2. Support and adapt to physical changes.
3. Participate in daily care and utilize measures to conceal body changes and appearance.
4. Report signs and symptoms of hormonal imbalance or central nervous system dysfunction.
5. Seek counseling if needed, occupational retraining if appropriate.

Nursing diagnosis

Knowledge deficit

Related factors: Lack of information about disease and care

Defining characteristics: Request for information about disease process, causes, treatments, preventive measures, and medical regimen; denial as result of absence of symptoms or alcohol abuse

OUTCOME CRITERIA

Short-term
Adequate knowledge, as evidenced by client's statement of status of disease and symptoms of worsening condition and of

need for compliance in medication and activity regimens and alcoholism rehabilitation (expected within 1 week)

Long-term

Adequate knowledge, as evidenced by compliance with requirements to maintain liver function and obtain optimal level of health (expected within 2 to 3 months)

NURSING INTERVENTIONS/INSTRUCTIONS

1. Assess life-style, abilities to learn and adapt to treatments, interests and diversional activities, family participation and support, and presence of alcoholism (first visit).
2. Perform abdominal assessment, including measurement for changes in abdominal girth indicating ascites, splenomegaly, hepatic level and hardness, and abdominal discomfort, and instruct client in performing this assessment (first visit and ongoing).
3. Assess complaints of nausea, vomiting, anorexia, weight loss or gain, constipation or diarrhea, fatigue, or pruritis, and instruct client to report these conditions to physician if they occur (each visit).
4. Assess for history of alcohol abuse, use of hepatotoxic drugs, exposure to chemicals, or gastrointestinal surgery (first visit).
5. Discuss and reinforce importance of alcohol abstinence (first visit and reinforce when needed).
6. Instruct client to schedule 6 to 8 hours of sleep per 24 hours and to schedule rest hours around meals and activities (first visit).
7. Instruct client to report any signs or symptoms of complications or worsening condition, including fever, bleeding, shortness of breath, increase in abdominal girth, weight or urinary output changes, edema, confusion or personality changes, abdominal pain, or jaundice (first week).
8. Instruct client to avoid exposure to toxic agents, medications, or environments and to possible infection (first visit).
9. Instruct client in medication administration, including vitamins, antipruritics, stool softeners, diuretics, electrolyte replacement, aldosterone-blocking agents, digestive enzymes, and others as ordered; inform client of dose, frequency, route, side effects, and food/drug/alcohol interactions (first visit and reinforce on second visit).

10. Advise client of importance of keeping appointments with physician and laboratory (first visit).
11. Provide information about community agencies and groups, such as Alcoholics Anonymous, (AA), for support, counseling, or educational materials (first visit).

CLIENT AND FAMILY/CARETAKER INTERVENTIONS

1. Comply with medical regimen and change life-style if needed.
2. Report signs and symptoms of complications.
3. Avoid alcohol and other substances toxic to liver.
4. Administer medications correctly and safely.
5. Avoid stressful situations; seek counseling if needed.
6. Schedule adequate rest and sleep and promote as part of daily routine.
7. Maintain physician and laboratory appointments.
8. Contact AA or other support groups for assistance.
9. Return to work and activities within limitations.

◣ Hepatitis

Hepatitis is the inflammation of the liver as the result of alcohol, drugs, or viruses. Viral hepatitis may be classified as hepatitis A, hepatitis B, or non-A, non-B hepatitis, depending on the viral strain. Hepatitis A is transmitted by the oral or fecal route, hepatitis B is transmitted by the parenteral route, and hepatitis non-A, non-B is transmitted through transfusions. The disease varies in severity, which determines the degree of liver cell injury and scarring and resolution or chronicity of the condition.

Home care is primarily concerned with proper testing and treatment necessary to prevent transmission and increased incidence of the disease in the community and with the teaching involved in the care and treatment of the acute stage of the disease and prevention of permanent liver damage.

Nursing diagnosis

Altered nutrition: less than body requirements

Related factors: Inability to ingest food; inability to digest foods because of biologic factors

Defining characteristics: Nausea; vomiting; anorexia; abdominal diarrhea; inability to store nutrients; inability to metabolize fats, proteins, and carbohydrates; excessive fluid losses; tenderness; weight loss

OUTCOME CRITERIA

Short-term
Adequate nutrition, as evidenced by consumption of increased carbohydrates and increased calories and by prescribed protein intake (expected within 3 days)

Long-term
Nutritional status optimal, as evidenced by intake of prescribed diet and by weight maintenance for health and functioning during course of disease (expected wtihin 1 to 2 months)

NURSING INTERVENTIONS/INSTRUCTIONS

1. Assess nutritional and gastrointestinal status, taking into consideration dietary preferences and restrictions or inclusions (see Gastrointestinal System Assessment, p. 17, for guidelines) (first visit).
2. Take height and weight and calculate weight requirements (first visit).
3. Measure abdominal girth, and determine weight on same scale, at same time of day with client wearing similar clothing (each visit).
4. Instruct client to keep food diary that includes types, portions, and preparation method of foods consumed (first visit).
5. Using these data as a basis for diet teaching, assist client in food selection for a high-carbohydrate, high-calorie diet; also should be high in protein in absence of edema (first visit and reinforce on second visit).
6. Instruct client to eat smaller, more frequent meals rather than three large meals; advise client to eat larger amounts during the day rather than in the evening (first visit).

7. Instruct client to drink 3000 ml of fluids per day (in absence of edema) and to estimate adequacy of output (first visit).
8. Suggest hard candy, sips of carbonated beverages, or dry food for nausea (first visit).
9. Instruct client in administration of prescribed antiemetic ½ hour before meals (first visit).

CLIENT AND FAMILY/CARETAKER INTERVENTIONS

1. Maintain a food/fluid diary.
2. Take and record weight, daily or as needed.
3. Maintain prescribed carbohydrate and caloric intake.
4. Spread meals over entire day, with most eaten early in the day, and intersperse meals with fluid intake.
5. Administer antiemetic before meals.
6. Perform oral care as needed.
7. Use hard candy and other dietary aids to control nausea.
8. Limit protein and fluids if edema is present

Nursing diagnosis

High risk for impaired skin integrity

Related factors: Internal factor of altered pigmentation

Defining characteristics: Jaundice, pruritis, dry skin, scratches or disruptions on skin

OUTCOME CRITERIA

Short-term
Skin intact and free from irritation, as evidenced by absence of rash, abrasions, excoriations, or disruptions (expected within 1 week)

Long-term
Skin integrity maintained, with optimal comfort and health achieved (expected within 1 month)

NURSING INTERVENTIONS/INSTRUCTIONS

1. Assess skin for color, temperature, integrity, and sensation; assess for presence of jaundice or pruritis and for evidence of scratching (see Integumentary System Assessment, p. 31, for guidelines) (each visit).

2. Instruct client in relief measures, such as cool-warm shower or cool compresses to area, mild soap for bathing, patting instead of rubbing dry, diversional methods, and use of emollients in water and topically (first visit).
3. Instruct client to maintain clean, short nails and to apply pressure to itchy areas instead of scratching (first visit).
4. Instruct client in use of antipruritics and antihistamine, including dose, time, frequency, and side effects; inform client of drug or alcohol interactions (first visit).
5. Inform client to wear loose clothing and to avoid tight, restrictive types of clothing, which might increase itching (first visit).

CLIENT AND FAMILY/CARETAKER INTERVENTIONS

1. Administer medications for relief of itching.
2. Use other relief measures to control pruritis.
3. Avoid scratching.
4. Notify physician if symptoms are not relieved or if breaks appear on skin.

Nursing diagnosis

Impaired social interaction

Related factors: Therapeutic isolation; body image disturbance

Defining characteristics: Verbalized discomfort in social participation, jaundiced appearance, fear of transmitting disease to others, stated lack of diversional activity and interactions

OUTCOME CRITERIA

Short-term
Minimal boredom, loneliness, and impaired body image, as evidenced by client's statement that body image is improving as condition resolves and by participation in activities to provide stimulation (expected within 1 week)

Long-term
Adaptation to temporary restrictions in social relationships to prevent transmission of disease and sensory deficits and by maintenance of optimal level of health and functioning (expected within 1 month)

NURSING INTERVENTIONS/INSTRUCTIONS

1. Instruct client in reasons for isolation precautions and length of time restrictions must be observed (first visit).
2. Instruct family to provide separate room and bathroom for client if possible (first visit).
3. Instruct family to spend time with client at intervals during day (first visit).
4. Inform client and family of precautions to take to prevent transmission, including hand washing, care of utensils and articles used for meals, and bowel elimination (first visit).
5. Encourage family to provide for diversional activities, such as books, cards, television, radio, newspaper, and telephone (first visit).
6. Inform client that jaundice is not permanent and disappears as disease is resolved (first visit)
7. Remove mirrors and cover body parts to preserve body image if jaundice is present (first visit).
8. Note negative attitudes and comments regarding skin color and pruritis, and provide support (each visit).

CLIENT AND FAMILY/CARETAKER INTERVENTIONS

1. Encourage visits from friends.
2. Maintain precautions to prevent transmission of disease.
3. Provide diversional activities when client is confined to room.
4. Promote and support positive attitude about temporary jaundice.

Nursing diagnosis

Knowledge deficit

Related factors: Lack of information about disease

Defining characteristics: Verbalization of need for information about disease and its transmission and about prevention of complications or relapse or recurrence

OUTCOME CRITERIA

Short-term
Adequate knowledge, as evidenced by client's stating methods of disease transmission, treatment, and prevention of compli-

cations and by client's compliance with diet, activity, and hygiene/sanitation regimens (expected within 3 days)

Long-term
Adequate knowledge, as evidenced by client's meeting requirements to achieve optimal level of liver function and absence of symptoms and complications or transmittal of disease to others (expected within 1 to 2 months)

NURSING INTERVENTIONS/INSTRUCTIONS

1. Assess life-style, ability and interest to learn, ability to adapt, and family participation and support (first visit).
2. Review history of flu-like symptoms: nausea, vomiting, anorexia, weight loss, fatigue, malaise, headache, myalgia, constipation or diarrhea; note also recent travel, transfusions, injections or sharing of needles, or exposure to toxins or to carriers (first visit).
3. Perform abdominal assessment (see Gastrointestinal System Assessment, p. 17, for guidelines) and note liver size and tenderness, enlarged nodes, presence of dark urine, clay colored stools, scleral icterus, jaundice (each visit).
4. Instruct client in causes, transmission, signs and symptoms, and treatment of disease (first visit).
5. Instruct client in hand-washing and isolation protocols, and emphasize washing hands especially after toileting (first visit).
6. Instruct client to avoid tiring self and to participate only in activity that is tolerated (first visit).
7. Instruct client to report edema in extremities or abdomen, unexplained weight gain, changes in personality or behavior, or evidence of bleeding (first visit).
8. Instruct client to avoid alcohol or toxins; review drug profile for hepatotoxic drugs (first visit).
9. Instruct client not to donate blood (first visit).
10. Instruct client to avoid sexual contact temporarily (first visit).
11. Instruct client to keep appointments with physician and for laboratory testing, and monitor laboratory results as available (each visit).
12. Initiate referral to appropriate health care facility for possible prophylactic care of household contacts and regular sexual partners (first visit).

13. Provide information on community agencies and groups, such as drug rehabilitation or counseling groups, for educational literature and support (first visit).

CLIENT AND FAMILY/CARETAKER INTERVENTIONS

1. Avoid transmission of disease by:
   - Proper hand washing
   - Proper disinfection of food utensils, clothing, and linens
   - Avoiding sharing of food, utensils, personal grooming items, toilet, clothing, or linens
   - Proper disposal of tissues
2. State cause, transmission, signs and symptoms, and treatment of disease.
3. Avoid alcohol, hepatotoxic drugs, and exposure to toxins
4. Avoid sexual contact.
5. Refrain from donating blood.
6. Avoid stressful situations; set aside rest periods during day.
7. Report signs and symptoms to physician as instructed.
8. Report for physician and laboratory appointments.
9. Have contacts report for prophylactic therapy.
10. Report pregnancy status to all health workers.
11. Contact support groups or counselor for assistance if appropriate.

◣ *Herniorrhaphy*

A hernia is a protrusion caused by a defect in the wall of the abdomen, scrotum inguinal area, or diaphragm. Bowel, peritoneum, fat, or bladder is forced through a weakened abdominal wall or other area. Etiologic factors include congentital malformations, trauma, aging, infection, obesity, or previous abdominal surgery. A herniorrhaphy is the repair and closure of the sac and the possible reinforcement of the area to prevent recurrence of the hernia.

Home care is primarily concerned with postoperative teaching to promote wellness and prevent recurrence of a hernia.

Nursing diagnosis

Knowledge deficit

Related factors: Lack of information about follow-up care

Defining characteristics: Request for information about prevention of recurrence, nutritional and elimination requirements, and activity restrictions

OUTCOME CRITERIA

Short-term
Adequate knowledge, as evidenced by client's stating measures and techniques to prevent recurrence, including activity restrictions and nutritional and elimination requirements (expected within 1 to 2 days)

Long-term
Adequate knowledge and compliance with postoperative care, as evidenced by resumption of activities of daily living (ADL) and return to employment or other activities involving minimal risk of recurrence (expected within 4 to 6 weeks)

NURSING INTERVENTIONS/INSTRUCTIONS

1. Instruct client to avoid heavy lifting or carrying, strenuous exercise, or straining (first visit).
2. Review occupational expectations and methods of minimizing strain with client, and instruct client in proper body mechanics (first visit).
   - When picking something up from floor, squat down, keeping back straight and knees and hips sharply flexed; straighten up using leg muscles. Or use long-handled grabbers.
   - When lifting, position load with wide base of support, with feet well apart; use stronger leg muscles rather than arm or abdominal muscles; keep back straight and load as close to body as possible.
3. Instruct client in ADL progression; may shower, resume ambulation and most activities; may resume full activity, including employment, in 3 to 6 weeks with physician recommendation (first visit).
4. Instruct client in normal stages of healing process, that inci-

sion should be kept clean and dry with edges well approximated, that it should change color from red toward pinkish, and that temperature should be similar to that of skin in other areas (first visit).

5. Instruct client to notify physician of changes in incision, including pain, redness, heat, swelling, or drainage (first visit).

6. Instruct client in dietary requirements and when to resume full diet; include caloric restrictions and options if obesity is a factor in etiology (first visit).

7. Instruct client to take stool softener to avoid straining during elimination, to include fiber in diet, and to maintain fluid intake of 8 to 10 glasses per day to avoid constipation (first visit).

CLIENT AND FAMILY/CARETAKER INTERVENTIONS

1. Resume ADL, using proper body mechanics and avoiding heavy lifting and strenuous activity.

2. Eat well-balanced diet.

3. Prevent constipation and straining with proper diet, fluids, and medication.

4. Maintain operative area dressings; change dressing when needed if soiled or damp.

5. Resume full activity following gradual progressive increases over time advised by physician.

6. Notify physican of any signs and symptoms of infection.

◣ *Peptic Ulcer*

A peptic ulcer is a sharp, circumscribed ulceration of the mucous membrane of the stomach (gastric: usually at the lesser curvature) or the duodenum (duodenal: usually at the point where the stomach contents enters the small intestine). The condition may be acute or chronic and may be caused by the effect on the mucosal barrier of drug ingestion, high levels of hydrochloric acid and enzyme secretions, prolonged illness, trauma or stress, or autoimmune disorders.

Home care is primarily concerned with the teaching involved in the healing of the ulcer and prevention of factors that are associated with chronicity or recurrence.

Nursing diagnosis

Pain

Related factors: Biologic/chemical/psychological injuring agents

Defining characteristics: Communication of pain descriptors (epigastric pain, burning, gnawing, aching, sore, occurs before or during eating); heartburn; indigestion; weight loss or gain; high level of stress; ingestion of drugs (steriods, antiinflammatories, antihypertensives)

OUTCOME CRITERIA

Short-term
Increased comfort, as evidenced by client stating that he or she feels better, that pain is decreased or absent (expected within 2 to 3 days)

Long-term
Absence of or minimal pain with decreased incidence of recurrence or relapse and achievement of optimal health and functioning (expected within 2 to 3 months)

NURSING INTERVENTIONS/INSTRUCTIONS

1. Assess abdomen (see Gastrointestinal System Assessment, p. 17, for guidelines); note vital signs, including temperature, type, intensity, and location of pain, radiation, bowel sounds, precipitating and alleviating factors (each visit).
2. Instruct client in administration of medications that will assist in relieving pain, such as antacids, sedatives, and histamine (H_2) blockers, if ordered (first visit).
3. When pain is minimal or relieved, review health regimen to include diet, rest/activity, and avoidance of stressors (each visit).

CLIENT AND FAMILY/CARETAKER INTERVENTIONS

1. Administer medications for pain correctly as instructed.
2. Avoid stressors and stressful situations.
3. Report new, increased, or uncontrolled pain to physician.

Nursing diagnosis

Knowledge deficit

Related factors: Lack of information about disorder

Defining characteristics: Verbalization of need for information about disease, causes, treatment (diet and medications), and importance of compliance

OUTCOME CRITERIA

Short-term

Adequate knowledge, as evidenced by client stating signs and symptoms of deteriorating condition or complication; diet, activity, and medication regimens; and life-style adaptations (expected within 3 days)

Long-term

Adequate knowledge, as evidenced by client meeting requirements to achieve optimal level of health and functioning (expected within 2 weeks)

NURSING INTERVENTIONS/INSTRUCTIONS

1. Assess nutritional status, food preferences, and cultural or religious restrictions (first visit).
2. Assess height and weight and calculate desired weight; instruct client to take and record weight weekly (first visit).
3. Instruct client on nutritionally adequate diet and prescribed modifications (first visit and reinforce on second visit).
   - Bland meals; eliminate food distressors such as black pepper, chili powder, raw, spicy, or fatty foods, fruit juices, and beverages containing caffeine
   - Smaller, more frequent meals (5 or 6 per day), including a bedtime snack; include protein source at each meal
   - Use skim rather than whole milk

4. Suggest that client rest before meals and that environment be quiet and pleasant during meals (first visit).

5. Instruct client to restrict alcohol and refrain from smoking (first visit and reinforce on second visit).

6. Instruct client in administration of antacids (tablet or liquid), sedatives, antianxiety agents, and histamine antagonists; include dose, route, frequency, side effects, and food/drug/alcohol interactions, and instruct client to avoid OTC drugs, especially aspirin or aspirin-containing drugs (first visit).

7. Assist client to identify and to explore sources of psychic stress and to develop methods to minimize or eliminate them (first and second visits).

8. Inform client of importance of compliance with treatment regimen and expected effects (first visit).

9. Instruct client to notify physician if hemorrhage occurs (weakness, apprehension, restlessness, vertigo/syncope, thirst, diaphoresis, dyspnea, tarry or bloody stools, vomiting with frank blood or coffee-ground appearance) (first visit).

10. Instruct client to notify physician if obstruction occurs (bloated feeling after meals, fullness after meals, absence of bowel elimination, anorexia, weight loss, vomiting large amounts, projectile vomiting, dehydration) (first visit).

11. Instruct client to call ambulance and go to emergency room if perforation occurs (sudden sharp epigastric or abdominal pain, pain radiation to shoulders, abdominal rigidity, diaphoresis, fever, rapid and shallow respirations, increased pulse rate) (first visit).

12. Encourage modification rather than complete life-style changes to increase compliance (first visit).

13. Suggest community resources and groups for smoking and stress and dietary counseling and support (first visit).

14. Encourage client to keep appointments with physician and for laboratory tests (first visit).

15. Instruct client to avoid aspirin and aspirin products.

CLIENT AND FAMILY/CARETAKER INTERVENTIONS

1. Eat a well balanced, bland diet in small and frequent meals; avoid dietary stressors.

2. Avoid alcohol, tobacco, and caffeine.

3. Avoid stress in environment and relationships and situations that may create stress.
4. Administer medications correctly and as instructed; avoid aspirin and nonsteroidal antiinflammatories.
5. Notify physician of signs and symptoms of complications if they occur.
6. Ask questions and clarify information when needed.
7. Seek out reinforcement and support in community groups that might be helpful.
8. Keep appointments with physician for follow-up care.

Nursing diagnosis

Anxiety

Related factors: Threat to or change in health status

Defining characteristics: Increased tension and apprehension about change in health and life-style, client's verbalization of inability to manage stress and symptoms of the disease

OUTCOME CRITERIA

Short-term
Decreased anxiety, as evidenced by more relaxed posture and facial expression, statements that anxiety has decreased and has been controlled, and decrease in symptoms as a result of compliance with health regimen (expected within 3 to 7 days)

Long-term
Anxiety minimal or controlled, as evidenced by client's acceptance of changes in life-style to achieve optimal health and functioning (expected within 4 weeks)

NURSING INTERVENTIONS/INSTRUCTIONS

1. Assess mental and emotional status (see Psychosocial Assessment, p. 41, for guidelines) (first visit).
2. Explore with client historical coping patterns and problem-solving ability; relate them to condition and pain episodes (first visit).
3. Assist client to develop effective coping and stress-reducing mechanisms (first visit and reinforce on second visit).
4. Include client in all aspects of planning care at home (each visit).

5. Provide continuing information about condition and progress (each visit).
6. Suggest counseling and/or relaxation techniques to reduce anxiety if chronic (first visit).

CLIENT AND FAMILY/CARETAKER INTERVENTIONS

1. Identify current coping mechanisms and explore options for improved coping and stress control.
2. Participate in planning of care, including adherence to dietary, activity, and medication regimens.
3. Perform relaxation exercises when feeling anxious.
4. Consult physician if unable to control anxiety.

◣ Ulcerative Colitis/Crohn's Disease

Inflammatory bowel diseases include ulcerative colitis, involving the large intestine, and Crohn's disease, involving any part of the intestinal tract but most usually the terminal ileum. Ulcerative colitis affects the mucous membranes, causing purulent exudate and bleeding. Segments or the entire colon may be affected, with periods of remission and exacerbation of inflammation. The disease may be confused with Crohn's disease. Crohn's disease affects all layers of the mucous membranes, and segments separated by normal bowel may be inflamed. Both diseases exhibit extracolonic manifestations as well as affect absorption of nutrients. Complications include intestinal obstruction, anemia, and nutritional and fluid and electrolyte imbalances.

Home care is primarily concerned with the teaching aspects of care and treatment for the disease and preventive measures to maintain health and avoid exacerbation.

Nursing diagnosis

Pain

Related factors: Biologic injuring agents of inflammatory disease

Defining characteristics: Verbalization of pain descriptors, groaning, abdominal guarding, restlessness, abdominal cramping

OUTCOME CRITERIA

Short-term

Pain minimal or controlled, as evidenced by client's statement that pain has subsided or disappeared, relaxed posture and facial expressions, and participation in activities of daily living (ADL) and other activities (expected within 3 to 4 days)

Long-term

Pain controlled or absent, as evidenced by return to normal gastrointestinal function; achieved as a result of compliance with medical regimen (expected within 2 to 4 weeks)

NURSING INTERVENTIONS/INSTRUCTIONS

1. Assess pain type, location, characteristics, duration, intensity, and relationship to diet, activity, and elimination (first visit).
2. Instruct client in medication administration, including analgesics and antiinflammatories prescribed (first visit).
3. Instruct client in relaxation exercises and guided imagery and to practice these techniques between episodes (first visit).
4. Instruct client to notify physician if pain is not relieved or increases in severity and if bloating, distention, vomiting, or abdominal rigidity is associated with increasing pain (first visit).

CLIENT AND FAMILY/CARETAKER INTERVENTIONS

1. Administer medication for optimal effects.
2. Practice diversional activities for relaxation and pain reduction.
3. Notify physician if pain persists or escalates or if new symptoms develop.

Nursing diagnosis

Altered nutrition: less than body requirements

Related factors: Inability to ingest or absorb nutrients because of biologic factors

Defining characteristics: Weight loss; inadequate intake of nutrients; anorexia; diarrhea; nausea

OUTCOME CRITERIA

Short-term
Adequate nutrition, as evidenced by client's statement of compliance with dietary requirements and regimen and by stabilization of weight (expected within 1 week)

Long-term
Adequate nutritional status, as evidenced by intake of required nutrients for optimal health and functioning (expected within 1 month and ongoing)

NURSING INTERVENTIONS/INSTRUCTIONS

1. Assess nutritional status, including food preferences, cultural and religious restrictions, and effect of different foods on illness (first visit).
2. Calculate ideal weight for size, sex, frame, and height (first visit).
3. Assess for nausea, vomiting, anorexia, weight loss, fatigue, malaise, and reactions to meals (each visit).
4. Instruct client to schedule rest periods after meals and to have 6 to 8 hours of sleep per night (first visit).
5. Inform client of measures that facilitate eating, including eliminating odors, providing a relaxed atmosphere and a quiet environment, eating smaller, more frequent meals, and taking antiemetics ½ hour before meals (first visit).
6. Include client in planning a bland, high-protein, reduced-fiber, low-residue, and possibly high-calorie diet, avoiding highly seasoned foods, raw fruits and vegetables, foods containing coarse cereals, bran, seeds, or nuts, milk, and fatty or fried foods (first visit).
7. Administer iron preparation intramuscularly as prescribed (any visit).
8. Initiate referral to nutritionist if indicated.

CLIENT AND FAMILY/CARETAKER INTERVENTIONS

1. Maintain or gain weight as determined.
2. Participate in planning and ingestion of a well-balanced diet with restrictions as determined.
3. Promote pleasant environment and dietary pattern that enhances intake.
4. Maintain rest and sleep schedule.
5. Avoid stress and irritants during meals.
6. Include increased calories and protein in diet plans.

Nursing diagnosis

Diarrhea

Related factors: Inflammation, irritation, or malabsorption of bowel

Defining characteristics: Abdominal pain; cramping; increased frequency; loose, liquid stools; urgency; mucus in stool; increased frequency of bowel sounds

OUTCOME CRITERIA

Short-term
Return of baseline bowel pattern, as evidenced by decrease in the frequency of bowel eliminations and by stool characteristics within baseline parameters (expected wtihin 1 week)

Long-term
Minimal or absence of diarrheal bowel eliminations, as evidenced by soft, formed stools eliminated according to baseline pattern (expected within 2 weeks)

NURSING INTERVENTIONS/INSTRUCTIONS

1. Assess bowel elimination patterns and stool characteristics (see Gastrointestinal System Assessment, p. 17, for guidelines) (first visit).
2. Instruct client to maintain a record of bowel movements, including number and when they occur and characteristics such as color, amount, consistency, odor, and presence of mucus, blood, or pus (first visit).
3. Monitor medication administration and instruct client in antidiarrheals and anticholinergics (each visit).

4. Instruct client to notify physician if diarrhea becomes more severe or frequent, if bleeding is noted, or if fatigue or weakness is noted (first visit).

CLIENT AND FAMILY/CARETAKER INTERVENTIONS

1. Monitor and record bowel elimination.
2. Administer medications correctly and as instructed.
3. Notify physician if diarrhea becomes worse and condition deteriorates or complications occur.

Nursing diagnosis

High risk for impaired skin integrity

Related factors: Excretions and secretions

Defining characteristics: Diarrhea; irritation, redness, or disruption of perianal area; perianal pain

OUTCOME CRITERIA

Short-term
Minimized risk for skin breakdown, as evidenced by appropriate care of perianal area, which should be free of maceration or excoriation caused by excretions (expected within 3 to 4 days)

Long-term
Skin integrity maintained, as evidenced by perianal area free of any irritation or breaks (expected within 1 week and ongoing)

NURSING INTERVENTIONS/INSTRUCTIONS

1. Assess perianal area for tissue integrity, color, and odor, and note presence of drainage, excoriation, maceration, abscess, fistula, or fissure formation (each visit).
2. Instruct client in perianal care to be done every morning and possibly after every bowel elimination, including sitz bath, cleansing with agent dispensed in a Peri-bottle, and application of protective ointment; advise client to continue care during periods of remission (first visit and reinforce on second visit).
3. Instruct client to notify physician if irritation is unrelieved and bleeding or drainage is noted (first visit).

CLIENT AND FAMILY/CARETAKER INTERVENTIONS

1. Provide perianal care daily or as needed.
2. Protect perianal area from irritation.
3. Maintain intact perianal tissue integrity.
4. Notify physician of severe excoriation or breakdown of perianal area.

Nursing diagnosis

High risk for fluid volume deficit

Related factors: Active fluid loss

Defining characteristics: Diarrhea, vomiting; diaphoresis; decreased urine output in relation to intake; dry skin and mucous membranes; weight loss; electrolyte imbalance (sodium, potassium)

OUTCOME CRITERIA

Short-term

Adequate fluid and electrolyte balance, as evidenced by absence of signs and symptoms of dehydration, balanced intake and output, and electrolyte levels within normal ranges (expected within 1 week)

Long-term

Fluid and electrolytes within balance, with optimal health and functioning achieved whether during remission or during exacerbation of disease (expected within 2 weeks and ongoing)

NURSING INTERVENTIONS/INSTRUCTIONS

1. Assess fluid needs according to age, weight, and estimated fluid losses (each visit).
2. Monitor for dehydration, including thirst, decreased urinary output, poor skin turgor, dry mucous membranes, and furrowed tongue (each visit).
3. Instruct client to take and record daily weights and estimated intake and output (first visit).
4. Instruct client to drink 8 to 10 glasses of fluid per day in small, spaced servings and to avoid fluids that are too hot or cold (first visit).

5. Instruct client in administration of potassium supplements and intake of foods containing potassium, including bananas, citrus juices, and dried fruits (first visit).
6. Monitor for electrolyte imbalance and instruct client in recognition of signs and symptoms, including muscle weakness, cramping, twitching, confusion, paresthesias, and pulse irregularities (first visit).
7. Monitor laboratory values for potassium, sodium, calcium, chloride, magnesium, hemoglobin, and hematocrit if available (any visit).

CLIENT AND FAMILY/CARETAKER INTERVENTIONS

1. Maintain fluid intake according to calculated needs and fluid losses.
2. Administer or increase intake of potassium replacement.
3. Weigh daily, compare intake and output of fluids in relation to diarrhea.
4. Report any signs and symptoms of dehydration or electrolyte decreases.

Nursing diagnosis

Ineffective individual coping

Related factors: Multiple life changes; chronic illness

Defining characteristics: Verbalization of inability to cope or ask for or seek out help; inability to problem solve and use defense mechanisms effectively; exacerbation of symptoms; chronic anxiety; depression

OUTCOME CRITERIA

Short-term
Improved coping ability, as evidenced by client's statement that recognizing and adapting to need for changes in life-style are necessary (expected within 1 week)

Long-term
Effective coping, as evidenced by compliance with treatment regimen and by changes in life-style to adapt to illness and to requirements for optimal health achievement (expected within 1 to 2 months and ongoing)

NURSING INTERVENTIONS/INSTRUCTIONS

1. Assess for developmental level and dependency needs, behavioral and emotional changes, use of defense mechanisms and their effectiveness, and ability to problem solve (first visit).
2. Establish a trusting relationship, and facilitate an open discussion to explore options and develop skills in coping and problem solving (each visit).
3. Indentify coping skills that work, and encourage positive feeling about success of any adaptation or changes (each visit).
4. Include client in all planning and formulation of realistic goals; assist if requested to do so (each visit).
5. Encourage expression of fears about possible surgery and threat to life.

CLIENT AND FAMILY/CARETAKER INTERVENTIONS

1. Share feelings, fears, and concerns with caretaker or family.
2. Plan and participate in own care and health promotion.
3. Set goals and strategies for remissions and exacerbations.
4. Participate in support group with persons who have similar condition.

Nursing diagnosis

Knowledge deficit

Related factors: Lack of information about disease and treatments

Defining characteristics: Request for information about disease, causes, signs and symptoms, medications, and need for compliance and for prevention of exacerbations

OUTCOME CRITERIA

Short-term

Adequate knowledge, as evidenced by client's statement of precipitating, aggravating, and alleviating factors in symptomatology and signs and symptoms of exacerbation or worsening condition (expected within 3 days)

Long-term
Adequate knowledge, as evidenced by client's meeting requirements to achieve optimal health and gastrointestinal functioning with reduction in exacerbations (expected within 1 to 2 months and ongoing)

NURSING INTERVENTIONS/INSTRUCTIONS

1. Assess client's life-style, learning and coping abilities, interests, and family participation and support (first visit).
2. Instruct client to maintain log of ADL that includes food diary, fluid intake, and descriptions of gastrointestinal episodes (first visit).
3. Assist client to identify characteristic trends and influencing factors that precipitate or alleviate symptoms; use data as a physiologic and psychologic baseline and a basis for teaching (first visit).
4. Instruct client to notify physician of any change in conditon that indicates complications or exacerbation (first visit).
5. Instruct client in correct medication administration, including vitamins, electrolyte replacement, antiemetics, antidiarrheals, steroids, immunosuppressants, antibiotics, and others prescribed; emphasize dosage, frequency, side effects, expected results, and interactions and to avoid OTC drugs without physician recommendation (first visit).
6. Instruct client to maintain scheduled physician appointments (first visit).
7. Provide information about agencies or groups for educational material, support or counseling, or new trends (first visit).

CLIENT AND FAMILY/CARETAKER INTERVENTIONS

1. Maintain log of progress and changes.
2. Monitor for influences of diet, fluids, activity, and stress.
3. Administer medications safely and correctly.
4. Notify physician of unremitting or escalating symptoms.
5. Participate in educational and support programs.
6. Carry out measures to prevent exacerbation.

Endocrine system

◢ Diabetes Mellitus

Diabetes mellitus is characterized by absence or inadequate production of insulin by the pancreas to meet body needs for carbohydrate, fat, and protein metabolism. Long-term effects include vascular changes, retinopathy, and neuropathy. The most common type found in adults is non–insulin dependent, or type II (NIDDM). A second type is insulin dependent, or type I (IDDM).

Home care is primarily concerned with the teaching aspects of medication regimens, monitoring glucose levels, and the measures to take for control of the disease to prevent complications.

Nursing diagnosis

Ineffective individual coping

Related factors: Multiple life changes; chronic illness and consequences

Defining characteristics: Chronic worry, anxiety, and complaints; tension; inability to cope with necessary life-style changes

OUTCOME CRITERIA

Short-term
Improvement in use of coping skills, as evidenced by use of coping mechanisms effectively and by verbalization of need to change life-style and request assistance when needed to meet needs (expected within 1 week)

Long-term
Effective coping with chronic illness, as evidenced by acceptable level of anxiety and concern and by adaptation to life-style changes (expected within 2 to 3 months)

NURSING INTERVENTIONS/INSTRUCTIONS

1. Assess for appropriate use of coping mechanisms, ability to problem solve, inner resources to manage anxiety and stress and support system (each visit).
2. Provide accepting, nonjudgmental attitude and environment when teaching and discussing needs and changes to be made in life-style (each visit).
3. Instruct to avoid events that produce stress or prevent use of constructive coping mechanisms or behavior (first visit).
4. Instruct client in coping, communication, and problem-solving skills (first and second visits).
5. Instruct client in relaxation and diversional techniques, such as music, muscle relaxation, and reading (first visit).
6. Encourage expression of concerns and mutual goal setting.

CLIENT AND FAMILY/CARETAKER INTERVENTIONS

1. Develop effective use of coping mechanisms.
2. Avoid stress-provoking events.
3. Engage in relaxation and diversional activities.
4. Request assistance when needed.
5. Reduce and/or control anxiety level.
6. Adapt to change in life-style to comply with medical regimen.

Nursing diagnosis

Altered nutrition: less than body requirements

Related factors: Inability to metabolize nutrients

Defining characteristics: Hyperglycemia; hypoglycemia; noncompliance with dietary, activity, and insulin regimens in controlling condition

OUTCOME CRITERIA

Short-term
Adequate nutrition, as evidenced by compliance with recommended American Diabetic Association (ADA) diet and absence of hyperglycemic or hypoglycemic states (expected within 1 week)

Long-term
Adequate nutritional intake and metabolic process, as evidenced by appropriate dietary planning and intake in relation to insulin production or administration and by blood and urinary glucose levels that are within normal ranges (expected within 1 month and ongoing)

NURSING INTERVENTIONS/INSTRUCTIONS

1. Assess nutritional status, including food preferences, religious and cultural restrictions, emotional factors related to food and eating, and actual and desired weight levels (first visit).
2. Instruct client to keep a diary of all foods consumed, amounts and methods of preparation, and weekly weights (first visit)
3. Instruct client about and review diabetic exchange lists and prescribed diet; use diary as a guide and make changes as needed; provide written instructions and information about diet (first visit and reinforce on second visit).
4. Instruct in ADA diets as prescribed, with reduced calories, sodium, and fat and cholesterol content if necessary; include avoidance of simple sugars (use sugar substitutes) and concentrated sweets and the importance of evenly spaced, regular meals and scheduled snacks; instruct client to eat all of meals and to avoid skipping or delaying a meal or bunching required foods in one meal to another (first visit and reinforce each visit).
5. Inform client of early signs and symptoms of hypoglycemia, including hunger, shakiness, palpitations, headache, weakness, irritability, nervousness, and visual disturbances (first visit).
6. Instruct client to carry candy or sugar at all times and, at first sign of hypoglycemic attack, to take milk (preferred) or fruit juice (sweetened), soft drink, or 4 teaspoons sugar or 4 or 5 pieces of hard candy or rub sugar preparation from a tube on gums (first visit and reinforce after any hypoglycemic episodes).
7. Inform client of signs and symptoms of hyperglycemia and possible ketoacidosis, including fatigue, malaise, flushed face, nausea and vomiting, marked thirst, fruity

(acetone) breath, hyperpnea, or changes in mentation (first visit).

8. Instruct client to notify physician if diet is not tolerated or foods cannot be retained or at first onset of any sign or symptom of high or low glucose levels or presence of ketones in urine (first visit).

9. Refer client to nutritionist for assistance in ADA diet and exchanges if needed (first visit).

10. Review activity and exercise in relation to prescribed diet.

CLIENT AND FAMILY/CARETAKER INTERVENTIONS

1. Maintain record of foods and weekly weight and incidence of dietary changes to accomodate test results of blood and urine.

2. Formulate meal menus and planning of dietary inclusions and restrictions.

3. Eat regularly scheduled meals following prescribed ADA diet and exchange lists.

4. Carry emergency sugar supply at all times.

5. Identify signs and symptoms of hypoglycemia and hyperglycemia.

6. Take extra nutrition before engaging in strenuous activities.

Nursing diagnosis

Knowledge deficit

Related factors: Request for information and instruction about disease and procedures to control disease and prevent complications

Defining characteristics: Verbalization of unfamiliarity with medication administration, dietary and exercise inclusions and restrictions, foot care, blood and urine testing for glucose, care of skin, teeth, and eyes, signs and symptoms of hyperglycemia and hypoglycemia, and measures to take to treat these conditions

OUTCOME CRITERIA

Short-term
Adequate knowledge, as evidenced by client verbalizations of medication administration, blood and urine testing, activity

regimen, care of feet, skin, and eyes, signs and symptoms of altered glycemic states, and treatment (expected within 4 to 7 days)

Long-term

Adequate knowledge, as evidenced by absence of complications following daily compliance with treatment regimen (expected within 1 month and thereafter)

NURSING INTERVENTIONS/INSTRUCTIONS

1. Assess all body systems for baselines; assess history of drug and hormone use and alcohol use (first visit).
2. Instruct client in and demonstrate self-administration of insulin, noting technique; rotation of sites; onset, peak, duration of action, and expected results of the insulin(s); possibility of local reaction to injection, and use and care of pump if applicable (first and second visits and ongoing as needed).
3. Instruct client in administration of oral hypoglycemics, noting dose, frequency, side effects, food/drug/alcohol interactions, and expected action and results (first visit).
4. Instruct client in and demonstrate blood collection and testing for glucose and use of glucometer; relate to insulin administration and diet; instruct client in urinary glucose and ketone testing to be done if blood glucose reaches a predetermined level (first visit and reinforce on second visit).
5. Assess activities of daily living and exercise pattern, and instruct client to exercise daily, implementing a consistent routine; instruct client in actions to take if exercise is increased (first visit).
6. Encourage client to stop smoking; suggest support groups (first visit).
7. Inform client of importance of complying with medication, exercise, and diet regimens to maintain glucose level within normal range, and instruct client to notify physician of continuous signs and symptoms of hypoglycemia or hyperglycemia (first visit).
8. Impress on client the importance of notifying physician if stress, trauma, or infection is present (first visit).
9. Instruct client in meticulous care of feet, with daily bathing in tepid water; rinse well and pat dry, especially between toes; see podiatrist for foot care; apply cream to

lower exremities; wear good-fitting shoes and cotton socks; check feet for cuts, scratches or blisters, ulcers, or delayed healing, and reduced sensation (first visit and reinforce on second visit).

10. Discuss sexual concerns (impotence, family planning) as appropriate (first visit).

11. Instruct client to inform all caregivers of diagnosis (dentist, surgeon) (first visit).

12. Instruct client to wear and/or carry identification indicating condition and medications (first visit).

CLIENT AND FAMILY/CARETAKER INTERVENTIONS

1. Administer insulin or hypoglycemic correctly and in timely manner.
2. Use insulin pump effectively if prescribed.
3. Test blood and urine at appropriate times, and analyze results for proper actions to take.
4. Exercise daily and maintain constant day-to-day program.
5. Cease smoking or join support group for assistance.
6. State signs and symptoms of hypoglycemia and hyperglycemia and appropriate actions to take.
7. State signs and symptoms of infection to report to physician.
8. Report any visual disturbances; participate in periodic eye examinations.
9. Note neuropathies and report any trauma to physician.
10. Perform consistent, meticulous foot care.
11. Follow up on sexual concerns to make informed decisions as indicated.
12. Wear or carry identification information.
13. Consult podiatrist, ophthamologist, and dentist for specific care.

Nursing diagnosis

Noncompliance

Related factors: Health beliefs and practices

Defining characteristics: Failure to adhere to medical regimen, with resulting development of complications or exacerbation of symptoms; failure to keep appointments or report to physician

OUTCOME CRITERIA
Short-term
Compliance with medical regimen, as evidenced by client identifying and performing dietary and activity modifications, medication regimen, blood and urine testing, and foot and skin care (expected within 1 week)

Long-term
Optimal and effective compliance, as evidenced by participation in all apsects of care, absence of complications, and functioning at a well level (expected within 2 to 3 months)

NURSING INTERVENTIONS/INSTRUCTIONS
1. Establish rapport and provide a nonthreatening, accepting environment for care and teaching (each visit).
2. Assess coping and learning abilities, developmental level and achieved tasks, economic level, support system; note perceived implications of disorder for life-style (each visit).
3. Evaluate knowledge and performance of dietary, activity, medication, and testing procedures and modifications (first visit).
4. Include client and significant others in planning and teaching of health care (each visit).
5. Help client to modify life-style with as few changes as possible; explore options and praise efforts and successes (each visit).
6. Suggest counseling or support groups such as the American Diabetic Association for information, supplies, and support.
7. Encourage expression of perception of disease.

CLIENT AND FAMILY/CARETAKER INTERVENTIONS
1. Participate in all aspects of health care; comply with requirements.
2. Accept support from family, friends, and agencies.
3. Demonstrate facility in performance of all procedures and planning of care for optimal health and functioning.

Hematologic system

◢ Acquired Immunodeficiency Syndrome (AIDS)

Acquired immunodeficiency syndrome is characterized by extreme immunosuppression, allowing for the development of malignancies and opportunistic infections caused by viruses, bacteria, fungi, and protozoa. It is a life-threatening illness whose cause is unknown. The disease demonstrates suppression of T helper cells and an increase in T cell suppressors, both of which decrease the body's ability to respond to an acute inflammatory reaction and depress a defensive response. AIDS is transmitted by administration of contaminated blood or blood products, sexual contact, use of contaminated needles, syringes, or instruments, or accidental exposure to contaminated blood through breaks in the skin or mucous membranes; perinatal transmission also occurs.

Home care is primarily concerned with the care and teaching aspects of infection prevention, activities of daily living, the medication regimen, and transmission prevention.

Nursing diagnosis

Anxiety

Related factors: Threat of death; change in health status

Defining characteristics: Presence of human immunodeficiency virus (HIV); presence of AIDS-related complex (ARC); apprehension and increased helplessness; absence of any effective treatment; fear of transmission to others

OUTCOME CRITERIA

Short-term
Decreased anxiety, as evidenced by client's statement of reduced fear and apprehension about change in health status and possible early death (expected within 1 week)

Long-term
Management or control of anxiety level, as evidenced by compliance with and acceptance of treatment regimen and change in life-style to prevent transmission of the disease to others (expected within 1 to 2 months and ongoing)

NURSING INTERVENTIONS/INSTRUCTIONS

1. Assess client's mental and emotional status in relation to life-threatening illness and associated stigma (see Psychosocial Assessment, p. 41, for guidelines) (first visit).
2. Encourage expression of fears and concerns in a supportive and nonjudgmental environment; instruct client in relaxation techniques (each visit).
3. Assist client to identify needed changes in life-style and methods to make necessary changes (first visit and thereafter as needed).
4. Inform client about activities allowed, treatments and tests to expect, and testing of contacts (first visit).
5. Initiate referral to counseling, support groups, or agencies that may assist with legal, economic, and health care needs (first visit).
6. Encourage expression of concerns and mutual goal setting.

CLIENT AND FAMILY/CARETAKER INTERVENTIONS

1. Develop coping for long-term treatment and possible outcome.
2. Maintain manageable level of anxiety.
3. Seek information that will reduce anxiety.
4. Express fears and concerns about necessary changes in life-style.
5. Contact and consult with support services available.

Nursing diagnosis

High risk for infection

Related factors: Inadequate secondary defenses

Defining characteristics: Immunodeficiency; potential for opportunistic infection, hyperthermia, prostration, change in breathing pattern (*Pneumocystis* pneumonia), change in thought process (cytomegalovirus) with dementia

OUTCOME CRITERIA

Short-term

Absence of infection, as evidenced by temperature and blood tests within normal ranges and by freedom from signs and symptoms of any opportunistic infection (expectation dependent on immune system status)

Long-term

Absence of infection with optimal functioning of all systems (expected as an ongoing finding)

NURSING INTERVENTIONS/INSTRUCTIONS

1. Perform complete physical assessment for data base and note any signs and symptoms associated with the disease (first visit).
2. Instruct client to monitor for and report presence of fever, malaise, night sweats, cough, dyspnea, headache, enlarged glands, epigastric or abdominal pain, vomiting or diarrhea, skin lesions, rashes, weakness, joint pain, or sensory or intellectual deficits (first visit).
3. Instruct client in preventive measures regarding infections, including hand washing, personal hygiene, and avoidance of crowds and persons with infection or who are ill (first visit).
4. Instruct client in administration of antiinfectives and specific preventive drugs for disease and to avoid any immunosuppressive drugs (first visit).
5. Encourage health promotion, including rest, nutritious diet, and stress management (each visit).

CLIENT AND FAMILY/CARETAKER INTERVENTIONS

1. Bathe daily and inspect for and report rashes, skin lesions or vesicles, or skin disruptions.
2. Perform hand washing after toileting, before meals, and before any procedures.
3. Take temperature if any symptoms appear, and report elevation.
4. Monitor for and report signs and symptoms of infection in any system.
5. Administer medications as instructed.
6. Avoid exposure to persons with infections.
7. Maintain healthy life-style that includes nutritious meals, 6 to 8 hours of sleep per night, and social and diversional activities.

Nursing diagnosis

Activity intolerance

Related factors: Generalized weakness

Defining characteristics: Verbalization of fatigue and weakness, inability to perform activities of daily living (ADL) and ambulate, repeated infections, malnutrition, wasting, lack of sleep

OUTCOME CRITERIA

Short-term
Increased activity and energy, as evidenced by performance of ADL and utilization of energy conservation techniques (expected within 1 week)

Long-term
Adequate activity within disease limitations, as evidenced by achievement of optimal level of self-care and general functioning (expected within 2 to 3 months as realistic)

NURSING INTERVENTIONS/INSTRUCTIONS

1. Assess client's ability to carry out ADL and energy and endurance levels; note strength, gait, posture, balance, presence of fatigue, general weakness, and sensory deficits (each visit).

2. Encourage rest after activity and at least 6 to 8 hours of sleep per night (first visit).
3. Assist client to identify activities that need pacing and in setting limits (first visit and reinforce on second visit).
4. Inform client of available energy-conserving aids to assist in dressing, bathing, grooming, toileting, and eating (first visit).
5. Assess support system; include support system in care planning and in care (first visit).
6. Coordinate social services and community resources for assistance and support (first visit).
7. Refer home health aide (HHA) to assist with ADL.

CLIENT AND FAMILY/CARETAKER INTERVENTIONS

1. Base rest and sleep on individual needs and condition.
2. Participate in activities within set limits.
3. Uses energy-saving devices in ADL.
4. Assist with any activity requiring support.
5. Utilize private and public resources for assistance.

Nursing diagnosis

Altered nutrition: less than body requirements

Related factors: Inability to ingest food and absorb nutrients

Defining characteristics: Anorexia, infection of oroesophageal tract, gastroenteritis, diarrhea, weight loss, wasting

OUTCOME CRITERIA

Short-term
Adequate nutrition, as evidenced by intake of nutritious and high-calorie foods and stable weight pattern (expected within 1 week)

Long-term
Optimal nutritional status, as evidenced by weight stability and by absence of disease manifestations that affect food intake necessary to maintain health and functioning (expected within 1 month and ongoing)

NURSING INTERVENTIONS/INSTRUCTIONS

1. Assess nutritional status, including height, actual and ideal weight, food preferences, and cultural and religious restrictions (first visit).
2. Perform gastrointestinal assessment (see Gastrointestinal System Assessment, p. 17, for guidelines); note presence of anorexia, nausea, vomiting, weight loss, persistent diarrhea, oroesophageal inflammation or lesions, and temperature elevation, and cross reference signs and symptoms with drug profile (each visit).
3. Instruct client in regular, scrupulous oral hygiene and in use of soft toothbrush, topical antifungal agents, mouthwashes, and topical anesthetics as prescribed in presence of oral inflammation or lesions (first visit).
4. Instruct client to eat high calorie, well balanced diet and to include foods that will prevent or minimize distressing manifestations (first visit).
5. Instruct client to eat smaller, more frequent meals that include commercially prepared supplements (first visit).
6. If nausea is present, suggest use of toast or dry crackers, choosing foods that are less aromatic and less strong in taste, and drinking beverages ½ hour before meals rather than with meals (first visit).
7. Instruct client to eat when rested and to rest ½ hour after meals with head elevated (first visit).
8. Instruct client to administer vitamin/mineral supplements daily (first visit).
9. Instruct client in administration of antidiarrheals and antiemetics if prescribed (first visit).
10. Inform client of alternative feeding methods such as tube feedings or total parenteral nutrition (TPN), and instruct client in procedures if implemented (applicable visit with reinforcement).
11. Initiate referral to nutritionist for consultation and to community resources for food preparation and delivery if needed (first visit).

CLIENT AND FAMILY/CARETAKER INTERVENTIONS

1. Perform and record daily weight, and report any significant, progressive losses.

2. Eat small, frequent, high-calorie meals that include preferences and nutritional requirements.
3. Perform mouth care after meals and if oral mucous membrane is impaired, and protect oral cavity from further trauma.
4. Treat nausea with dry foods and timely intake of fluids.
5. Supplement meals with foods and beverages of high nutrient value.
6. Administer vitamin/mineral supplements, antidiarrheals, antifungals, antibiotics, and topical anesthetics as instructed.
7. Monitor tube feedings or TPN if present, and perform procedures for administration and care of these methods of feeding if capable of managing them.
8. Consult with nutritionist.
9. Utilize community resources for food service.

Nursing diagnosis

Impaired social interaction

Related factors: Therapeutic isolation; inability to engage in satisfying personal relationship

Defining characteristics: Stigma associated with AIDS and unaccepted social behavior (drug abuse, sexual preference), fear of transmission of disease, fear of loss of confidentiality and loss of or rejection by significant others and community as result of diagnosis

OUTCOME CRITERIA

Short-term
Involvement in social interaction, as evidenced by verbalization of behaviors resulting from isolation and of options to reverse these and to adapt to requirements for meaningful relationships (expected within 1 week)

Long-term
Optimal social relationships, as evidenced by participation in social activities with significant others and support group (expected within 1 month)

NURSING INTERVENTIONS/INSTRUCTIONS

1. Provide continuity of care by providing same professional caregiver for treatment and care (each visit).

2. Use therapeutic communication, including touch (each visit).
3. Identify type and amount of support available in home and community (first visit).
4. Provide an understanding, nonjudgmental environment (each visit).
5. Facilitate individual and group interaction; note that behavior or personality changes may be the result of neurologic dysfunction (each visit).
6. Provide a range of diversional options, including books, games, collecting, and visits from friends (first visit).
7. Refer to AIDS support group or counseling as needed (any visit).

CLIENT AND FAMILY/CARETAKER INTERVENTIONS

1. Occupy time with diversional activities.
2. Accept visits from friends.
3. Verbalize understanding of social fears and lack of knowledge regarding disease.
4. Interact with support groups and services.
5. Consult counseling or agencies for assistance.

Nursing diagnosis

Anticipatory grieving

Related factors: Perceived potential loss of physiopsychosocial well-being

Defining characteristics: Expression of distress at potential loss; anger; guilt; denial of potential loss; sorrow; choked feelings; changes in sleep, eating, and activity patterns

OUTCOME CRITERIA

Short-term
Progress in grieving, as evidenced by attitude and behavior changes manifested by stage in process (expected within days)

Long-term
Grief process resolving, as evidenced by resumption of lifestyle with or without changes as needed and by integration of grieving stage into life-style and activities (expected within 2 to 3 months and ongoing)

NURSING INTERVENTIONS/INSTRUCTIONS

1. Assess degree and stage of grief (each visit).
2. Inform client of stages of grieving process and that behavior is acceptable for specific stage and that resolution will be final stage (first visit).
3. Allow expression of feelings and perceptions about disabilities and potential loss and death in a nonjudgmental environment (each visit).
4. Initiate referral for psychological and spiritual counseling and hospice care as appropriate (any visit).

CLIENT AND FAMILY/CARETAKER INTERVENTIONS

1. Progress through grief process to resolution.
2. Seek counseling as needed.
3. Verbalize stages and behaviors during grief process.

Nursing diagnosis

Knowledge deficit

Related factors: Lack of exposure to information

Defining characteristics: Request for information about change in sexual patterns and social behavior necessary to prevent transmission of disease, legal and medical rights and assistance, and community resources available

OUTCOME CRITERIA

Short-term
Adequate knowledge, as evidenced by client's statements regarding disease progression and transmission and treatments (expected within 3 days)

Long-term
Adequate knowledge, as evidenced by compliance in meeting requirements of changed life-style, with limitiations imposed by condition, to achieve optimal level of functioning (expected within 1 month)

NURSING INTERVENTIONS/INSTRUCTIONS

1. Carry out Centers for Disease Control (CDC) universal precautions in all aspects of nursing care (each visit).

2. Include significant others in instruction; allow for active participation in care planning (each visit).
3. Assess for and instruct client in recognition of opportunistic infection, recurrence, reinfections, neoplasms, and neurologic manifestations and in treatment available for these conditions (each visit).
4. Instruct client in transmission modes, and stress that disease is not transmitted by casual contact or living with others but by sexual contact, exchange of needles in drug use, administration of blood or blood products, or sharing of razors or other items that might contain the virus (first visit).
5. Instruct client in general cleaning and disinfection methods; bleach solution (1:10) may be used to clean contaminated materials (first visit).
6. Advise client of need for testing sexual contacts or high-risk contacts in addition to concurrent counseling about transmission (first visit).
7. Instruct client in options for sexual activity, including abstinence, use of latex condom lubricated with nonoxynol 9, and birth control planning (first visit and reinforce second visit).
8. Encourage rehabilitation of intravenous drug users; instruct them not to share needles or paraphernalia and to wash syringes with soap and water and then cleanse with bleach and rinse thoroughly after each use (each visit).
9. Instruct client in administration of zidovudine, pentamidine, antibiotics and anti-infectives, psychotropics, anticonvulsants, immunomodulators, analgesics, antipyretics, and chemotherapy as prescribed, including dose, route, frequency, side effects, and interactions; inform client of possible resources for medications (first visit and reinforce as needed).
10. Instruct client not to donate blood or organs (first visit).
11. Instruct client to inform all nursing, medical, and laboratory personnel of condition (first visit).
12. Assist client in organizing health care information; provide written instructions and reminders for care, medications and schedules, and resource and emergency telephone numbers (first visit).
13. Inform client of importance of follow-up with physician and laboratory visits (first visit).

14. Refer client to community groups, resources, and organizations for support, information, and financial and legal needs (first visit).

CLIENT AND FAMILY/CARETAKER INTERVENTIONS

1. Monitor and report any signs and symptoms of opportunistic infections.
2. Prevent transmission to others.
3. Report contacts to be tested.
4. Administer medications as prescribed and instructed; utilize a written plan and schedule.
5. Avoid activities that will spread disease, and verbalize how disease is transmitted and measures to take to protect others from disease
6. Inform those who need to know diagnosis, with assurance of confidentiality.
7. Seek out support services available for persons with AIDS.

Nursing diagnosis

High risk for caregiver role strain

Related factors: Severity of illness of the care reciever; complexity and number of caregiving tasks

Defining characteristics: Caregiver's report of not having enough resources to provide care (emotional and physical strength; help from others) and of difficulty in performing specific caregiving activities (bathing, cleaning up after incontinence, managing client's weakened condition and discomforts)

OUTCOME CRITERIA

Short-term
Potential for caregiver role strain identified, as evidenced by caregiver's verbalization of difficulties encountered in performing care and concern about ability and conflicts in giving care (expected within 1 week)

Long-term
Prevention of caregiver role strain, as evidenced by continued safe and appropriate care provided without compromise to own physical and emotional needs (expected within 1 month and ongoing)

NURSING INTERVENTIONS/INSTRUCTIONS

1. Assess severity of illness and care needs of the receiver of care and ability of caregiver to perform role (first visit).
2. Assess relationship between care receiver and caregiver before illness and stressors placed on the relationship by the illness (first visit).
3. Assist caregiver to monitor continued ability to perform care and treatments,changes in day-to-day needs, changes in stressors and strains, maintenance of routines, and need for additional resources (aides, homemaker, respite care, friends, family) (first visit).
4. Discuss role performance and whether expectations are realistic, flexibility of role, and decision-making process (first visit).
5. Initiate referral to IIIIA, social worker, or psychological counseling to assist with economic and mental or physical health needs (any visit).

CLIENT AND FAMILY/CARETAKER INTERVENTIONS

1. Develop ability to cope with caregiver role and flexibility in day-to-day functioning.
2. Explore financial, legal, and physical assistance sources, and consider a referral to these services.
3. Maintain own health and well-being in caregiver role.
4. Maintain ongoing care and treatment regimen.

🔺 *Anemia*

Anemia is a condition characterized by decreases in red blood cell, hemoglobin, and hematocrit levels. It may be caused by excessive blood loss (hypovolemic), a decrease in production of red blood cells by bone marrow (aplastic), a decrease in production of red blood cells from inadequate intake of iron and folic acid (iron deficiency), a decrease in the development of red blood cells because of the lack of the instrinsic factor needed for vitamin B_{12} absorption (pernicious), or the destruction of red blood cells (hemolytic). Whatever the type, the decrease in red blood cells affects the transport of oxygen in the body, with severity dependent on the degree of decrease.

Home care is primarily concerned with iron deficiency and pernicious anemias and the teaching aspects for compliance with the medical regimen to control the disorder and prevent relapses.

Nursing diagnosis

Altered nutrition: less than body requirements

Related factors: Inadequate intake of iron and folic acid

Defining characteristics: Reduced intake of food containing iron and folic acid, weight loss, weakness, anorexia, nausea, vomiting, glossy red tongue, lesions on oral mucosa, shortness of breath, pallor, headaches, irritability, dysphagia, fissures at angles of tongue

OUTCOME CRITERIA

Short-term
Adequate nutrition, as evidenced by consumption of a well-balanced diet, with necessary supplementation, and maintenance of appropriate weight for height, frame, and age (expected within 4 days)

Long-term
Adequate nutritional status achieved, as evidenced by daily requirements and supplemental therapy maintained, with optimal level of health and physiologic functioning (expected within 1 month)

NURSING INTERVENTIONS/INSTRUCTIONS

1. Review history and focus on source and remediation of deficiency, including increased iron requirements, inadeqaute intake, decreased or inadeqaute absorption, or chronic blood loss (first visit).
2. Assess hematologic, cardiovascular, neurologic, integumentary, gastrointestinal, and endocrine systems for status and effect of anemic condition on them (see specific system assessments for guidelines) (first visit).
3. Assess nutritional status, including food preferences and cultural or religious and medical restrictions (first visit).

4. Instruct client to take and record weights weekly (first visit).

5. Instruct client to maintain a food diary for 1 week that includes all foods comsumed and amounts and methods of preparation; use data as a basis for dietary teaching (first visit).

6. Instruct client in a well-balanced diet that includes snacks and foods that will supply deficiency; inform client that more frequent, smaller meals are recommended if nausea/vomiting or fatigue interferes with intake (first visit and reinforce on second visit).

7. Instruct client (and supply list) in sources of dietary iron, including red meat, organ meats, egg yolk, green leafy vegetables, dried legumes, enriched breads and cereals, and dried fruits (first visit).

8. Instruct client in good oral hygiene, especially after meals and if mouth is sore (first visit).

9. Instruct client in administration of iron preparation and vitamin C, and inform client that stools may turn dark green or black and that milk and antacids will decrease absorption of iron (first visit).

10. Suggest bland diet and to avoid irritating, hot, spicy foods if tongue is sore or in presence of gingival or mouth irritation or lesions (first visit).

11. Refer client to nutritionist or counselor if needed (any visit, based on evaluation).

CLIENT AND FAMILY/CARETAKER INTERVENTIONS

1. Take and record weekly weight using same scale and clothing and at same time of day.

2. Maintain daily log of intake and review each week for possible changes.

3. Eat a well-balanced diet that includes sources of iron and folic acid.

4. Maintain oral hygiene; apply lubricant to lips if needed.

5. Administer medications safely and as instructed.

6. Modify diet if oral discomfort occurs.

7. Consult with nutritionist if needed.

Nursing diagnosis

Activity intolerance

Related factors: Generalized weakness; imbalance between oxygen supply and demand

Defining characteristics: Decreased red blood cells and hemoglobin; hypoxia; fatigue; inability to carry out activities of daily living (ADL); decreased stamina; weakness; loss of positional and vibratory senses; numbness and tingling of extremities

OUTCOME CRITERIA
Short-term
Tolerance and endurance improved, as evidenced by modification of ADL and increased participation in activities (expected within 1 week)

Long-term
Optimal activity tolerance, as evidenced by increased energy and endurance and independence in ADL and mobility for optimal or higher level of health and functioning (expected within 1 month)

NURSING INTERVENTIONS/INSTRUCTIONS
1. Assess client's ability to perform ADL by having client demonstrate several typical activities and noting vital signs afterwards for increases in pulse or dyspnea (first visit).
2. Instruct client to personalize and pace activities and to schedule rest periods between these activities; include work as well as home schedules (first visit).
3. Instruct client to change position slowly and to sit down if dizzy (first visit).
4. Instruct client to request assistance in ADL and ambulation if needed, especially if there are sensory changes in extremities (first visit).
5. Encourage self-care with use of aids if they promote independence (first visit).
6. Instruct client to elevate head of bed to facilitate respirations and to administer supplemental oxygen if needed, with instructions about hazards associated with this therapy (first visit).
7. Refer home health aide to assist with ADL as needed.

CLIENT AND FAMILY/CARETAKER INTERVENTIONS

1. Follow plan for rest and activity.
2. Perform ADL independently with increasing endurance.
3. Obtain assistance or aids as needed.
4. Administer supplemental oxygen as instructed.
5. Sleep with head elevated; take steps to eliminate dyspnea associated with activity by resting.

Nursing diagnosis

Knowledge deficit

Related factors: Lack of exposure to information

Defining characteristics: Request for information about medical regimen, maintenance therapy, and prevention of recurrence of signs and symptoms of anemia

OUTCOME CRITERIA

Short-term
Adequate knowledge, as evidenced by client stating precautions needed for specific anemia being treated, medication regimen and implications, course of disease and treatment, and complications if not treated (expected within 3 days)

Long-term
Adequate knowledge, as evidenced by compliance with medication, dietary, and activity regimens and other treatment to prevent recurrence of anemia and complications (expected within 1 month)

NURSING INTERVENTIONS/INSTRUCTIONS

1. Instruct client to inform all physicians and dentists of disorder (first visit).
2. Inform client that, for pernicious anemia, parenteral vitamin B_{12} must be administered monthly for life, and instruct client in administration if warranted (first and second visit).
3. Instruct client to avoid infections by hand washing, good personal hygiene, and avoiding exposure to persons with upper respiratory infections; encourage client to update immunizations (first visit).
4. Instruct client to report any presence of infection with fever

to physician; any recurrence of skin color changes (pallor), changes in motor or sensory responses in expremities, presence of dizziness, or dyspnea should also be reported (first visit).

5. Instruct client to keep warm with extra clothing and blankets, if needed, and to avoid heating pads and hot water bottles (first visit).

6. Instruct client in skin care, including use of mild soap, gentle massage, and use of emollients; note pressure points for erythema and reduced sensation (first visit).

7. Inform client of measures to avoid trauma to skin if vasomotor disturbance or peripheral neuropathies exist (first visit).

8. Inform client that diet inclusions and several medications may be used for anemia, including iron, pyridoxine, vitamain B_{12}, and folic acid, and to avoid all OTC medications unless approved by physician (first visit).

9. Instruct client to keep physician and laboratory appointments, and emphasize need for compliance as symptoms decrease (first visit).

CLIENT AND FAMILY/CARETAKER INTERVENTIONS

1. Maintain dietary and medication regimens for specific anemia.

2. Follow personal hygiene practice; avoid contact with possible infection; maintain immunizations.

3. Maintain warmth and avoid injury to skin and dry, irritated skin.

4. Notify physician of signs and symptoms of infection or recurrence of condition.

5. Comply with physician and laboratory visits for injection of vitamin B_{12} and assessment of condition.

6. Wear clothes and shoes that maintain warmth and prevent trauma to extremities.

7. State cause of disorder and reason for treatment regimen.

Musculoskeletal system

◣ *Amputation*

An amputation is the surgical removal of all or part of an extremity. The procedure may be performed at a joint or in the middle of a limb to treat a malignancy, severe infectious process, circulatory impairment, traumatic event or injury, or congenital defect. Care management includes the use of a prosthesis as part of the rehabilitative program as well as treatment for the underlying condition that is associated with the amputation.

Home care is primarily concerned with the teaching aspects of stump care, prosthesis care, and compliance with the rehabilitative phase of the medical regimen.

Nursing diagnosis

Impaired physical mobility

Related factors: Intolerance to activity; musculoskeletal impairment (lower extremity amputation)

Defining characteristics: Inability to purposefully move within physical environment; reluctance to attempt movement and ambulation; improper prosthesis fit; inadequate healing and conditioning of stump

OUTCOME CRITERIA

Short-term
Adequate mobility, as evidenced by progressive independence in ambulation with prosthesis without falls or trauma (expected within 1 week)

Long-term
Adequate mobility achieved, as evidenced by effective use of prosthesis for ambulation and activities of daily living (ADL) with independence and optimal functioning (expected within 2 to 3 months)

NURSING INTERVENTIONS/INSTRUCTIONS

1. Assess client's mobility and activity status, effectiveness of use of prosthesis for ambulation, balancing difficulties, and use of assistive aids for walking (see Musculoskeletal System Assessment, p. 25, for guidelines) (first visit and each visit as needed).

2. Assess prosthesis fit, healing and conditioning of stump, and presense of pain when client is using prosthesis (each visit).

3. Instruct client in use of crutches, cane, or walker with or without prosthesis as appropriate (first visit).

4. Instruct client to balance on one leg without support and to ambulate with extension of stump (first visit).

5. Instruct client to ambulate with proper gait, using prosthesis as taught (first visit).

6. Provide and instruct in range-of-motion (ROM) exercises for unaffected joints (first visit).

7. Instruct client in exercises to tighten gluteal and abdominal muscles and to transfer from bed to sitting or standing position and back to bed (first and second visits).

8. Instruct client in prescribed exercises to legs, using weights, push-ups, knee bends, and standing or walking with one foot (each visit).

9. Instruct client to progress in ambulation from 5-minute periods to daily increases as tolerated and within restrictions; advise client to have assistance until stability and coordination are achieved (first visit).

10. Instruct client in arranging pathways and in furniture arrangement that promotes support in ambulation and prevents accidents from bumping or falling and injuring operative or other site (first visit).

11. Inform client of resources for purchasing or renting supplies and equipment (first visit).

12. Initiate or reinforce physical therapy (any visit).

13. Refer home health aide (HHA) for assistance in mobility and ADL.

CLIENT AND FAMILY/CARETAKER INTERVENTIONS

1. Perform daily progressive muscle and joint exercises.
2. Ambulate safely with or without use of prosthesis.
3. Provide safe environment for ambulation without trauma.

4. Use aids such as crutches, cane, and walker as needed.
5. Perform prescribed physical rehabilitation as instructed by therapist.
6. Avoid strain, fatigue, and falls while using prosthesis.
7. Achieve independence in mobility with use of prosthesis, including transfer and position changes.
8. Comply with appointments for physical therapy.

Nursing diagnosis

Self-care deficit (bathing/hygiene, dressing/grooming, feeding, toileting)

Related factors: Impaired mobility and activity ability (upper or lower extremity amputation)

Defining characteristics: Inability to wash body parts, put on or take off clothing, maintain appearance, bring food to mouth for ingestion, use toilet or commode, and carry out toilet hygiene

OUTCOME CRITERIA

Short-term

Adequate participation in ADL, as evidenced by progressive independence in daily activities with use of prosthesis (expected within 1 week)

Long-term

Adequate participation in ADL achieved, as evidenced by effective use of prosthesis for all personal care, with optimal functioning and independence (expected within 2 to 3 months)

NURSING INTERVENTIONS/INSTRUCTIONS

1. Assess client's activity status, ability to perform ADL with or without prosthesis, and ability to use assistive aids for bathing, grooming, dressing, toileting, and eating (see Functional Assessment, p. 43, for guidelines) (first visit).
2. Assess prosthesis fit (artificial arm, hook, cosmetic hand) and healing and condition of stump (any visit).
3. Instruct client in use of one arm or hand and aids for cooking, personal care, and other activity needs (each visit).
4. Instruct in ROM exercises for unaffected joints and prescribed exercises for arm and shoulder, including frequen-

cy, length of time, and progressive increases (first and second visits).
5. Initiate or reinforce physical and/or occupational therapy (any visit).
6. Refer HHA to assist with ADL as needed (first visit).

CLIENT AND FAMILY/CARETAKER INTERVENTIONS

1. Perform daily progressive ADL with or without prosthesis.
2. Use aids to assist with toileting, eating, bathing, dressing, grooming, cooking, working in home, and returning to occupation.
3. Avoid accidents and fatigue during use of prosthesis for ADL.
4. Perform prescribed physical and occupational rehabilitation as instructed by therapists.
5. Achieve independence in ADL with use of prosthesis.
6. Comply with appointments for occupational therapy.

Nursing diagnosis

High risk for impaired skin integrity

Related factors: External mechanical factor of pressure

Defining characteristics: Weight bearing on stump; improper fit of prosthesis; improper care of stump and improper conditioning; redness, pain, edema, and irritation at stump site

OUTCOME CRITERIA

Short-term
Preservation of skin integrity, as evidenced by intactness at stump surgical site and by absence of irritation, pain, or edema (expected within 1 week and after prosthesis use)

Long-term
Absence of skin damage or breakdown, as evidenced by maintenance of optimal skin integrity for health and prosthesis use (expected ongoing)

NURSING INTERVENTIONS/INSTRUCTIONS

1. Assess stump site for redness, tenderness, irritation, edema, flabbiness, fit of prosthesis, and pressure against stump (see

Integumentary System Assessment, p. 31, for guidelines) (first visit and each visit thereafter.)

2. Instruct client to assess stump and report changes to physician or prosthetist (first visit).
3. Instruct client in cleansing and gentle drying of stump and in massaging and exposing to air for 20 minutes (first visit).
4. Instruct client in removal and reapplication of dressing/bandage, with proper wrapping (first and second visits).
5. Instruct client to avoid use of powders or lotions on stump; instruct client in application of stump sock after cleansing and drying and to change daily (first visit).
6. Instruct client to pad pressure areas on skin and stump (first visit).
7. Instruct client to discontinue use of prosthesis if skin is red or irritated and to have prosthesis checked for fit if this occurs (first visit).
8. Advise client to seek assistance from prosthetist for problems of fit or use of prosthesis, whether for arm or leg (first visit).

CLIENT AND FAMILY/CARETAKER INTERVENTIONS

1. Maintain integrity and cleanliness of stump skin.
2. Protect stump from pressure of prosthesis.
3. Avoid skin damage from improper fit of prosthesis.
4. Use proper stump sock, mild soap and warm water, and thorough drying in stump care.
5. Bandage or wrap stump properly.
6. Secure services of prosthetist when needed.

Nursing diagnosis

Body image disturbance

Related factors: Biophysical factor of amputation procedure

Defining characteristics: Verbal response to change in structure and function of body part or to loss of body part; negative feelings about body; feelings of helplessness or powerlessness; change in social involvement

OUTCOME CRITERIA

Short-term
Improved body image adaptation, as evidenced by statement of feelings and concerns about changes in appearance and limitations imposed by loss of body part and need to change life-style (expected within 1 week)

Long-term
Optimal adaptation to body image, as evidenced by improvement in role performance and interpersonal relationships and by willingness to change functional patterns and integrate them into life-style (expected within 2 to 3 months)

NURSING INTERVENTIONS/INSTRUCTIONS

1. Assess client's life-style, roles, and ability to adapt to changes (first visit).
2. Allow client to express fears and concerns about ability to resume normal life (each visit).
3. Allow time for questions and clarifications; provide accepting, nonjudgmental environment (each visit).
4. Instruct client to encourage visits from friends, clergy, and other amputees (any visit).
5. Encourage client to express strengths, and inform client of options for life-style changes, including sexual activity, ADL, social and occupational interactions, and recreational and leisure activities (any visit).
6. Inform client of and refer to sex therapist, occupational rehabilitation, counseling services, and driving instruction (first visit).
7. Inform client of clothing that deemphasizes lost limb (first visit).

CLIENT AND FAMILY/CARETAKER INTERVENTIONS

1. Verbalize concerns and feelings about loss.
2. Allow for grieving over loss.
3. Participate in all aspects of care independently.
4. Return to work or enter vocational rehabilitation.
5. Adapt to limitations imposed by loss of limb.
6. Resume close relationships with others and actvities, interests, and social interactions with others.

Nursing diagnosis

Knowledge deficit

Related factors: Lack of information about condition and care

Defining characteristics: Request for information about prosthesis care, medical regimen for progressive rehabilitation, and signs and symptoms of complications

OUTCOME CRITERIA

Short-term

Adequate knowledge, as evidenced by client's statement of treatment regimen, care of prosthesis, and signs and symptoms to report (expected within 4 days)

Long-term

Adequate knowledge, as evidenced by compliance with medical regimen and prevention of complications to achieve optimal level of health and functioning (expected within 2 to 3 months)

NURSING INTERVENTIONS/INSTRUCTIONS

1. Assess life-style changes, ability to adapt, learning ability and interest in learning, and family participation and support (first visit)

2. Instruct client to assess for complications, including swelling, color change, pain, purulent drainge from stump site, temperature elevation, and pulse and respiration changes and to report these signs and symptoms to the physician (first visit).

3. Inform client that pain in the amputated limb (phantom pain) is a normal response (first visit).

4. Instruct client in washing and drying socket of prosthesis, application of prosthesis, wearing proper shoes with prosthesis for proper gait, and having prosthesis checked for fit or adjustment as needed (first visit and each visit thereafter as needed).

5. If medication is prescribed, instruct client in administration, including dose, frequency, time, food and drug interactions, and side effects (first visit).

6. Instruct client to keep all appointments with physican, laboratory, prosthetist, and therapists (first visit).
7. Inform client of community agencies and support groups for information and securing equipment and supplies (any visit).

CLIENT AND FAMILY/CARETAKER INTERVENTIONS

1. Assess and monitor stump and remaining limbs for signs and symptoms of complications, and report to physician.
2. Clean stump and prosthesis, and apply prosthesis correctly.
3. Administer medications correctly and safely, with desired results.
4. Adapt to change in life-style.
5. Comply with medical regimen, and keep appointments with interdisciplinary professionals.
6. Contact agencies, clubs, and groups for assistance, equipment, information, and support.

◣ *Osteoarthritis and Rheumatoid Arthritis*

Arthritis includes conditions that affect and cause damage to joints, cartilage, and connective tissue and result in activity and mobility limitations. Osteoarthritis is a chronic degenerative disease that is localized and progressive; it results in cartilage erosion and most commonly affects weight-bearing joints. Rheumatoid arthritis is a chronic inflammatory disease; it is systemic and progressive and affects the synovial joints and related structures.

Home care is primarily concerned with the care of the involved joints and with teaching aspects of the medical regimen, prevention of injury to the joints, and progression of the disease.

Nursing diagnosis

Chronic pain

Related factors: Chronic physical disability

Defining characteristics: Verbal report of pain experienced for more than 6 months; fear of reinjury; altered ability to continue previous activities; guarded movement; physical and social withdrawal; depression

OUTCOME CRITERIA

Short-term
Minimal pain or reduction in pain, as evidenced by client's statements that pain medication and measures to increase comfort are effective in controlling pain (expected within 3 days)

Long-term
Absence or control of pain, as evidenced by optimal mobility and activity necessary for functioning, socialization, and performing activities of daily living (ADL) independently (expected within 2 to 3 weeks)

NURSING INTERVENTIONS/INSTRUCTIONS

1. Assess pain and characteristics, including remissions and exacerbations or, if the pain is continuous, factors that relieve or precipitate pain (each visit).
2. Instruct client in administration of analgesics, antirheumatics, and steroid and nonsteroidal antinflammatories, including dose, action of drug, times, frequency, side effects (especially steroids), to take drugs continuously regardless of improvement, and to avoid abrupt discontinuation of steroid therapy (first visit).
3. Instruct client to coordinate medication for pain with activities and to avoid overwork or activities that cause stress to joints (first visit).
4. Instruct client to avoid stressful situations, damp, moist, environments, or extremes in environmental temperatures (first visit).
5. Instruct client to avoid prolonged activities, including walking, standing, and sitting, as well as sudden movements (first visit).

6. Instruct client in use of bed cradle, footboard, and bed board (first visit).
7. Instruct client in application of heat treatments, including warm baths and showers, electric blanket, and warm, wet compresses, and inform client of possible paraffin application during physical therapy session (first visit and reinforce on second visit).
8. Instruct client in application of splints to reduce pain by immobilization of the joints, including when to remove and reapply them (first visit).
9. Suggest relaxation techniques, methods of distraction, and use of transcutaneous electrical nerve stimulator (TENS) (first visit).

CLIENT AND FAMILY/CARETAKER INTERVENTIONS

1. Assess and administer analgesic for pain.
2. Place affected joints in position of comfort.
3. Apply heat treatments as instructed.
4. Administer medications as instructed; observe and report side effects.
5. Apply splints, footboard, soft linens, pillows, bed cradle, or other devices as appropriate to control pain and support joints.
6. Employ relaxation and diversional activities during painful episodes.
7. Avoid overactivity, stress, and environmental changes that affect joints.
8. Apply and use TENS correctly and safely.
9. Report time, intensity, duration, and site(s) of pain.

Nursing diagnosis

Impaired physical mobility

Related factors: Pain and discomfort; musculoskeletal impairment

Defining characteristics: Reluctance to attempt movement, inability to purposefully move within physical environment, limited range of motion, imposed restrictions of movement

OUTCOME CRITERIA

Short-term

Adequate activity and mobility, as evidenced by progressive ambulation and movement, within restrictions or limitations imposed by the disease process, and participation in ADL (expected within 1 week)

Long-term

Optimal achievement of physical mobility, as evidenced by ability to maintain health and functioning and by performance of ADL within restrictions without complications (expected within 1 to 2 months)

NURSING INTERVENTIONS/INSTRUCTIONS

1   Assess ability to ambulate and to participate in ADL, limitations of joint movement, presence of pain on movement, and need for assistive aids (see Musculoskeletal System Assessment, p. 25, for guidelines) (first visit).
2. Instruct client in prescribed limitations in use of joints, 1 hours rest periods throughout day to rest affected parts, and scheduling of activities to avoid fatigue and joint injury (first and second visits).
3. Instruct client to allow plenty of time to perform all activities and to take pain medication prior to exercises if drug is not too potent (first visit).
4. Instruct client in correct body alignment and in body mechanics for transferring, lifting, reaching, stooping, bending, pushing, and ambulating as well as in resting position (first visit and reinforce on second visit).
5. Instruct client in use of assistive aids and supportive devices, such as crutches, braces, corrective shoes, cane, walker, and wheelchair, and in use of helps to perform ADL, such as long-handled pickups, Velcro closures, holders for mirrors, books, etc., and zippered clothing (first visit).
6. Instruct client in exercises for involved and uninvolved joints, including type and frequency of range-of-motion (ROM) and muscle-setting exercises (each visit as needed).
7. Instruct client in joint protection during activities and in the use of immobilization aids to rest joints when needed (first visit).

8. Encourage client to participate in ADL and diversional activities within restrictions (first visit and as needed).

9. Instruct client in skin protection for areas under splints and at enlarged joint areas since these are susceptible to breakdown (each visit).

10. Initiate referral to physical therapist for exercise regimen and occupational therapist for ADL and fine-motor exercises (any visit).

11. Refer home health aide to assist with ADL as needed.

CLIENT AND FAMILY/CARETAKER INTERVENTIONS

1. Perform planned exercises and activities, with progressive increases daily or weekly.

2. Perform ambulation, transferring, reaching, and position changes using proper body mechanics and maintaing body alignment.

3. Participate in ADL as able, with progress until independence is achieved.

4. Provide rest periods throughout day as needed to avoid overactivity.

5. Use assistive and supportive aids for joint protection.

6. Adjust work hours according to activity tolerance.

7. Use assistive aids for ADL, toilet seat, eating aids, reaching aids, and dressing and grooming aids as needed.

8. Report to physician any prolonged pain that is not controlled and that limits activity and exercise.

9. Maintain physical and occupational therapy regimens with changes as indicated.

10. Administer analgesic prior to activity or ambulation as appropriate.

Nursing diagnosis

Ineffective individual coping

Related factors: Personal vulnerability, multiple life changes

Defining characteristics: Verbalization of inability to cope with chronic illness or ask for help; inability to meet basic needs and role expectations; chronic worry and anxiety; chronic fatigue; inability to problem solve; immobility; chronic pain; social isolation

OUTCOME CRITERIA

Short-term
Improved coping skills, as evidenced by client's statement of chronic nature of the disease and knowledge of need to develop new coping and problem-solving skills for compliance with long-term treatments (expected within 1 week)

Long-term
Positive coping with chronic illness, as evidenced by optimal participation in care and willingness to adapt to life style changes to achieve maximum health and functioning status (expected within 2 months)

NURSING INTERVENTIONS/INSTRUCTIONS

1. Assess mental and emotional status, ability to adapt, level of anxiety, and coping mechanisms used and their effect (first visit).
2. Provide accepting environment, and allow expressions of fears, concerns, and feelings regarding deformity and effect on body image (each visit).
3. Allow client to control planning of care and to make decisions for mutual goal setting (each visit).
4. Assist client to identify desires and ways to change lifestyle, as well as which coping mechanisms work and which are destructive (each visit).
5. Instruct client in methods to develop new coping skills and to try changes without fear of failing (first visit).
6. Initiate psychotherapy, support group assistance, or counseling if indicated (any visit).
7. Refer to social worker if social services and mental health assistance are needed (any visit).

CLIENT AND FAMILY/CARETAKER INTERVENTIONS

1. Develop coping and problem-solving skills that are effective.
2. Verbalize feelings and concerns about body image and long-term disability with family members, and request assistance when needed.
3. Identify negative and positive behaviors, and maintain productive coping methods.
4. Utilize significant others, groups, and agencies for help and support.

5. Join and participate in the Arthritis Foundation.
6. Manage own care effectively, and maintain a positive attitude.

Nursing diagnosis

Knowledge deficit

Related factors: Lack of information about care and preventive measures

Defining characteristics: Request for information about disease process, cause, and treatment; risk of falls/injury in an unsafe environment; signs and symptoms of complications; need to modify life-style

OUTCOME CRITERIA
Short-term
Adequate knowledge, as evidenced by client's statement of cause, treatment, measures to prevent injury/trauma, signs and symptoms to report, and medication regimen (expected within 1 week)

Long-term
Adequate knwoledge, as evidenced by client's complying with medical regimen and meeting requirements of modified life-style necessary to achieve optimal health and musculoskeletal functioning (expected within 1 to 2 months)

NURSING INTERVENTIONS/INSTRUCTIONS

1. Assess life-style, ability to adapt to change and disabilities, learning ability and interest, and family participation and support (first visit).
2. Inform client of cause and chronicity of disease, remissions and exacerbations; need for long-term consistent therapy; and progressive joint weakness and instability (first visit).
3. Instruct client in fluid, nutritional, and rest plan and in need to avoid weight gain (first and second visits).
4. Instruct client in signs and symptoms of complications to report, including uncontrolled pain, redness, swelling, and inability to move joint (first visit).
5. Inform client of prevalence of advertised quack cures and misinformation (first visit).

6. Inform client of alternative timing and positioning for sexual closeness (any visit).

7. Instruct client to provide safe environment to reduce injury from falls, including removal of small rugs, use of night-lights and hand rails, use of cane or walker, wearing good-fitting sturdy shoes, and clearing all pathways (first visit).

8. Instruct client fully in medication administration, including analgesics, steroids, salicylates, and gold injections, with action, dosage, frequency, side effects, results to expect, and food and drug interactions (first visit and reinforce each visit thereafter).

9. Inform client of need for and importance of all physical therapy recommendations and of need to keep appointments for laboratory work and with physician (first visit).

10. Instruct client to adjust daily schedules and change activities that are not tolerated well and to take 1-hour rest periods frequently during the day (first and each visit as needed).

11. Initiate referral to community agencies and support groups, such as the Arthritis Foundation, for literature and for places to acquire supplies and equipment (any visit).

CLIENT AND FAMILY/CARETAKER INTERVENTIONS

1. State cause, prescribed treatments, fluid and dietary requirements, rest needs, and signs and symptoms to report to physician.

2. Assess daily for changes that are positive and negative in terms of progress.

3. Administer medications correctly, and report any untoward responses.

4. Avoid stressful situations when possible.

5. Adjust sexual activities as needed.

6. Avoid unrecognized treatments that may cause disappointment or injury.

7. Maintain therapy regimens, laboratory testing schedule, and appointments with physician or other referrals.

8. Participate in and accept assistance from agencies and support groups as needed.

9. Adapt to life-style changes in a realistic manner.

◢ *Fractured Hip; Hip or Knee Prosthesis or Replacement*

Hip fractures include fractures of the head, neck, and trochanter parts of the femur. They usually result from osteoporosis or falls. The surgical procedure for hip/knee replacement includes the removal of the ball and socket of the hip joint and insertion of a prosthesis or the replacement of the surfaces of the tibia and femur with a prosthesis. Either procedure is done to correct damage caused by fracture, deformity, or rheumatoid or degenerative arthritis.

Home care is primarily concerned with the teaching of the medical and rehabilitative regimen to ensure optimal mobility.

Nursing diagnosis

Impaired physical mobility

Related factors: Musculoskeletal impairment

Defining characteristics: Inability to purposefully move within environment; reluctance to attempt movement; limited range of motion; fear of dislocating prosthesis

OUTCOME CRITERIA
Short-term
Adequate activity and mobility, as evidenced by progressive ambulation and movement within imposed limitations (expected within 1 week)

Long-term
Optimal physical mobility and independence in activities of daily living (ADL) achieved within restrictions to maintain health and functioning without complications (expected within 1 month)

NURSING INTERVENTIONS/INSTRUCTIONS

1. Assess ability to participate in ADL, mobility status, and need for assistive aids for ambulation and self-care (see Musculoskeletal System Assessment, p. 25, for guidelines) (first visit and as needed).
2. Instruct client in transfer and pivoting techniques to get into car, bed, wheelchair, toilet, shower, or other places (first and second visits).
3. Instruct client in muscle-strengthening exercises to prepare for use of devices for ambulation and ADL; instruct client in use of walker, cane, or crutches as appropriate (each visit).
4. Instruct client in range-of-motion (ROM) exercises as permitted and instruct client to perform them on all functioning joints, including number of times and frequency (first visit and reinforce on second visit).
5. Instruct client in and encourage him or her to perform all personal care and to increase ambulation daily (each visit).
6. Instruct client in weight-bearing limitation on operative side (first visit).
7. Initiate referral to physical therapist, occupational therapist, and vocational therapist (any visit).
8. Refer home health aide to assist in ADL as needed.
9. Arrange for equipment in home, including hospital bed, wheelchair, walker, or other (first visit).

CLIENT AND FAMILY/CARETAKER INTERVENTIONS

1. Perform daily planned exercise regimen, including ROM exercises and ambulation using appropriate assistive aids.
2. Progress in independence in walking and in transfer techniques.
3. Use assistive aids for ADL, including raised toilet seat, long-handled tongs for reaching or picking up articles, and others, depending on needs associated with dressing, meal preparation, and bathing.
4. Participate in physical therapy program.
5. Carry out prescribed physical rehabilitation as instructed by therapist.

Nursing diagnosis

High risk for trauma

Related factors: Internal factors of surgical procedure affecting movement; external factors of unsafe environment

Defining characteristics: Weakness; reduced weight bearing; reduced movement of limb; lack of safety precautions; inability or refusal to use assistive aids

OUTCOME CRITERIA

Short-term

Absence of falls or injury, as evidenced by ability to move without pain and weakness and by increased weight bearing using assistive aids (expected within 1 week)

Long-term

Ongoing absence of trauma, as evidenced by maintenance of optimal health and functioning, with length of extremity maintained without injury (expected within 1 month and ongoing)

NURSING INTERVENTIONS/INSTRUCTIONS

1. Assess for signs of prosthesis dislocation, such as shortening of or inability to move or bear weight on operative extremity and severe pain and spasms during movement, and instruct client to observe for these signs and symptoms (each visit).
2. Instruct client to maintain weight-bearing restrictions and to avoid hip flexion, elevation of knees, stooping, crossing legs, twisting of the limb, and positions during intercourse that cause hip to turn inward or rotation of the knee (first visit).
3. Instruct client to use assistive aids for ambulation and holding bars to assist with movement and provide stability (first visit).
4. Instruct client to turn only on side as instructed when in bed and to avoid lifting heavy objects (first visits).
5. Instruct client to provide clear pathways, to remove rugs, cords, furniture, or other objects, to avoid stairways, and to take plenty of time for all activities (first visit).
6. Instruct client to take rest periods and avoid activities when fatigued (first visit).

CLIENT AND FAMILY/CARETAKER INTERVENTIONS

1. Provide clear pathways, good lighting, and assistive aids to prevent falls.
2. Avoid positions, turning, weight bearing, sitting, lifting, and stooping as instructed, to prevent dislocation.
3. Avoid strain and fatigue as result of activity.
4. Follow recommendations for positioning during sexual intercourse.
5. Allow sufficient time for activities.
6. Report to physician any signs or symptoms indicating displacement.

Nursing diagnosis

Knowledge deficit

Related factors: Lack of information about postoperative care

Defining characteristics: Request for information about medical regimen and rehabilitation requirements

OUTCOME CRITERIA

Short-term

Adequate knowledge, as evidenced by client's statement of signs and symptoms of complications to report and ability to perform postoperative wound care and administer administration correctly (expected within 1 week)

Long-term

Adequate knowledge, as evidenced by achievement of optimal health and return of functioning within prescribed limits (expected within 2 to 3 months)

NURSING INTERVENTIONS/INSTRUCTIONS

1. Assess life-style and ability to adapt, learning abilities, and family assistance and support (first visit).
2. Inform client of signs and symptoms of complications, including persistent or increased pain in extremity, numbness in extremity, bleeding, edema, redness, or pain at incision site, and continued difficulty in bearing weight on extremity, and instruct client to report to physician (first visit).

3. Instruct client in administration of analgesics and antibiotics, including action, dose, frequency, route, and side effects (first visit).
4. Instruct client in sterile dressing changes and allow for return demonstration; instruct client to note drainage characteristics and report (first visit and reinforce on second visit).
5. Encourage client to participate in diversional activities according to interests (first visit).
6. Instruct client to report any changes in elimination pattern (constipation) for advice in taking stool softener or for changing fluid and nutritional intake (first visit).
7. Inform client of importance of compliance with physical and occupational rehabilitation program (any visit).

CLIENT AND FAMILY/CARETAKER INTERVENTIONS

1. Administer medications correctly as prescribed.
2. Provide care to surgical site as needed, using sterile technique.
3. Establish and maintain bowel elimination pattern.
4. Monitor for complications and report to physician if present.
5. Comply with rehabilitation program with satisfaction.
6. Participate in diversional and stress-reducing activities.

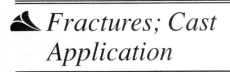

Fractures; Cast Application

A fracture is a break in a bone caused by trauma (falls or accidents) or disease (osteoporosis with pathologic fracture). It is usually accompanied by contusion of the surrounding soft tissue. Fractures may be complete or incomplete, simple or compound, and may affect any bone in the body. A fracture is corrected by closed reduction or open reduction and immobilization of the part by casting, splinting, or traction.

Home care is primarily concerned with the teaching of care for the affected body part, ensuring immobilization

and healing of the fracture, and preventing complications of the fracture.

Nursing diagnosis

Pain

Related factors: Physical injuring agents of bone fracture

Defining characteristics: Verbal descriptors of pain; guarding and protective behavior; alteration in muscle tone

OUTCOME CRITERIA

Short-term

Minimal pain or absence of pain, as evidenced by client's statement that pain has been reduced or controlled and that measures to promote comfort are effective (expected within 3 days)

Long-term

Absence of pain, as evidenced by achievement of optimal comfort level and mobility for health and functioning in presence of casted body part (expected within 1 week or when cast removed)

NURSING INTERVENTIONS/INSTRUCTIONS

1. Assess, and instruct client and family to assess, type of fracture and associated pain, tight cast (insert finger between cast and skin), swelling, pallor or cyanosis, coolness of skin, loss of sensation, and decreased peripheral pulse in casted extremity; assess every 30 minutes for 24 hours and then every 3 to 4 hours (first visit).
2. Instruct client to handle involved extremity gently, with smooth movement, especially first 24 hours, and to elevate on pillow for comfort (first visit).
3. Instruct client in administration of analgesic, including dose, frequency, and relief to expect (first visit).
4. Instruct client to participate in diversional activities and relaxation exercises to reduce pain (music, reading, TV, imagery) (first visit).
5. Instruct client to change position every 2 hours to prevent pressure of cast to one area (first visit).

CLIENT AND FAMILY/CARETAKER INTERVENTIONS

1. Assess pain and administer analgesic accordingly.
2. Provide comfort measure to reduce pain.
3. Utilize diversional methods and interactions to relieve pain.

Nursing diagnosis

High risk for impaired skin integrity

Related factors: External factors of pressure of cast and physical immobilization

Defining characteristics: Redness, swelling, irritation of skin at cast edges or bony prominences; immobility of injury part

OUTCOME CRITERIA

Short-term
Skin integrity preserved, as evidenced by intactness at pressure areas (expected within 2 to 3 days)

Long-term
Absence of skin damage, as evidenced by maintenance of optimal skin integrity and by return to normal functioning (expected ongoing)

NURSING INTERVENTIONS/INSTRUCTIONS

1. Assess skin at edges of cast, splint, or other device used to immobilize fractured bone; note redness, irritation, breaks, or pain, and instruct client to assess and report these signs and symptoms if they are present (first visit).
2. Petal edges of cast or device with soft adhesive, and inform client of rationale and of procedure to replace petaling (first visit).
3. Instruct client to avoid sticking things into cast to scratch itchy areas (first visit).
4. Encourage client to change positions frequently (first visit).

CLIENT AND FAMILY/CARETAKER INTERVENTIONS

1. Maintain skin integrity at areas prone to irritation.
2. Protect skin from rough edges of cast or rubbing from device.
3. Avoid skin damage caused by foreign objects in cast.

Nursing diagnosis

Impaired physical mobility

Related factors: Pain and discomfort; musculoskeletal impairment

Defining characteristics: Inability to purposefully move within physical environment; imposed restriction of movement by cast or splint; ability to use assistive aids and provide self-care

OUTCOME CRITERIA

Short-term

Adequate activity and mobility within limitations of cast or splint, as evidenced by movement with use of assistive aids (expected within 2 to 3 days)

Long-term

Optimal physical mobility and independence in activities of daily living (ADL) achieved within restrictions to maintain health and functioning without complications (expected within 1 week or at time of cast removal)

NURSING INTERVENTIONS/INSTRUCTIONS

1. Assess mobility status with cast and ability to progress daily with or without assistive aids; assess for mobility with leg cast or for ADL with arm cast (see Musculoskeletal System Assessment, p. 25, for guidelines) (first and second visits).
2. Instruct client in use of walking cast, crutches, or arm sling as appropriate (first visit or when weight bearing is allowed).
3. Instruct client in transfer to bed, chair, car, and toilet and in use of aids for bathing, dressing, grooming, and personal hygiene activities as needed (first visit).
4. Instruct client to arrange furniture and clear pathways for ambulation and to place articles within easy reach and for convenience (first visit).
5. Instruct client in range of motion (ROM) exercises for uncasted parts and to move unaffected body parts frequently while progressing in ADL and other activities; include digits on casted extremity (first visit).
6. Initiate referral to physical therapist if needed (any visit).

7. Refer home health aide to assist in ADL as appropriate (first visit).

CLIENT AND FAMILY/CARETAKER INTERVENTIONS

1. Ambulate and participate in ADL at earliest possible time using assistive aids.
2. Ambulate when weight bearing is allowed; apply sling properly; avoid activities that might damage cast.
3. Provide and promote activities that require use of all muscles and independence in ADL.
4. Perform ROM and other strength-maintenance muscle exercises.
5. Maintain clear, safe pathways and safe environment to prevent falls and injury and bumping or damage to cast.

Nursing diagnosis

High risk for peripheral neurovascular dysfunction

Related factors: Fracture; mechanical compression (cast)

Defining characteristics: Pallor; cyanotic color and coolness of skin at cast edges; decreased peripheral pulses; change in sensation or feeling proximal to cast edges; numbness or loss of sensation at cast site

OUTCOME CRITERIA

Short-term
Neurovascular function preserved, as evidenced by digits or areas proximal to cast warm and pink and perception to touch present (expected within 2 to 3 days)

Long-term
Absence of neurovascular dysfunction in presence of cast, as evidenced by optimal color, temperature, sensation, and peripheral pulses until cast removed and fracture healed (expected for period of cast application[s])

NURSING INTERVENTIONS/INSTRUCTIONS

1. Assess skin at cast edges and on digits for color, presence of pain or numbness, peripheral pulses and capillary refill,

and warmth or coolness, and instruct client to assess and report any changes to physician (first visit).

2. Instruct client in monitoring neurovascular status of casted part by noting swelling; taking peripheral pulses bilaterally and comparing them; placing pressure on digits to note capillary refill when pressure is released; and noting color of skin, which may be pink, red, pallid, or cyanotic, and temperature of skin, which may be cool or warm to touch; inform client of frequency (possibly twice daily) of assessment (first visit).

3. Position casted part for comfort, usually elevated; instruct client to avoid trauma or pressure to casted areas to prevent injury (each visit).

CLIENT AND FAMILY/CARETAKER INTERVENTIONS

1. Assess neurovascular status of casted area at least daily.
2. Provide positioning and comfort to casted area.
3. Report signs and symptoms of neurovascular complications of fracture and/or cast application.

Nursing diagnosis

Knowledge deficit

Related factors: Lack of information

Defining characteristics: Request for information about cast care and safety precautions to prevent falls or complications

OUTCOME CRITERIA

Short-term

Adequate knowledge, as evidenced by client's statement of measures to care for cast and prevent complications of cast application (expected within 1 week)

Long-term

Adequate information, as evidenced by client's meeting requirements of modified life-style resulting from fracture and casted part to achieve optimal health and functioning as healing is completed (expected within 4 to 6 weeks or until cast removed)

NURSING INTERVENTIONS/INSTRUCTIONS

1. Assess client's life-style, ability to adapt to change and temporary disability, learning ability and interest, and family participation and support (first visit).
2. Inform client of cause and type of fracture and type and function of cast (first visit).
3. Instruct client to handle wet cast with palms of hands for at least 24 hours until cast is completely dry; use fan to dry cast by placing it 18 to 24 inches from the cast; expose all parts to air for drying, and avoid covering cast until dry (first visit).
4. Instruct client to wear comfortable, loose clothing to fit over cast (first visit).
5. Instruct client to maintain skin integrity (clean, dry, and free of irritants) and to assess for complications to report, including foul, musty odor from cast, evidence of staining that comes from wound under cast, elevated temperature, pallor or cyanotic color and cool skin, decreased peripheral pulse, change in sensation or feeling, and increasing pain (first visit).
6. Instruct client to decrease itching by using alcohol swabs or blowing cool air into cast with fan and to avoid use of powders or lotion under cast (first visit).
7. Instruct client to petal cast edges with soft tape or to pad edges to prevent irritation of skin (first visit).
8. Instruct client to cover cast with a plastic bag while bathing or taking a shower (first visit).
9. Instruct client to clean cast with a damp cloth if soiled (first visit).
10. Instruct client to protect cast from damage or breakage by avoiding weight bearing or activities until cast is completely dry (first visit).
11. If medications are prescribed, instruct client in administration, including dose, frequency, time, side effects, and food and drug interactions (first visit).

CLIENT AND FAMILY/CARETAKER INTERVENTIONS

1. Assess for and report signs and symptoms of complications of fracture and cast application, including circulatory, neurologic, or skin symptoms or presence of infectious process.

2. State purpose and importance of cast and immobilization of body part.
3. Maintain dry, intact cast; clean with damp cloth or shoe polish.
4. Protect skin at edges of cast with pedaling.
5. Avoid inserting anything into cast or allowing cast to get wet.
6. Administer medications correctly and safely.
7. Secure rental or purchase of equipment and supplies.

◢ *Laminectomy/Spinal Fusion, Lumbar or Cervical*

A laminectomy is the surgical removal of the posterior arch of a vertebra to treat a herniated nucleus pulposus (bulging disk), tumor, or bone fragment that creates pressure on the spinal nerve roots and causes chronic pain. The procedure is usually performed on a cervical or lumbar vertebra. The fusion of bone fragments from the iliac crest may be performed to provide stability for the spine if degenerative disease is present.

Home care is primarily concerned with the teaching aspects of postoperative care to promote healing and function, prevent complications, and achieve a successful outcome of the surgery.

Nursing diagnosis

Impaired physical mobility

Related factors: Pain and discomfort; neuromuscular and musculoskeletal impairment

Defining characteristics: Reluctance to attempt movement of legs or arms; limited range of motion; decreased muscle strength and control; difficulty in performing activities of daily living

OUTCOME CRITERIA
Short-term
Adequate activity and mobility within prescribed limits, as evidenced by progressive ambulation within imposed limitations and movement within proposed restrictions (expected within 3 days)

Long-term
Return to optimal physical mobility and self-care activities within restrictions to maintain health and functioning without complications (expected within 2 to 3 weeks)

NURSING INTERVENTIONS/INSTRUCTIONS
1. Assess ability to participate in activities of daily living (ADL), body alignment, ambulation limitations, and knowledge of prescribed restrictions (see Musculoskeletal System Assessment, p. 25, for guidelines) (first visit and as needed).
2. Instruct client to apply brace and collar before ambulation, to stabilize surgical site (first visit).
3. Instruct client in logrolling, ambulation, sitting, bending, and stooping using proper body mechanics (first visit and reinforce on second visit).
4. Instruct client to sit in straight-backed chair and seat for driving and to splint back when sitting or rising from chair (first visit).
5. Instruct client in range-of-motion and other exercises as permitted (first visit and reinforce on second visit).
6. Advise client to sleep on firm mattress with hips and knees flexed or in proper body alignment (first visit).
7. Instruct client in use of assistive aids for ADL within recommended restrictions (each visit).
8. Initiate referral to physical therapist (first visit).
9. Refer to home health aide to assist with ADL as needed (first visit).

CLIENT AND FAMILY/CARETAKER INTERVENTIONS
1. Perform progressive ambulation, ADL, and other activities allowed, using proper body mechanics.
2. Participate in exercise regimen as instructed.
3. Apply cervical collar, corset, and brace correctly, and wear as prescribed.

4. Limit or avoid sexual activity, driving, and lifting as instructed.
5. Take rest periods as needed; stop activity if weak or tired or if painful response occurs.
6. Change mattress if necessary; utilize aids in turning in bed or getting up.
7. Participate in physical therapy program.
8. Resume work on a part-time basis, or consider the need for a change in occupation.

Nursing diagnosis

Knowledge deficit

Related factors: Lack of information about postoperative care

Defining characteristics: Request for information about postoperative activity restrictions, wound care, urinary and bowel elimination, medication regimen

OUTCOME CRITERIA

Short-term
Adequate knowledge, as evidenced by client's statement of postoperative care requirements and performance of postoperative procedures (expected within 1 week)

Long-term
Adequate knowledge, as evidenced by compliance with postoperative medical regimen and meeting requirements to return to optimal health and functioning (expected within 4 to 6 weeks)

NURSING INTERVENTIONS/INSTRUCTIONS

1. Assess life-style, ability to adapt, learning ability and interest, and family participation and support (first visit).
2. Inform client of cause of vertebral abnormality and surgical procedure done to correct it (first visit).
3. Instruct client in administration of analgesics and muscle relaxants as ordered, including times, dosage, frequency, side effects, and food and drug interactions (first and second visits).
4. Instruct client in wound care, including dressing change using sterile technique, and to report pain, redness, or

swelling at site; allow for return demonstration of dressing change (first and second visits).

5. Instruct client to report leg or arm pain or numbness or weakness in leg or arm (first visit).

6. Inform client of bowel and bladder elimination changes and their causes and of use of stool softener, fluid intake, and exercises to assist in return to normal pattern (first visit).

7. Inform client of importance of compliance with activity/exercise regimen proposed and of avoiding activities that place stress on operative area (changing position, lifting, pushing, pulling, stooping) (first visit).

8. Instruct client in padding brace, cast, neck collar, or any other device, to protect skin from rough edges or excessive tightness; check skin for changes caused by pressure when removing device (first visit).

9. Instruct client to comply with follow-up appointments with physician (first visit).

CLIENT AND FAMILY/CARETAKER INTERVENTIONS

1. Administer medications correctly as prescribed.

2. Provide care to surgical site as needed, using sterile technique.

3. Assess skin under collar, brace, or other immobilizing device, and provide skin care to prevent irritation and breakdown.

4. Participate in prescribed activities safely and within restrictions imposed by surgery.

5. Establish and maintain bowel and urinary elimination pattern.

6. Report adverse effects of medications, treatments, and surgical intervention if appropriate.

◤ *Lyme Disease*

Lyme disease is an acute, recurrent systemic inflammatory disease thought to be transmitted by a tick. A spirochete is either injected into the skin or bloodstream via the tick saliva or deposited in fecal material on the skin. Symptoms occur in episodes that recur every one to several weeks and that last about one week. Symptoms include erythema and skin lesions, local inflammation and swelling of large joints (arthritis), cardiac conduction abnormalities, and neurologic abnormalities (meningitis, Bell's palsy).

Home care is primarily concerned with the teaching aspects of symptomatic treatment and care and associated conditions.

Nursing diagnosis

Pain
Related factors: Biologic injuring agent

Defining characteristics: Communication of pain descriptors; guarding and protective behavior toward painful parts; headache; backache; swollen, hot joint

OUTCOME CRITERIA
Short-term
Reduction in pain, as evidenced by decreased swelling in joints and absence of exacerbation that involves other joints (expected within 1 week)

Long-term
Absence or control of musculoskeletal pain, as evidenced by client's statements that pain has been relieved and that optimal function of joints has been achieved (expected within 1 to 2 months)

NURSING INTERVENTIONS/INSTRUCTIONS
1. Assess for temperature elevation, joint or muscle pain, swollen joints, and remissions and exacerbations involving other joints (each visit).
2. Instruct client to elevate and immobilize affected part and in how to handle gently and position for comfort (first visit).
3. Instruct client in medication administration (analgesics, antibiotics, nonsteroidal antiinflammatory drugs), including dose, frequency, side effects, food and drug interactions, and response to expect (first visit).

CLIENT AND FAMILY/CARETAKER INTERVENTIONS

1. Maintain protective measures for affected part.
2. Comply with medication administration, with desired effects.
3. Report exacerbation of pain and joint involvement.

Nursing diagnosis

Knowledge deficit

Related factors: Lack of information about condition and complications

Defining characteristics: Request for information about medication regimen and about protection from skin, cardiac, or neurologic manifestations

OUTCOME CRITERIA

Short-term
Adequate knowledge, as evidenced by client's statement of medical regimen and measures to prevent complications (expected within 1 week)

Long-term
Adequate knowledge, as evidenced by compliance with medical regimen to achieve health and functioning and by prevention of exacerbations (expected within 2 to 3 months)

NURSING INTERVENTIONS/INSTRUCTIONS

1. Assess life-style and ability to adapt, interest and willingness to learn, and family participation and support (first visit).
2. Assess for presence of changes in tick bite site and development of multiple, smaller lesions, pruritis, burning and warmth to touch, and if lesion is slowly disappearing; instruct client to avoid rubbing or scratching lesions or using strong or irritating substances on skin (first visit and each visit thereafter).
3. Instruct client in taking temperature and reporting elevations or chills (first visit).
4. Inform client of risk for cardiac involvement and instruct client to report any dyspnea, chest pain, syncope, palpitations, or reduced pulse rate that occurs within 1 month after

rash, although these complications are not common (first visit).

5. Inform client of risk for neurologic complications, and instruct client to report neuritis, palsies, or frequent headaches that occur within 11 weeks after skin rash (first visit).

6. Instruct client in medication administration to prevent infection after skin rash disappears and in the addition of steroids and aspirin if cardiac or neurologic symptoms appear (each visit).

7. Inform client of characteristic tendency toward remissions and exacerbations, with the main manifestations occurring in the musculoskeletal system (first visit).

8. Instruct client to use insect repellant on clothing and to cover bare body parts if visiting parks or woods or known tick-infested areas (first visit).

9. Instruct client to contact National Lyme Borreliosis Foundation for information and support (first visit or as needed).

CLIENT AND FAMILY/CARETAKER INTERVENTIONS

1. Administer medications safely and montor effects.
2. Protect skin from infection and tick bites.
3. Monitor for complications of the disease, and report to physician any signs or symptoms indicating cardiac or neurologic involvement or exacerbation of musculoskeletal involvement.
4. Maintain remission with preventive measures and health-seeking behaviors.
5. Seek out assistance and information from community and national agencies and foundations.

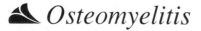 Osteomyelitis

Osteomyelitis is an infection of the bone and may be acute or chronic. It may occur as a result of surgery or compound fractures, in which case the infectious agent is introduced directly into the bone, or the bloodstream may carry an infectious agent to the bone from infected soft tissue or joints. The infection may spread through the marrow, cortex, and periosteum. Causative agents include *Staphylococcus aureus* (most common), *Streptococcus* group A, *Escherichia coli, Pseudomonas,* and *Klebsiella.*

Home care is primarily concerned with symptomatic treatment and with teaching of the medication regimen and prevention of secondary infection or transmission of infection to others.

Nursing diagnosis

Pain

Related factors: Biologic injuring agents (infection)

Defining characteristics: Communication of pain descriptors; guarded or protective behavior toward painful part

OUTCOME CRITERIA

Short-term
Pain minimized or controlled, as evidenced by client's statement that pain is relieved by initiation of measures to prevent discomfort; relaxed posture and expressions (expected within 3 days)

Long-term
Absence of pain and achievement of optimal functioning without pain (expected within 2 weeks)

NURSING INTERVENTIONS/INSTRUCTIONS

1. Assess, and instruct client to assess, pain and characteristics, as well as precipitating and alleviating factors, with an emphasis on early recognition of onset (first visit).
2. Assess pain for type, location over long bones with redness and edema, sudden onset, intensity, and duration (first visit).
3. Instruct client in administration of analgesics and antibiotics as ordered to control pain and reduce infectious process causing pain (first visit and reinforce on second visit).
4. Immobilize part with pillows and splints to prevent increased pain, and instruct client in need for bed rest and in methods to immobilize limb (first visit).

5. Instruct client in use of bed cradle and in supporting limb and handling gently when moving in bed, to prevent pressure or further injury to limb (first visit).
6. Maintain body alignment and correct positioning of limb (each visit).

CLIENT AND FAMILY/CARETAKER INTERVENTIONS

1. Maintain bed rest and position of comfort.
2. Administer analgesic and monitor response in controlling pain.
3. Perform measures to prevent pain and injury to limb.
4. Maintain immobilization of part during acute phase.

Nursing diagnosis

Impaired physical mobility

Related factors: Pain and discomfort; intolerance to activity

Defining characteristics: Limited range of motion; imposed restrictions of movement by splint or traction; reluctance to attempt movement; decreased muscle strength

OUTCOME CRITERIA

Short-term
Increasing tolerance to activity, as evidenced by increased endurance and participation in activities of daily living (ADL) within imposed restrictions (expected within 1 week)

Long-term
Optimal mobility, energy, endurance, and participation in activities, as evidenced by performance of ADL and progressive ambulation (expected within 1 month)

NURSING INTERVENTIONS/INSTRUCTIONS

1. Assess discomfort, weakness, muscle strength or atrophy, range of motion (ROM) in all joints, and presence of traction or splints (see Musculoskeletal System Assessment, p. 25, for guidelines) (first visit).
2. Perform ROM exercises within limitations set by physicians as healing allows, and instruct client to perform ROM and muscle exercises (first and second visits).
3. Progressively allow ambulation with use of assistive aids as

needed when healing allows, and encourage client to comply daily as instructed while limiting activity (each visit).
4. Refer home health aide to assist in ADL until healing allows self-care (first visit).

CLIENT AND FAMILY/CARETAKER INTERVENTIONS

1. Perform ROM exercises, ADL, and ambulation daily, with increases as endurance and healing allow.
2. Perform ADL with assistance and eventual independence.
3. Apply and use splint for ambulation.
4. Prevent muscle wasting and contractures.
5. Plan activities around rest periods.
6. Use assistive aids or device for ambulation if needed.

Nursing diagnosis

High risk for secondary infection

Related factors: Inadequate primary defenses (traumatized tissue)

Defining characteristics: Altered bone integrity with fracture or risk of fracture; spread of infectious agent; redness, swelling, drainage at entry site of catheter used for medication administration (right atrial); septicemia; meningitis

OUTCOME CRITERIA

Short-term
Prevention of infection spread, as evidenced by normal range of temperature and vital signs and by absence of purulent drainage (expected within 1 week)

Long-term
Maintenance of infection-free state, as evidenced by the absence of septicemia, meningitis, or pathologic fracture (expected within 1 to 2 months)

NURSING INTERVENTIONS/INSTRUCTIONS

1. Assess temperature for elevation; note amount and characteristics of drainage if present (each visit).
2. Instruct client to avoid heat application to the area or exercises that would increase circulation to the part and stimulate the spread of infection (first visit).

3. Instruct client in antiinfective adminsitration, including dose, frequency, method, route, food and drug interactions, and side effects, for oral administration and topical administration via dressing if applicable (first visit).
4. Instruct client in sterile dressing change (dry, wet) and in disposal of soiled dressings using universal precautions; allow for return demonstration (first visit).
5. Instruct client to avoid exposure to persons with infections or illnesses that might be transmitted to client (first visit).

CLIENT AND FAMILY/CARETAKER INTERVENTIONS

1. Administer antiinfective for 6 to 8 weeks as prescribed.
2. Perform hand washing and sterile dressing changes.
3. Take temperature daily and if chilled or drainage becomes purulent, and report to physician.
4. Provide light clothing and linens in a comfortable, cool environment.
5. Avoid exposure to persons with infections; prevent transmission of pathogens to client.
6. Use proper precautions in disposal of contaminated articles and supplies.

Nursing diagnosis

Knowledge deficit

Related factors. Lack of information about treatment measures

Defining characteristics: Request for information about medication regimen, nutrition, fluids, and activity requirements

OUTCOME CRITERIA

Short-term
Adequate knowledge, as evidenced by client's statement of medical regimen requirements and adaptive life-style behaviors necessary to achieve optimal health (expected within 1 week)

Long-term
Adequate knowledge, as evidenced by compliance with medical regimen and meeting the requirements to achieve return to health and optimal functioning with absence of recurrent infection (expected within 1 to 2 months)

NURSING INTERVENTIONS/INSTRUCTIONS

1. Assess life-style; adapting abilities, learning interest, abilities, and readiness; and family participation and support (first visit).
2. Instruct client in high-protein and vitamin C diet inclusions to facilitate healing, and inform client of need for more than normal nutritional requirements; offer a list and sample menus that include preferences and meet the recommended standards for height and weight; instruct client to weigh weekly on same scale, at same time, and with similar clothing (first visit and second visit if needed).
3. Instruct client in administration of antiinfective, analgesic, and antipyretic, following guidelines and a schedule that are mutually planned (first visit).
4. Inform client of activity restriction and rationale (first visit).
5. Instruct client in daily requirements of fluid intake, especially if temperature is elevated (first visit).
6. Instruct client in skin protection and care if splints or traction is used and prolonged rest and immobilization are advised; instruct client in massage of bony prominences and in position changes and to report any reddened areas (first and second visits).
7. Discuss effect of disease process on self-concept and body image when long-term care is necessary and possible deformity occurs; allow client to express feelings and explore coping strategies (first visit).

CLIENT AND FAMILY/CARETAKER INTERVENTIONS

1. Administer medications correctly, and record any side effects.
2. Comply with dietary and fluid requirements, and increase protein and vitamin C intake.
3. Adapt to long-term immobilization and restriction in activity.
4. Maintain intact skin, with protection to pressure points.
5. Display optimistic attitude for a recovery without deformity.

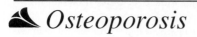 Osteoporosis

Osteoporosis is a condition characterized by reduced bone mass or density resulting from increased bone resorption. It is associated with liver or renal diseases, menopause, hyperthyroidism, hyperparathyroidism, and Cushing's syndrome. Reduced mobility and inadequate dietary calcium contribute to the disorder. Bone fracture and deformity are common results of long-term osteoporosis.

Home care is primarily concerned with the teaching of the medical regimen to prevent or control the progression of bone mass loss and subsequent fractures.

Nursing diagnosis

High risk for trauma

Related factors: Bone weakness from reduced bone mass

Defining characteristics: Falls, spontaneous fractures

OUTCOME CRITERIA

Short-term
Minimal risk for trauma, as evidenced by client's compliance with safety measures to prevent falls and with treatment regimen (expected within 4 to 7 days)

Long-term
Absence of bone fracture, as evidenced by intact skeletal system and achievement of mobility and activities of daily living for optimal health and functioning (expected within 1 month and ongoing)

NURSING INTERVENTIONS/INSTRUCTIONS

1. Assess environment for safety hazards; assess client for weakness, past falls and fractures, and presence of back pain (first visit).
2. Instruct client to remove small rugs, obstructed pathways, and water on floors and to install hand grips, holding bars, and antislip equipment, to have adequate lighting and sturdy chairs, and to use low bed or footstool (first visit).

3. Instruct client to use cane, walker, or other method of support (first visit).
4. Instruct client in activity needs, daily walking and exercises, and other activities to maintain bone density (first visit and reinforce on second visit).
5. Inform client of and recommend therapist for weight-bearing exercises (first visit).

CLIENT AND FAMILY/CARETAKER INTERVENTIONS

1. Perform daily exercise regimen, including recommended frequency and number of times for each exercise.
2. Join activity group for exercises if appropriate.
3. Wear corset to prevent vertebral collapse.
4. Maintain mobility and activities of daily living without falls.
5. Maintain a hazard free environment to prevent trauma.
6. Provide aids to maintain safe mobility and self-care.

Nursing diagnosis

Knowledge deficit

Related factors: Lack of information

Defining characteristics: Request for information about causes, treatment, and measures to prevent condition

OUTCOME CRITERIA

Short-term
Adequate knowledge, as evidenced by client's verbalization of cause, medication regimen, and complications of the disease (expected within 3 days)

Long-term
Adequate knowledge, as evidenced by client's compliance with requirements for health and functioning and prevention of complications (expected within 2 weeks and ongoing)

NURSING INTERVENTIONS/INSTRUCTIONS

1. Assess client's life-style, ability to adapt, learning abilities and interest in health maintenance, and family participation and support (first visit).

2. Assess client's history to determine underlying cause of condition, including diabetes mellitus, cirrhosis of liver, kidney disease, hyperthyroidism, or hyperparathyroidism (first visit).
3. Instruct client in cause of disease, effects of bone loss, and risk for deformity or pathologic fracture (first visit).
4. Instruct client in prescribed medication regimen, including estrogen therapy and calcium and vitamin D supplements, with action, dose, frequency, time, side effects, and drug/food/alcohol interactions; calcium injection if prescribed (first visit and reinforce on second visit).
5. Inform client of foods containing calcium and vitamin D to include in diet if supplements are not prescribed (first visit).
6. Inform client of importance of follow-up x-ray studies and bone-density procedures if ordered (first visit).
7. Instruct client to report to physician bone pain or inability to move any part of the body (first visit).

CLIENT AND FAMILY/CARETAKER INTERVENTIONS

1. Verbalize cause, treatment, and complications of the disease.
2. Administer prescribed medications accurately as instructed.
3. Include foods high in calcium and vitamin D in dietary intake.
4. Comply with requirement of 1000 mg/day of calcium and estrogen therapy if postmenopausal.
5. Maintain appropriate follow-up appointments with physician and diagnostic laboratory.

Renal/urinary system

▲ Kidney Transplantation

Kidney transplantation is the surgical placement of a donor kidney (from a cadaver or from a family member) into a matching-tissue-type recipient with end-stage renal disease. Recipients of a kidney transplant require immunosuppression to prevent rejection. The advisability of transplantation is dictated by the client's age and health problems, the availability of a donor kidney, and the client's preference for the procedure rather than relying on dialysis. Graft rejection may be acute or chronic, with the least acute response resulting from the most adequately matched donor and recipient.

Home care is primarily concerned with teaching the client about immunosuppressive therapy and monitoring for signs and symptoms of rejection

Nursing diagnosis

Anxiety

Related factors: Threat to or change in health status

Defining characteristics: Verbalization of fear of organ rejection; apprehension; uncertainty; fear of consequences of rejection; focus on self

OUTCOME CRITERIA

Short-term
Decreased anxiety, as evidenced by client's statement of increased interest in care, increased participation by client in care, and relaxed posture and facial expression (expected within 3 days)

Long-term
Optimal level of anxiety or control of anxiety, as evidenced by client's compliance with and acceptance of treatment and by positive treatment response (expected within 1 month)

NURSING INTERVENTIONS/INSTRUCTIONS

1. Assess client's mental and emotional status (see Psychosocial Assessment, p. 41, for guidelines) (first visit).
2. Provide an accepting environment, and allow for expression of fears and concerns about organ rejection (each visit).
3. Provide continuing information about progression to wellness; explain that one or more rejection episodes may occur within several months of transplant but they do not mean that kidney will be lost (each visit).
4. Initiate referral to counseling or support group if indicated (last visit).

CLIENT AND FAMILY/CARETAKER INTERVENTIONS

1. Seek information that will reduce anxiety.
2. Develop coping strategies for possibility of rejection.
3. Maintain manageable level of anxiety.
4. Consult with counselor or support group for control of anxiety.

Nursing diagnosis

Altered family processes

Related factors: Situational crisis of transplant surgery

Defining characteristics: Family system unable to meet needs of donor and recipient, both physical and emotional; inappropriate level and direction of energy; inability to accept or receive help; inability of family to adapt to situation

OUTCOME CRITERIA

Short-term
Beginning progress toward family's acceptance of and adaptation to organ transplant, as evidenced by open communication, mutual support, and participation in care (expected within 1 week)

Long-term
Return of family to former positive interactions and support as client returns to wellness (expected within 1 to 2 months)

NURSING INTERVENTIONS/INSTRUCTIONS

1. Assess family interaction, dynamics, and supportive behaviors (see Family Assessment, p. 46, for guidelines) (first visit).
2. Include family members in teaching in a nonjudgmental environment; allow family members to ask questions (each visit).
3. Encourage openess among family members; inform them of importance of maintaining own health and social activities (first visit).
4. Suggest family counseling or support groups, rehabilitative services, or financial resources as needed (first visit).

CLIENT AND FAMILY/CARETAKER INTERVENTIONS

1. Verbalize feelings and concerns.
2. Identify problems in family and ways to solve them together.
3. Resolve life-style changes together.
4. Seek out and participate in support group activity.
5. Participate in rehabilitation.
6. Enter into family activities and contribute to family harmony.

Nursing diagnosis

Knowledge deficit

Related factors: Lack of exposure to information about medical regimen

Defining characteristics: Request for information about immunosuppressive therapy, signs and symptoms of rejection to report, health-promotion behaviors

OUTCOME CRITERIA

Short-term
Adequate knowledge, as evidenced by client's statement of treatment protocols, compliance with intensive medication regimen, and active participation in preventive health care (expected within 7 to 10 days)

Long-term
Adequate knowledge, as evidenced by client's meeting requirements for changed life-style and achievement of optimal level of health and functioning (expected within 4 to 6 weeks)

NURSING INTERVENTIONS/INSTRUCTIONS

1. Instruct client in progressive resumption of activity; emphasize avoidance of contact sports or any activity that might be traumatic to operative site (first visit).
2. Assess operative area for size, color, temperature, approximation of edges, and presence of drainage, and instruct client to notify physician of any changes in site (first visit).
3. Instruct client in administration of immunosuppressive agents, steroids, and antacids, including dose, frequency, multiple side effects, and possible interactions with OTC drugs, foods, and alcohol (first visit).
4. Assess client for side effects of drug therapy, including gastrointestinal irritation and bleeding, hepatotoxicity, cushingoid body changes, decreased wound healing, visual changes, and personality changes (each visit).
5. Instruct client in monitoring of weight, intake and output, and vital signs; demonstrate and have client return demonstration; instruct client to keep log on results (first visit and reinforce on second visit).
6. Inform client of possible signs and symptoms of organ rejection, including flu-like symptoms, difficult urination, oliguria, weight gain, edema, increased blood pressure, and pain or tenderness over operative site; instruct client to report any of these signs to physician. (first visit and reinforce each visit).
7. Instruct client to avoid active, live-virus immunization and children with recent immunization (oral polio) (first visit).
8. Instruct client in proper collection of random, midstream, or 24-hour urine specimens (whichever is ordered), and stress importance of delivery to laboratory (first visit).
9. Inform client of importance of keeping physician appointments and laboratory testing for complete blood count, drug levels, electrolytes, renal function tests, urinalysis, and culture and sensitivities (first visit).

10. Instruct client to wear or carry identification and medical information, including surgery and date, medications, and physician's name and telephone number (first visit).
11. Initiate referral to nutritionist, dentist, and specialist physician as appropriate (first visit).

CLIENT AND FAMILY/CARETAKER INTERVENTIONS

1. Resume activities within limitations and avoid trauma to site.
2. Administer prescribed medications correctly and consistently, and monitor for side effects to report.
3. Monitor and record daily or weekly weight, vital signs, and intake and output.
4. List signs and symptoms of graft rejection, and report to physician if they occur.
5. Engage in multisystem regimen to avoid infection, and report any signs and symptoms of renal/urinary or respiratory infection.
6. Maintain clean wound, with progressive healing stages.
7. Maintain appointments with physicians and laboratory.
8. Wear identifying medical information at all times.
9. Consult with health professionals for regular health maintenance and advice.

◣ *Prostatic Hypertrophy/ Prostatectomy*

Benign prostatic hypertrophy is the enlargement of the prostate gland, which is thought to be caused by an imbalance between the male and female sex hormones that occurs in men over the age of 50 years. The condition results in partial or complete obstruction of the urethra or incomplete emptying of the bladder. Prostatectomy, the partial or complete surgical removal of the prostate gland, can be done to relieve obstruction caused by compression on the urethra (suprapubic or transurethral) or to remove a malignant mass (perineal or retropubic). The surgical approach is dependent on age, size and location of the obstruction or mass, and severity of symptoms.

Home care is primarily concerned with the maintenance of urinary elimination before and after surgery, wound care after surgery, and the teaching of medical or surgical regimens and prevention of complications as applicable.

Nursing diagnosis

Urinary retention

Related factors: Blockage

Defining characteristics: Bladder distention; small, frequent voiding; absence of urinary output; dribbling; dysuria; residual urine; overflow incontinence; pain with bladder fullness and overdistention; small urinary stream; hesitancy in urinating

OUTCOME CRITERIA

Short-term

Distress associated with urination minimized, as evidenced by client's statement of relief of retention with use of palliative measures (evidenced within 2 days)

Long-term

Urinary bladder distention and symptoms controlled, with optimal urinary elimination (expected within 1 to 2 weeks and ongoing)

NURSING INTERVENTIONS/INSTRUCTIONS

1. Assess renal/urinary and reproductive systems (see Renal/Urinary System Assessment, p. 28, and Reproductive System Assessment, p. 33, for guidelines), and note decreased size and force of urinary stream, difficulty in starting to urinate, urgency, frequency, dribbling, nocturia, hematuria, inability to completely empty bladder, and presence of overflow incontinence (first visit).
2. Assess for suprapubic distention by palpation and for possible complete retention with anuria and suprapubic pain (each visit).
3. Instruct client to note times and amounts of urinary elimination and to compare with times and amounts of fluid intake (first visit).

4. Instruct client to maintain hydration with intake of 8 to 10 glasses water per day and to avoid alcohol and caffeine-containing beverages (first visit).

5. Instruct client to notify physician if client is unable to void or if signs and symptoms of urinary elimination problems escalate (first visit).

6. Instruct client to avoid straining at bowel elimination; instruct client in administration of stool softener if needed (each visit).

7. Instruct client to take sitz baths to facilitate voiding and decrease distress (first visit).

8. Instruct client to empty bladder every 2 to 3 hours and not to delay voiding when urge is present (first visit).

9. Instruct client in administration of antispasmodics and analgesics as ordered, including dose, frequency, side effects, and food/drug/alcohol interactions (first visit).

10. Catheterize client using aseptic technique if ordered and when voiding has been absent for 6 to 8 hours (any visit).

CLIENT AND FAMILY/CARETAKER INTERVENTIONS

1. Record changes in urinary elimination patterns and signs and symptoms of distress in a diary.

2. Notify physician of failure of relief measures to control signs and symptoms.

3. Avoid constipation and straining by administration of stool softener

4. Maintain fluid intake of 2 to 3 liters per day; avoid fluids that increase diuresis.

5. Empty bladder at designated times and when urge is present.

6. Take medications prescribed for specific complaints.

Nursing diagnosis

High risk for infection

Related factors: Inadequate primary defenses (stasis of urine, broken skin)

Defining characteristics: Invasive procedure (surgery); surgical wound with redness, edema, pain, purulent drainage; urinary retention; positive wound or urinary culture; cloudy, foul-smelling urine

OUTCOME CRITERIA

Short-term
Reduction in infection potential, as evidenced by decreased urinary retention and by proper care of surgical site (expected within 3 to 4 days)

Long-term
Absence of infection, as evidenced by temperature and white blood count within normal ranges, surgical site clean and healing, urine clear, and urination without symptoms (expected within 4 to 6 weeks)

NURSING INTERVENTIONS/INSTRUCTIONS

1. Assess temperature, pulse, respiration, and blood pressure, and instruct client to report chills and fever over 100° F to physician (each visit).
2. Assess incisional drains and operative wounds as applicable for pain, color, temperature, swelling, drainage, and approximation of edges (each visit).
3. Perform sterile wound care and catheter or meatal care (each visit).
4. Instruct client in care of catheter, placement and emptying of drainage bag, and use of leg bag (first visit).
5. Instruct client to inform physician of changes in urine characteristics, including cloudiness and foul odor (first visit).
6. Monitor for hematuria and assess client's ability to empty bladder after catheter removed (each visit).
7. Instruct client to administer antibiotics and urinary antiseptics as ordered for treatment or prophylaxis (first visit).

CLIENT AND FAMILY/CARETAKER INTERVENTIONS

1. Monitor vital signs and temperature and report changes.
2. Report changes in urine characteristics, hematuria, or changes in appearance of wound.
3. Maintain closed drainage system for indwelling catheter.
4. Perform wound and catheter care using sterile technique.
5. Maintain adequate hydration.
6. Administer antibiotics for full course and other medications for urinary bladder treatment.

Nursing diagnosis

Sexual dysfunction

Related factors: Altered body function

Defining characteristics: Impotence; decreased libido; erectile dysfunction following surgery; sterility

OUTCOME CRITERIA

Short-term
Temporary dysfunction progressing to normal function, as evidenced by client's statement of understanding of surgical outcome and changes that can be expected in sexual functioning (expected within 1 week)

Long-term
Optimal sexual functioning within physiologic limitations resulting from surgical procedure (expected within 1 month)

NURSING INTERVENTIONS/INSTRUCTIONS

1. Provide a nonjudgmental, nonthreatening environment for client to have time and opportunity to ask questions or discuss sexual function according to comfort level (each visit).
2. Inform client of sexual implications of surgery and possibility of sterility or impotence (first visit).
3. Inform client of change in urine clarity after intercourse if transurethral procedure is done (first visit).
4. Inform client that sexual intercourse may resume 6 to 8 weeks after surgery, and provide information about alternate methods of gratification for partner (first visit).
5. Inform client about possible aids available to assist with penile erection if applicable (first visit).
6. Initiate referral for sexual counseling if indicated or requested (last visit).

CLIENT AND FAMILY/CARETAKER INTERVENTIONS

1. Express feelings and concerns about sexuality for resolution.
2. Communicate needs and abilities to perform sexual intercourse and response of partner.
3. Consult sex therapist with or without partner.
4. Explore use of aids for impotence.

Nursing diagnosis

Anxiety

Related factors: Threat to health status; threat to change in role functioning

Defining characteristics: Urinary incontinence, blood in urine; change in role and relationships; altered body image if dribbling or incontinence is chronic or with use of retention catheter; urgency and inability to reach bathroom

OUTCOME CRITERIA

Short-term

Decreased and manageable anxiety level, as evidenced by client's statements of knowledge of postoperative course and improved bladder control (expected within 3 days)

Long-term

Anxiety controlled, as evidenced by maintenance of improved urinary elimination pattern and by improved body image (expected within 1 month)

NURSING INTERVENTIONS/INSTRUCTIONS

1. Assess client's coping abilities and ability to adapt to changes in health status; assist in identification and utilization of positive and effective coping mechanisms and problem-solving skills (each visit).
2. Instruct client to avoid heavy lifting or carrying a heavy object or prolonged sitting or driving for 3-6 weeks (first visit).
3. Inform client that some blood may remain in urine for several weeks (first visit).
4. Instruct client to become acquainted with locations of bathrooms when away from home and to refrain from fluid intake before going out and at bedtime (first visit).
5. Inform client that postoperative dribbling and some incontinence are common and may be minimized by exercising; instruct client in perineal exercises (first visit).
6. Assist client to formulate an exercise schedule that is progressive in frequency and number of times (first visit).

CLIENT AND FAMILY/CARETAKER INTERVENTIONS

1. Utilize positive coping strategies that reduce anxiety and improve body image.
2. Avoid activities postoperatively that cause complications.
3. Verbalize normal postoperative course and expectations.
4. Perform perineal exercises daily to strengthen sphincter tone.
5. Reduce embarrassment of dribbling and incontinence by limiting fluids and wearing waterproof undergarment.
6. Use bathroom as frequently as needed, at least every 2 hours.

◣ Renal Failure, Chronic (CRF)

Chronic renal failure is the progressive, gradual deterioration of kidney function, resulting in decreased glomerular filtration rate (GRF), renal blood flow, resorption ability, and function of the tubules. The condition is irreversible as it progresses toward uremia but may be controlled by dietary and fluid restrictions. As the kidneys lose the ability to maintain fluid and electrolyte balance, the client is provided with renal dialysis. Diseases that predispose a person to the development of CRF are immunologic (glomerulonephritis), infectious (pyelonephritis, tuberculosis), urinary obstructive (prostatic hypertrophy, renal calculi), metabolic (diabetes mellitus), congenital (polycystic disease), vascular (hypertension), or nephrotoxic (drugs). All organs of the body are affected by CHF.

Home care is primarily concerned with providing for activities of daily living as needed, administration of peritoneal dialysis if appropriate, and teaching the client about dietary and fluid restrictions, compliance with hemodialysis, and prevention of complications of the disease.

Nursing diagnosis

Anxiety

Related factors: Threat of death; threat to or change in health status

Defining characteristics: Apprehension; uncertain outcome; increased helplessness and tension; possible future kidney dialysis or transplant; changes in life-style

OUTCOME CRITERIA

Short-term
Decreased anxiety, as evidenced by client's statement of reduced fear and apprehension about change in health status and possible dialysis and transplant availability (expected within 3 days)

Long-term
Management or control of anxiety level, as evidenced by compliance with and acceptance of treatment regimen and change in life-style (expected within 1 to 2 months)

NURSING INTERVENTIONS/INSTRUCTIONS

1. Assess client's mental and emotional status regarding life-threatening illness (see Psychosocial Assessment, p. 41, for guidelines) (first visit).
2. Encourage expressions of fears, concerns, and questions regarding therapy and its effects in an accepting environment (each visit).
3. Assist client to identify needed changes in life-style and methods for making necessary changes (first visit and reinforce each visit).
4. Inform client of all activities, treatments, and tests and effects to expect (first visit).
5. Initiate referral to counseling or support group (any visit).

CLIENT AND FAMILY/CARETAKER INTERVENTIONS

1. Develop coping mechanisms for long-term treatment and possible outcome.
2. Maintain manageable level of anxiety.

3. Seek information that will reduce anxiety.
4. Express fears and concerns about necessary changes in life-style.
5. Consult with counselor, clergy, or support group.

Nursing diagnosis

Fluid volume excess

Related factors: Compromised regulatory mechanism

Defining characteristics: Edema; weight gain; decreased urinary output; electrolyte imbalance, (potassium, sodium, calcium, magnesium, phosphorus); increased blood pressure and pulse; decreased specific gravity; increased blood urea nitrogen and creatinine

OUTCOME CRITERIA
Short-term
Balanced intake and output, as evidenced by decreasing edema, compliance with fluid and electrolyte restrictions, and stable weight and blood pressure (expected within 1 week)

Long-term
Adequate renal function, as evidenced by optimal intake and output ratio and by maintenance of renal status within limitations imposed by disease (expected within 1 to 2 months)

NURSING INTERVENTIONS/INSTRUCTIONS
1. Assess client's renal status (see Renal/Urinary System Assessment, p. 28, for guidelines); evaluate baseline weight, hydration, peripheral edema, vital signs, output trends, and urine characteristics (each visit).
2. Instruct client in techniques for taking blood pressure and weight and for monitoring edema and intake and output, and allow for return demonstration (first visit).
3. Instruct client in fluid restriction as prescribed: generally previous day's urinary output plus 500 to 800 ml over intake; include allotment and measurement of fluids, rationale for therapy, and how to distribute fluids over 24 hours (first visit and reinforce on second and third visits).
4. Instruct client to restrict sodium intake by avoiding addition of table salt and eating of cold cuts, processed, canned,

or convenience foods, and other foods high in sodium (first visit).

5. Instruct client to restrict potassium intake by avoiding citrus products, dried fruits, and bananas (first visit).

6. Instruct client to notify physician of increasing weight gain and edema, decreased urinary output, or increased blood pressure (first visit).

7. Instruct client, and reinforce instruction, in need for continual kidney dialysis, procedure for peritoneal dialysis in the home, and performance of procedure by client or family member if realistic and possible (first visit and ongoing visits).

8. Instruct client in administration of diuretics and antihypertensives, including dose, frequency, route, side effects, possible interferences with OTC drugs, and possible reactions with foods (first visit).

CLIENT AND FAMILY/CARETAKER INTERVENTIONS

1. Monitor and record blood pressure, weight, intake and output, and edema daily.

2. Restrict fluid; use ice chips, and spread limited fluids over 24 hours; measure fluids at mealtime, snack time, and medication time.

3. Restrict foods containing large amounts of sodium or potassium.

4. Administer medications correctly and as instructed.

5. Report signs and symptoms of increasing failure or increased sodium or potassium levels.

6. Participate in hemodialysis, and perform peritoneal dialysis as appropriate in home.

Nursing diagnosis

Altered nutrition: less than body requirements

Related factors: Inability to ingest foods

Defining characteristics: Anorexia, dietary protein restriction, nausea, vomiting, hiccups

OUTCOME CRITERIA

Short-term
Adequate nutrition, as evidenced by absence of anorexia and by ingestion of protein-restricted diet (expected within 1 week)

Long-term
Optimal nutrition, as evidenced by compliance with special dietary restrictions throughout illness, including achievement of caloric, electrolyte, and protein requirements (expected within 1 month)

NURSING INTERVENTIONS/INSTRUCTIONS

1. Assess nutritional status and eating patterns, including food preferences and cultural and religious adaptations; note presence of anorexia, nausea, vomiting, stomatitis, bad taste in mouth, or tissue wasting (each visit).
2. Instruct client in protein restricted diet if client is not on dialysis; emphasize proteins with high biologic value (each visit).
3. Instruct client in adequate foods to increase caloric intake, derived primarily from carbohydrates and unsaturated fats; integrate information about fluid and electrolyte requirements/restrictions into instruction (each visit).
4. Instruct client in administration of vitamin supplements, phosphorus-binding agents, and calcium supplements (first visit).
5. Instruct client in oral hygiene, especially after meals; encourage client to brush teeth and use mouthwash, hard candy, or sour candy for breath control (first visit).
6. Instruct client to eat smaller, more frequent meals and to take antiemetics half-hour before eating if nauseated (first visit).
7. Provide written instructions, sample menus, and recipes, and emphasize that compliance with dietary regimen will ease distressing symptoms of anorexia, nausea, vomiting, fatigue, and edema (each visit).

CLIENT AND FAMILY/CARETAKER INTERVENTIONS

1. Adjust eating schedule to rest periods and to antiemetic administration.

2. Perform mouth care frequently during day.
3. Follow restrictions in diet (protein, sodium, potassium) using planned menus.
4. Eat smaller, more frequent meals.
5. Administer vitamin and mineral supplements and other medications as instructed.
6. Maintain ideal weight as closely as possible.
7. Read labels on foods and avoid foods containing large amounts of sodium or potassium; note caloric value of purchased foods.

Nursing diagnosis

High risk for impaired skin integrity

Related factors: External factors of immobility; internal factors of urea deposits and peripheral neuropathy

Defining characteristics: Pruritis; yellow pigmentation; scratching with breaks in skin; redness at pressure points; buildup of uremic frost on skin; dryness of skin; numbness in feet and legs

OUTCOME CRITERIA

Short-term
Skin integrity intact, as evidenced by decreased pruritis and by compliance with skin care regimen (expected within 4 days)

Long-term
Skin integrity maintained, as evidenced by absence of skin disruption with skin in optimal condition (expected within 1 month and ongoing)

NURSING INTERVENTIONS/INSTRUCTIONS

1. Assess skin (see Integumentary System Assessment, p. 31, for guidelines), and note color, turgor, integrity, temperature, presence of scratch marks, and presence of uremic frost or pruritis (each visit).
2. Instruct client to bathe daily and to use a superfatted soap and emollients if itching is present (first visit).
3. Instruct client to maintain nails in short and clipped condition and to cut them straight across when trimming (first visit).

4. Instruct client to avoid scratching or rubbing skin (first visit).
5. Instruct client in perineal care after toileting (first visit).
6. Instruct client in use of antipuritics, oral and topical (first visit).
7. Instruct client in hand-washing technique.

CLIENT AND FAMILY/CARETAKER INTERVENTIONS

1. Bathe daily; use lotion, moisturizer, emollients; pat skin and avoid rubbing.
2. Perform perineal care after toileting.
3. Avoid scratching; maintain nails in short, clean condition.
4. Administer medications for pruritis as instructed.
5. Report skin breaks, rashes, or scratches to physician.

Nursing diagnosis

High risk for activity intolerance

Related factors: Deconditioned status, generalized weakness

Defining characteristics: Verbalization of fatigue and weakness; activity restrictions; inability to produce erythropoietin, causing anemia; defect in platelet function; faulty bone metabolism

OUTCOME CRITERIA

Short-term
Adequate activity, as evidenced by participation in activities of daily living (ADL) within limitations (exepcted within 1 week)

Long-term
Mobility and self-care in ADL achieved for optimal level of functioning, within limintations imposed by illness (expected within 1 month)

NURSING INTERVENTIONS/INSTRUCTIONS

1. Assess client's level of participation in ADL, endurance, muscle strength, gait, peripheral neuropathy, and fatigue with activity (first visit).
2. Encourage independence in ADL; instruct client to prioritize and pace activities, to use aids to conserve energy, and to schedule rest periods between activities (first visit).

3. Instruct client in measures to take to protect feet and legs from trauma (first visit).
4. Initiate referral to physical and/or occupational therapy if indicated (any visit).
5. Refer home health aide to assist with ADL when appropriate.

CLIENT AND FAMILY/CARETAKER INTERVENTIONS

1. Schedule rest periods, and pace activities according to endurance and energy.
2. Participate in ADL.
3. Wear sturdy, well-fitted shoes and clean socks.
4. Avoid injury caused by limited energy and fatigue.
5. Equip environment with holding bars and aids for washing, dressing, grooming, toileting, and eating.

Nursing diagnosis

Altered thought processes

Related factors: Physiologic changes

Defining characteristics: Drowsiness, inability to concentrate, memory deficit, hallucinations, seizures, high level of nitrogenous wastes

OUTCOME CRITERIA

Short-term
Minimal changes in thought processes, as evidenced by appropriate attitude, behavior, and communication (expected within 1 week)

Long term
Thought processes maintained intact, as evidenced by optimal level of mental functioning within disease limitations (expected within 1 month and ongoing)

NURSING INTERVENTIONS/INSTRUCTIONS

1. Assess client's mental and orientation status, and compare findings with previous profiles (each visit).
2. Adapt communication style and instruction to client's needs and abilities (each visit).
3. Reinforce need for compliance with dietary restrictions and

medication administration and dialysis to maintain thought processes (first visit and reinforce when needed).
4. Provide stimulating and diversional experiences, including reality-based experiences (each visit).

CLIENT AND FAMILY/CARETAKER INTERVENTIONS
1. Comply with medical regimen.
2. Participate in reality-based activities, utilizing aids to reinforce orientation.
3. Comply with dialysis protocol.
4. Use aids to assist with remembering medications, dietary, and fluid schedules.

Nursing diagnosis

Ineffective family coping: compromised

Related factors: Prolonged, progressive disease that exhausts supportive capacity of significant people

Defining characteristics: Less than satisfactory supportive behaviors and results; client's expression of concerns about response to health needs by others; expressed need by family for knowledge and understanding of client needs

OUTCOME CRITERIA
Short-term
Improved coping by family, as evidenced by family's acknowledgement of disabling effects of disease and required life-style changes and by family's cooperation and participation in treatment regimen (expected within 1 week)

Long-term
Optimal level of participation and support of family menbers to facilitate client life-style and improvement in health status (expected within 1 to 2 months)

NURSING INTERVENTIONS/INSTRUCTIONS
1. Assess family interactions, coping abilities, strengths of individual members, level of participation and support, and resources available and utilized by family (see Family Assessment, p. 46, for guidelines) (first visit).

2. Provide accurate information to family about treatment regimen and progress; allow time for questions and clarifications (each visit).
3. Encourage family to discuss strengths and options for change and to identify coping mechanisms used (each visit).
4. Include family members in teaching and planning of care (each visit).
5. Inform client of government and community agencies available for support and assistance (first visit).
6. Encourage family to contact counselor and to arrange for hospice care if appropriate (any visit).

CLIENT AND FAMILY/CARETAKER INTERVENTIONS

1. Verbalize concerns and feelings about burden of caring for family member with long-term disorder.
2. Seek assistance if needed
3. Participate in planning and implementing care.
4. Adapt to limitations of client and integrate them into family activity.
5. Support dialysis program.
6. Continue family activities and open communication.

Nursing diagnosis

Anticipatory grieving

Related factors: Perceived potential loss of physiopsychosocial well-being

Defining characteristics: Altered sleep and communication patterns; sorrow; expression of distress at potential loss

OUTCOME CRITERIA

Short-term
Progress in grieving, as evidenced by verbalization, attitude, and behavior changes manifested by stage in process (expected within days)

Long-term
Grief process resolving, as evidenced by resumption of lifestyle with or without changes as needed and by integration of

grieving stage into life-style and activities (expected within 2 to 3 months and ongoing)

NURSING INTERVENTIONS/INSTRUCTIONS

1. Assess degree and stage of grief; include suicide potential (each visit).
2. Inform client of stages of grief and that client's behavior is acceptable for specific stage and that resolution will be final stage (first visit).
3. Allow expression of feelings about disabilities and potential loss and implications for the future (each visit).
4. Provide open communication and accepting environment for interactions (each visit).
5. Initiate referral for psychological or spiritual counseling (any visit).

CLIENT AND FAMILY/CARETAKER INTERVENTIONS

1. Progress through grieving process to resolution.
2. Seek counseling as needed.

Nursing diagnosis

Knowledge deficit

Related factors: Lack of exposure to information about medical regimen

Defining characteristics: Request for information about dialysis and about care of abdominal site or arteriovenous fistula site

OUTCOME CRITERIA

Short-term
Adequate knowledge, as evidenced by compliance with medication regimen, identification of signs and symptoms to report, and demonstration of shunt care or care of abdominal site for dialysis (expected within 1 week)

Long-term
Adequate knowledge, as evidenced by client's meeting requirements for a modified life-style without complications and maintaining optimal health and functioning within disease limitations (expected within 1 to 2 months)

NURSING INTERVENTIONS/INSTRUCTIONS

1. Instruct client in administration of prescribed drugs, including diuretics, exchange resins, sodium bicarbonate or citrate, antibiotics, and clofibrate; include dose, route, frequency, side effects, and fluid allotment (first visit).

2. Instruct client in measures for preventing constipation, including high-fiber diet and exercise (first visit).

3. Instruct client in measures to prevent infection, including hand washing, catheter care, avoiding persons with upper respiratory infections, and using sterile technique in shunt or peritoneal dialysis site care (first visit and reinforce on second visit).

4. Assess for cardiovascular changes (increased blood pressure, dysrhythmias, visual changes), respiratory changes (decreased breath sounds, crackles, wheezes, chest pain, dyspnea, fever, restlessness), neurologic changes (lassitude, apathy, decreased mental acuity, paresthesias, muscle cramps, twitching, irritability, confusion), and hematologic changes (fatigue, pallor, easy bruising, petechiae, purpura, bleeding from any site) (each visit).

5. Assess for signs of hypocalcemia, including confusion, emotional lability, numbness, tingling or twitching of fingers or toes, Chvostek sign or Trousseau sign, muscle weakness, and stupor (each visit).

6. Instruct client to notify physician if symptoms increase in severity or any complications occur (first visit).

7. Instruct client in arteriovenous shunt/fistula care (first and second visits):
   - Avoid taking blood pressure or blood samples from affected arm.
   - Avoid carrying purse or heavy item over affected arm.
   - Avoid wearing tight clothing over affected arm.
   - Avoid tugging, pulling, or lying on affected arm.

8. Instruct client in dressing change at abdominal peritoneal site, and allow for return demonstration (first visit).

9. Instruct client to monitor patency of external shunt, including presence of bright red blood and a thrill or bruit on auscultation over site (first visit).

10. Instruct client to monitor patency of internal fistula, including checking pulsations at site (first visit).

11. Inform client of importance of compliance with total care

regimen and of incorporation of regimen into daily activities (each visit).

12. Instruct client to follow up with physician and laboratory visits as scheduled; inform client of importance of dialysis schedule (each visit).

13. Instruct client to wear or carry identification information at all times, including condition and physician's name and telephone number (first visit).

CLIENT AND FAMILY/CARETAKER INTERVENTIONS

1. Comply with medication regimen.
2. Manage constipation with diet and medication.
3. Use measures to prevent infection and other complications.
4. Report deteriorating condition or presence of signs and symptoms of complications associated with dialysis access site.
5. Maintain patency of access site; take measures to avoid injury to site.
6. Maintain dialysis, physician, and laboratory appointments.
7. Wear identification information for emergency care.
8. Comply with total medical regimen and integrate into lifestyle.

▲ Urinary Tract Infection (UTI)

Infection of the lower urinary tract (cystitis) is caused by gram-positive or gram-negative organisms that gain access to the bladder by sexual intercourse, urethral trauma, poor personal hygiene, or an indwelling catheter or by stasis of urine as a result of obstructive conditions, neurogenic bladder, or kidney disease. The condition is more common in women because of the proximity of the urethra to the vagina and anus. Cystitis may become chronic as microorganisms become resistant to therapy. Chronic cystitis is particularly common in elderly people who have indwelling catheters for long periods of time.

Home care is primarily concerned with the teaching of medication regimens to prevent or control recurrent bladder infections and possible spread to the kidneys.

Nursing diagnosis

Pain

Related factors: Biologic injuring agents (bacterial infection)

Defining characteristics: Communication of pain descriptors; urine culture positive for infectious organism; dysuria; cloudy and foul-smelling urine

OUTCOME CRITERIA

Short-term
Minimal pain or decrease in pain, as evidenced by client's statement of compliance with urinary tract analgesic and antibiotic therapy (expected within 2 days)

Long-term
Absence of pain, as evidenced by completion of antibiotic regimen and increased comfort in lower abdomen and during urination (expected within 10 days)

NURSING INTERVENTIONS/INSTRUCTIONS

1. Assess client's pain, including site, duration, intensity, aggravating and alleviating factors, and characteristics associated with voiding (each visit)
2. Instruct client in administration of systemic antibiotics, urinary antiseptics, or urinary tract analgesics, including dose, frequency, side effects, and food/drug/alcohol interactions; inform client that phenazopyridine may turn urine orange or orange-red and stain undergarments (first visit).
3. Instruct client in use of heating pad over suprapubic area or low back region and in use of sitz bath (first visit).

CLIENT AND FAMILY/CARETAKER INTERVENTIONS

1. Administer medications as instructed and for proper length of time.
2. Apply heat for symptomatic relief.

Nursing diagnosis

Altered urinary elimination patterns

Related factors: Mechanical trauma of bladder infection

Defining characteristics: Dysuria; frequency; nocturia; urgency; urinary retention and stasis; small, frequent voidings

OUTCOME CRITERIA

Short-term
Minimal urinary alteration, as evidenced by resumption of normal micturition pattern (expected within 2 days)

Long-term
Urinary elimination pattern within baseline and free from any abnormal changes (expected within 2 weeks)

NURSING INTERVENTIONS/INSTRUCTIONS

1. Perform renal and reproductive assessment (see Renal/Urinary System Assessment, p. 28, and Reproductive System Assessment, p. 33, for guidelines); note temperature and assess for history of UTI or renal problems, or presence of sexually transmitted diseases (first visit).
2. Instruct client to monitor pattern and frequency of voidings and characteristics of urine and to note pain or burning on urination, urgency, hesitancy, and force of flow (each visit).
3. Encourage client to consume up to 3000 ml of fluid per day if allowed (first visit).
4. Instruct client in acid-ash diet, including meat, fish, poultry, eggs, cheese, corn, cereals, cranberries, plums, and prunes; instruct client to avoid alcohol, caffeine, and pepper, since they aggravate symptoms (first visit).

CLIENT AND FAMILY/CARETAKER INTERVENTIONS

1. Record all output and characteristics of urine, with symptomatology if present.
2. Drink 8 to 10 glasses of water or juice at regular intervals.
3. Include or avoid specific foods that affect condition.

Nursing diagnosis

Knowledge deficit

Related factors: Lack of exposure to information about infection

Defining characteristics: Request for information about medication administration and measures to prevent recurrence of infection

OUTCOME CRITERIA

Short-term
Adequate knowledge, as evidenced by identification of and compliance with hygienic practices and medication regimen (expected within 3 days)

Long-term
Adequate knowledge, as evidenced by completion of medical regimen and hygienic measures to prevent recurrence (expected within 10 days)

NURSING INTERVENTIONS/INSTRUCTIONS

1. Instruct client in absolute necessity of taking full course of antibiotics even if symptoms disappear (first visit).
2. Instruct client in hygienic practices (first visit):
   - Wash with soap and water daily.
   - Void when urge is felt; do not delay, and void every 2 hours if possible.
   - Women should wipe from front to back.
   - Urinate after intercourse.
3. Instruct client to notify physician if symptoms persist or escalate or if flank pain or fever is present (first visit).
4. Suggest showers instead of tub baths (first visit).
5. Instruct female client to avoid use of feminine sprays and to wear cotton undergarments (first visit).
6. Advise client to have follow-up urine cultures if symptoms recur (last visit).

CLIENT AND FAMILY/CARETAKER INTERVENTIONS

1. Follow hygienic preventive procedures.
2. Administer all medications as prescribed.

3. Maintain consistency in daily care; avoid allowing irritating substances to come into contact with genital area.
4. Collect midstream urine specimen and take to laboratory if symptoms escalate or recur.

Integumentary system

◣ Burns

Burns are injuries that destroy layers of the skin and, in some cases, underlying tissues. Types of burn injuries include thermal, chemical, and electrical. Burns are classified as partial thickness, which may be superficial (first degree) or deep (second degree) and which involve the dermis and epidermis, with potential for epithelial regeneration, and full thickness (third or fourth degree), which involve all skin layers, including nerve endings, and well as muscles, tendons, and bones, with scarring and loss of function, and which require skin grafting. With full thickness burns, all systems are affected: cardiovascular (impaired circulation and occluded blood supply), respiratory (edema and obstruction of the airway), renal (reduced blood flow to kidneys with ischemia), musculoskeletal (formation of scar tissue with contractures), neurologic (disorientation, withdrawal), gastrointestinal (stress ulcer), and endocrine (stress diabetes). The most important treatments in the initial and acute phase of burn care include fluid replacement, wound care, and pain and infection control.

Home care is primarily concerned with the rehabilitation phase of burn care and includes teaching the client about the care and treatment of the healing wounds and supporting the client's compliance with the physical therapy regimen.

Nursing diagnosis

Pain

Related factors: Biologic injuring agents

Defining characteristics: Verbalization of pain descriptors; pain during physical therapy

311

OUTCOME CRITERIA

Short-term

Pain minimized, as evidenced by performance of physical therapy with reduced pain (expected within 1 week)

Long-term

Absence of pain, as evidenced by ultimate restoration of function and by increased comfort level during physical therapy (expected within 3 months or depending on extent of treatment)

NURSING INTERVENTIONS/INSTRUCTIONS

1. Assess pain severity during exercises and effect of pain on therapy in achieving function (first visit).
2. Assess itching of healing areas as pain subsides (first visit).
3. Administer analgesic and instruct client to take analgesic before therapy (first visit and when needed).

CLIENT AND FAMILY/CARETAKER INTERVENTIONS

1. Administer analgesic correctly as needed for pain and before physical therapy sessions.
2. Support client in long-term, painful physical therapy regimen.

Nursing diagnosis

Impaired skin integrity

Related factors: External factor of burn

Defining characteristics: Disruption of skin surface; destruction of skin layers; sensitivity of newly healed skin to slight pressure or trauma; itching and flaking during healing

OUTCOME CRITERIA

Short-term

Preservation of skin integrity, as evidenced by healing with newly formed skin and nerve regeneration (expected within 1 week and ongoing)

Long-term

Absence of skin impairment, as evidenced by gradual return of function and new skin development (expected within 2 to 3 months, depending on extent of injury)

NURSING INTERVENTIONS/INSTRUCTIONS

1. Assess skin and grafted area for sensitivity to cold, heat, or touch; itching that occurs with healing; flaking; and formation of blisters with slight trauma (each visit).
2. Instruct client to apply topical antihistamine cream and palliative creams to itchy, dry, flaking skin on healed areas (first visit).
3. Instruct client to avoid direct sunlight and restrictive clothing (first visit).
4. Inform client of healing process, including discoloration and development of scar tissue with contours (first visit).
5. Instruct client in application of Jobst pressure garments for maintaining gentle pressure on the healed burn area and to wear 24 hours a day for possibly as long as 1 year (first visit).
6. Inform client that healing is usually complete within 6 weeks, with mature healing and return of suppleness and normal coloring within 6 to 12 months (first visit).
7. Instruct client in wound care and dressing changes for unhealed open areas on skin, using sterile technique (first and second visits).

CLIENT AND FAMILY/CARETAKER INTERVENTIONS

1. Protect healing skin from trauma and from sensitivity reactions to cold, heat, sun, and excessive pressure or constriction.
2. Apply topical medication to allay itching.
3. Wear pressure garment continuously, as instructed.
4. Perform dressing changes using sterile technique; note and report any drainage at wound edge or fluid under the graft.

Nursing diagnosis

Impaired physical mobility

Related factors: Pain and discomfort, musculoskeletal impairment, severe anxiety

Defining characteristics: Reluctance to attempt movement; limited range of motion; decreased muscle strength; muscle atrophy; contractures of major joints

OUTCOME CRITERIA

Short-term
Adequate mobility, as evidenced by minimal discomfort during physical therapy and reduced risk for contracture formation of skin and underlying tissues (expected within 1 week)

Long-term
Adequate mobility and activity performance, as evidenced by skin healing and maturity, with the absence of contractures of major joints, skin, ligaments, and tendons and client's acceptance of physical therapy as a part of daily living (expected within 2 to 3 months and ongoing)

NURSING INTERVENTIONS/INSTRUCTIONS

1. Assess client's ability for movement of all joints and muscles and ability to ambulate and perform activities of daily living (ADL) without assistance; note especially skin at neck area, axillae, antecubital spaces, fingers, groin, popliteal area, and ankles, as appropriate, for developing skin contractures and shortening of tendons and ligaments during healing (each visit).
2. Perform and instruct client to perform active range-of-motion exercises, muscle stretching, and ambulation progressively and concurrently with physical therapy (first visit and reinforce each visit).
3. Inform client of inportance of continuous long-term physical therapy, depending on extent of burn injury and tissue damage, to achieve optimal function (first visit).
4. Provide referral to physical therapy and encouragement to comply with physical therapy program and to correlate with ADL and social and diversional activities (first and second visits).
5. Refer home health aide to assist with ADL as needed.

CLIENT AND FAMILY/CARETAKER INTERVENTIONS

1. Comply with daily rehabilitaton program requirements and self-care activities, using assistive aids for eating, toileting, bathing, grooming, and dressing as needed.
2. Perform joint and muscle exercises as instructed by therapist and reinforced by home nurse; take analgesic prior to exercises.

3. Note and report pain or resistance to exercising to therapist and possibly physician.

Nursing diagnosis

Body image disturbance

Related factors: Biophysical factor of effect of burns

Defining characteristics: Verbal and nonverbal response to change in body structure and function; negative feelings about body, scarring, deformity, disfigurement, discoloration, and contour of scarring; social isolation

OUTCOME CRITERIA

Short term

Improved adaptation to body image change, as evidenced by client's statement of feelings about changed appearance and limitations imposed by condition and need to change life-style until restoration of function is achieved (expected within 1 to 2 weeks)

Long-term

Optimal adaptation to body image change, as evidenced by client's statement of acceptance of appearance and by client's expression of ability to cope with life changes and meet needs for optimal health and functioning (expected within 2 to 3 months)

NURSING INTERVENTIONS/INSTRUCTIONS

1. Assess client's life-style, roles, and ability to adapt to and integrate long-term rehabilitation into treatment regimen (first visit).
2. Allow client to express feelings about appearance, loss of function, presence of any deformity or disfigurement, loss of control over life situations, and inability to meet role expectations (each visit).
3. Reassure client that feelings, anxiety, and expressions of concern are a normal part of adjustment to the changes in life-style that occur (first visit).
4. Encourage client to ask for help when needed, to identify strengths, and to suggest options for changing life-style, including ADL, social and occupational interactions, and recreation and leisure activities (any visit).

5. Assist client to identify coping mechanisms that work and that have a positive effect on adjustment to body image changes (any visit).
6. Emphasize the positive aspects of the rehabilitation and adjustment process and what is achieved instead of what is not achieved (each visit).
7. Assist client to identify clothing that will cover scarring or deformity as appropriate (first visit or as needed).
8. Refer client to counseling, occupational therapist, or social services as needed (any visit).
9. Refer to social worker for long-term planning and counseling (any visit).

CLIENT AND FAMILY/CARETAKER INTERVENTIONS

1. Verbalize concern and feelings about appearance.
2. Allow grieving over change in body image.
3. Adapt to life-style change and frustrations of long-term treatment.
4. Utilize positive coping mechanisms with success.
5. Adapt to change in appearance and limitations imposed by disability.
6. Resume close relationships, social, family, and occupational.
7. Utilize counseling and/or other professional services as needed.

Nursing diagnosis

Knowledge deficit

Related factors: Lack of information about long-term therapy

Defining characteristics: Request for information about risk of complications, nutritional needs, and long-term health maintenance

OUTCOME CRITERIA

Short-term
Adequate knowledge, as evidenced by client's statement of basic needs for health promotion (expected within 1 week)

Long-term
Adequate knowledge, as evidenced by compliance with requirements to maintain optimal health and functioning (expected ongoing)

NURSING INTERVENTIONS/INSTRUCTIONS

1. Assess for daily basic needs based on progression toward wellness and past patterns (first visit).
2. Instruct client in need for scheduled rest periods, especially before or after physical therapy (first visit).
3. Instruct client in high-protein, high-calorie diet as appetite improves, to enhance the healing process; refer client to dietitian if appropriate (first visit and reinforce on second visit).
4. Instruct client to assess for and report any redness, swelling, pain, or drainage at burn/healing site (first visit).
5. Inform client that cosmetic or reconstructive surgery may be needed if burn is extensive and tissue destruction is major; information should reinforce physician notification only (any visit).
6. Arrange visits from other burn victims for support if appropriate (any visit).

CLIENT AND FAMILY/CARETAKER INTERVENTIONS

1. Assess and monitor wound for infectious process and report to physician.
2. Provide suggested dietary inclusions and rest and sleep opportunities.
3. Promote morale and optimism during long-term therapeutic regimen.
4. Express and fulfill daily basic needs for health maintenance.

◣ *Cellulitis*

Cellulitis is the localized acute inflammation of tissues. The condition may follow disruptions in the skin and is most commonly caused by group A beta-hemolytic streptococci, which produce enzymes that affect deeper subcutaneous tissue. Cellulitis may be a primary infection or a secondary infection as a complication of another disorder. The infection may become gangrenous if not treated.

Home care is primariy concerned with the teaching of antibiotic therapy to control infection and with local treatments to reduce inflammation and pain.

Nursing diagnosis

Pain

Related factors: Biologic injuring agents of inflammation

Defining characteristics: Communication of pain descriptors; guarding and protective behavior of site; hot, tender, reddened, edematous area

OUTCOME CRITERIA

Short-term

Reduction in pain, as evidenced by client's verbalization of pain relief and by relaxed expression and posture (expected within 7 days)

Long-term

Optimal comfort level, as evidenced by complete relief from pain at the infection site and by compliance with medication regimen (expected within 2 weeks)

NURSING INTERVENTIONS/INSTRUCTIONS

1. Assess client's pain for type, intensity, location, and duration (each visit).
2. Immobilize affected area, generally lower extremity, upper extremity, or face, and position client for comfort (each visit).
3. Apply, and instruct client to apply, cool, possibly wet pack for comfort (first visit).
4. Intruct client in administration of analgesics; include dose, route, frequency, food/drug/alcohol interactions, and side effects (first visit).

CLIENT AND FAMILY/CARETAKER INTERVENTIONS

1. Immobilize, position, and protect affected part.
2. Apply cool packs as instructed; avoid placing ice directly on skin.
3. Administer medications as prescribed.

Nursing diagnosis

Hyperthermia

Related factors: Illness of infection

Defining characteristics: Increase in body temperature above normal range; warm to touch; malaise

OUTCOME CRITERIA

Short-term
Reduction in hyperthermia, as evidenced by progressively decreasing body temperature and resolution of inflammatory manifestations (expected within 3 to 7 days)

Long-term
Absence of hyperthermia, as evidenced by afebrile state, temperature within normal range, and complete resolution of inflammatory process (expected within 2 weeks)

NURSING INTERVENTIONS/INSTRUCTIONS

1. Assess affected area for heat, local erythema, edema, peau d'orange appearance, and loss of function; note also presence of lymphadenopathy, vesicles, or bullae (each visit).
2. Instruct client in technique for taking temperature orally and recording every 4 hours while awake as needed (first visit).
3. Instruct client in measures to maintain hydration; instruct client to increase fluid intake to 2 to 3 liters per day (first visit).
4. Instruct client in administration of antipyretics and antibiotics, including dose, time, frequency, side effects, and how to take; instruct client to complete the full course of antibiotics (first visit).

CLIENT AND FAMILY/CARETAKER INTERVENTIONS

1. Take and record temperature every 4 hours and if feeling chilled, and maintain a log of the readings.
2. Provide consistent, adequate fluid intake.
3. Administer complete course of antibiotics; take antipyretic as instructed.

Nursing diagnosis

Knowledge deficit

Related factors: Lack of information about infection

Defining characteristics: Request for information about infectious process, cause, treatment, and care

OUTCOME CRITERIA

Short-term
Adequate knowledge, as evidenced by client's identification of and compliance with treatments and care (expected within 2 to 7 days)

Long-term
Adequate knowledge, as evidenced by compliance with and completion of treatments and by resolution of the inflammatory/infectious process (expected within 2 weeks)

NURSING INTERVENTIONS/INSTRUCTIONS

1. Assess client's history to determine underlying cause of condition; include any thermal, mechanical, or chemical injury, cutaneous infection or abnormality, past surgeries and resulting scars, endocrine disorders, or impaired defenses (first visit).
2. Assess client's life-style and ability to adapt, interest in learning to care for infection, and need for family participation (first visit).
3. Instruct client to note condition of skin and local condition of infection, size, odor, induration, and drainage and to change the dressings using sterile technique; instruct to maintain elevation of extremity (first visit and reinforce on second visit).
4. Instruct client in hand-washing technique, which client should perform before giving care to affected area; instruct client in disposal of infectious articles (first visit).
5. Instruct client in signs and symptoms of systemic infection and to report these to physician immediately (first visit).

CLIENT AND FAMILY/CARETAKER INTERVENTIONS

1. Wash hands before caring for infection and after touching dressings or soiled materials.
2. Perform measures to prevent transmission of infectious agent or spread of infection in client.
3. Report increased temperature or pulse, headache, malaise, anorexia, nausea, or altered mental status to physician.

◤ *Decubitus Ulcer*

Decubitus ulcer (pressure sore, bedsore) is caused by the breakdown of the epidermal and underlying structures as a result of excessive pressure or shearing forces. Areas usually affected are the bony prominences. The risk for decubitus ulcer is increased in those who are immobilized or malnourished or who have altered sensation or circulation or fecal or urinary incontinence. The persons most commonly affected are the elderly.

Home care is primarily concerned with the care and teaching aspects of decubitus ulcer prevention and control and with the healing of existing ulcers.

Nursing diagnosis

Impaired skin integrity

Related factors: External factors of pressure, shearing; internal factors of nutrition, circulation, level of consciousness, sensation

Defining characteristics: Redness, warmth at pressure area; disruption of skin, with pain, swelling, heat, induration, drainage, and tissue necrosis, depending on stage of decubitus

OUTCOME CRITERIA
Short-term
Reduction in skin impairment, as evidenced by absence of blanching, hyperemia, or disruption in skin over stress areas (expected within 2 weeks)

Long-term
Absence of skin impairment despite immobilization, negative
nitrogen balance, incontinence, or impaired innervation or circulation (expected within 1 month and ongoing)

NURSING INTERVENTIONS/INSTRUCTIONS

1. Assess skin, creases, folds, and bony prominences, including color, temperature, tone, turgor, and integrity; note
   presence of edema, irritation, maceration, excoriation,
   induration, ulceration, drainage, or necrosis (see
   Integumentary System Assessment, p. 31, for guidelines)
   (each visit).
2. Locate and measure decubiti, and document degree of
   breakdown (each visit).
3. Instruct client in hygienic measures, including personal and
   skin care, bathing and cleansing after toileting, and taking
   sponge bath in bed (first visit).
4. Instruct client in postitioning in bed or sitting (first visit).
5. Instruct client in active and passive range-of-motion
   (ROM) exercises and in use of prophylactic and palliative
   measures, including pillows, heel and elbow guards, sheep-
   skin, and air or fluid mattress and pads (each visit).
6. Apply protective topical agent and dressing as prescribed;
   irrigate decubitus with sterile saline, and apply debriding
   agent as prescribed; instruct client in medication and dressing changes (each visit).
7. Massage bony prominences; avoid pulling or sliding client
   in bed if client is on bed rest (each visit).

CLIENT AND FAMILY/CARETAKER
INTERVENTIONS

1. Maintain clean, dry skin; bathe daily with mild soap; rinse
   well and pat dry.
2. Pad and protect heels, elbows, back of head, iliac crests,
   sacrococcygeal area; apply emollient to intact skin.
3. Maintain clean bed, free of wrinkles and crumbs.
4. Use foot board and bed cradle as appropriate.
5. Position self hourly using overhead bar if able.
6. Position every 2 hours; massage pressure areas; perform
   ROM exercises.
7. Expose decubitus to air, light, and heat for prescribed
   intervals.

8. Avoid shearing forces when moving client; lift and roll instead of pulling or sliding.

Nursing diagnosis

Knowledge deficit

Related factors: Lack of information about care and prevention of decubitus ulcer

Defining characteristics: Request for information about cleansing, dressing, heat application, and preventive measures to avoid new decubitus formation or further breakdown of existing decubitus

OUTCOME CRITERIA

Short-term
Adequate knowledge, as evidenced by client's statement about causes of skin breakdown and care to prevent or treat decubitus (expected within 1 week)

Long-term
Adequate knowledge, as evidenced by client's compliance with medical regimen and meeting requirements for adaptation of activities of daily living to achieve optimal health and skin integrity (expected within 1 month)

NURSING INTERVENTIONS/INSTRUCTIONS

1. Assess client's nutrition and neurologic status for obesity or thinness, state of consciousness, paralysis, incontinence of urine/stool, immobility, and use of sedatives or tranquilizers (each visit).
2. Assess client's weight weekly and compare with actual and ideal weight (any visit).
3. Encourage and instruct client in high-calorie, high-protein diet with adequate fluid intake (2 liters per day) as appropriate (first visit).
4. Institute bowel and bladder training program if indicated (each visit).
5. Instruct client in prescribed treatments for skin area and their frequency, such as massage, padding, heat application, cleansing and dressing area, and postition changes (first visit and reinforce on second visit).

6. Inform client of use and availability of cushions, egg crate or alternating pressure mattresses, or rice/bean bags to relieve pressure on skin (first visit).

CLIENT AND FAMILY/CARETAKER INTERVENTIONS

1. Maintain hydration and well-balanced meals that include protein and vitamin C; take supplements as needed for calories.
2. Avoid medications that affect awareness and consciousness.
3. Offer toileting every 2 to 3 hours while client is awake; provide measures to prevent urine or bowel incontinence, or apply device to prevent exposure to the skin.
4. Report progressive skin breakdown that occurs in spite of preventive measures.
5. Change position and utilize aids to reduce pressure on skin.

◤ *Herpes Zoster*

Herpes zoster is an acute, viral central nervous system infection that involves the dorsal root ganglia; it is characterized by painful skin eruptions in areas supplied by peripheral sensory nerves that arise in the affected ganglia. The condition may be associated with systemic diseases or immunosuppressive therapy. Most commonly, the eruptions start on the thorax area and spread unilaterally.

Home care is primarily concerned with the relief of pain and discomfort and with teaching the client about medication administration and treatment of prolonged neuralgia.

Nursing diagnosis

Pain

Related factors: Biologic injuring agents

Defining characteristics: Communication of pain descriptors (severity, location, duration); guarding and protective behavior toward affected area(s); self-focusing; restlessness

OUTCOME CRITERIA

Short-term
Increased comfort, as evidenced by client's statement that pain is decreased or absent (expected within 2 to 3 days)

Long-term
Absence of or minimal pain, with decreased incidence of recurrent episodes and achievement of optimal health and functioning without pain (1 to 2 months)

NURSING INTERVENTIONS/INSTRUCTIONS

1. Assess pain, burning, or neuralgia on side of trunk or other area; assess severity of pain before and during outbreak of vesicles (first visit).
2. Instruct client in administration of oral medications to reduce pain (analgesics), inflammation (steroids), and itching (antihistamines), including dose, frequency, action, side effects, and food and drug interactions (first visit).
3. Instruct client in application of topical medication to reduce itching and promote healing and comfort (calamine lotion, zinc oxide, benzoin, steroids) (first visit).
4. Apply wet, cool compresses or cool sprays, and instruct client in application (first visit).
5. Instruct client to take warm tub baths with Burow's solution and to avoid rubbing skin dry, extremes in temperature or pressure against painful areas, and tight clothing around area (first visit).
6. Instruct client in diversional therapy, such as music, relaxation techniques, and guided imagery (each visit).
7. Instruct client to avoid lying on affected area (first visit).

CLIENT AND FAMILY/CARETAKER INTERVENTIONS

1. Administer medications orally and topically correctly and effectively.
2. Report prolonged pain to physician.
3. Maintain calm environment including diversion from pain.
4. Avoid actions that cause or trigger pain, including rubbing, pressure or temperature extremes, and scratching.

Nursing diagnosis

Knowledge deficit

Related factors: Lack of information about disease

Defining characteristics: Expressed need for information about disease causes and treatment and prevention of complications

OUTCOME CRITERIA

Short-term
Adequate knowledge, as evidenced by client's statement of cause, treatments, and prognosis for the disease (expected within 1 week)

Long-term
Adequate knowledge, as evidenced by client's meeting requirements to achieve optimal level of health by compliance with the treatment regimen (expected within 1 month)

NURSING INTERVENTIONS/INSTRUCTIONS

1. Assess client's life-style and ability to adapt, learning abilities and interests, readiness to learn, and family participation and support (first visit).
2. Inform client of cause of the disease, course of the disease, unpredictability of the disease, and exacerbations in clear, honest language (first visit).
3. Instruct client in care of lesions and to prevent infection by avoiding scratching, touching, picking, or squeezing lesions (first visit).
4. Instruct client in hand washing and precautions to take (skin and protective isolation) if needed (first visit and thereafter).
5. Inform client of rest requirements and that inadequate rest may lengthen course of illness; instruct client to schedule rest periods and provide a stress-free, quiet environment (each visit).
6. Inform client of importance of nutrition and fluid requirements; instruct client to note and report weight loss (first visit).
7. Instruct client in antibiotic therapy to prevent or treat infection (first visit).

CLIENT AND FAMILY/CARETAKER INTERVENTIONS

1. Maintain measures to prevent infection and to meet fluid, nutrition, and rest requirements for healing lesions.
2. Comply with medication regimen correctly.
3. Provide restful, stress-free environment.
4. Verbalize cause of the disease, methods of transmission, and methods for control of disease manifestations and prevention of exacerbations or sequelae.
5. Provide care for lesions, and take measures to prevent infection of lesions.

◢ *Psoriasis*

Psoriasis is a non-inflammatory chronic dermatologic condition in which many silvery, scaley-appearing red papules and plaques appear at bony prominences. The condition may affect any part of the body, including hands, feet, ears, nails, back, buttocks, and scalp. In addition to the most common psoriasis form, vulgaris, guttate, pustular, and erythrodermic forms exist. Psoriasis may be associated with rheumatoid-like arthritis and commonly develops between 10 and 40 years of age. Recurrence may result from local trauma, environmental factors, withdrawal from systemic corticosteroids, emotional stress, or infection.

Home care is primarily concerned with the teaching aspects of treatments, resulting in comfort and prevention of exacerbation of the condition.

Nursing diagnosis

Impaired skin integrity

Related factors: Alterations in skin by dermatitis

Defining characterstics: Scales and plaques over any part of body; possible itching or scratching; disruption of skin surfaces

OUTCOME CRITERIA

Short-term
Minimal skin impairment from eruptions, as evidenced by client's compliance with prescribed skin care and reduction of symptoms (expected within 1 week)

Long-term
Absence of skin impairment, as evidenced by adaptive lifestyle changes to minimize recurrences, continued compliance with prescribed skin regimen, and intact and lesion-free integument (expected within 4 to 6 weeks)

NURSING INTERVENTIONS/INSTRUCTIONS

1. Assess skin for color, integrity, and presence of papules, plaques, or pustules; include location, extent and distribution (see Integumentary System Assessment, p. 31, for guidelines) (each visit).
2. Relate skin manifestations to implications of prescribed drug use (each visit).
3. Instruct client in skin care and application of topical petrolatum-based emollients and combinations of topical corticosteroids, salicylic acid, crude coal tar, or anthralin preparations as prescribed (first visit and reinforce on second visit).
4. Instruct client in scalp care, including loosening and removal of scales, use of tar shampoo, and application of topical steroids (first visit).
5. Instruct client in medication administration, including time, dose, interval, route, side effects, method, and areas of application (first visit).
6. Apply and instruct client in application of occlusive wraps, avoiding exposure of eye or other sensitive area to medications (first visit).
7. Inform client of methods to minimize staining of garments (first visit).
8. Administer and instruct in alternate therapies, such as light therapy alone or in conjunction with medication, photochemotherapy, and protection of sensitive areas (first visit).
9. Instruct client in practices regarding teratogenic drugs and effect of systemic antimetabolites or oral retinoids on hepatic, renal, and hematopoietic systems; monitor for toxicities (each visit).

10. Provide clear written instructions for all skin care and medication protocols (first visit and review on second visit).

CLIENT AND FAMILY/CARETAKER INTERVENTIONS

1. Take tub baths instead of showers for 15 to 20 minutes daily, and apply topical preparations to damp skin.
2. Use written protocol for scheduling time, type, and method of topical medications, and administer only as directed.
3. Apply salicylic acid to affected areas on scalp at bedtime; sleep with shower cap on.
4. Loosen scales on scalp in morning, shampoo with tar preparation, and follow with topical steroid preparation.
5. Use salicylic acid on affected areas only; avoid use of plastic occlusive wrap with coal tar or anthralin application.
6. Apply topical steroid with occlusive plastic dressing; modify vinyl jogging suit for fuller body coverage.
7. Apply anthralin with gloves to affected area only with a downward motion, and wear old clothes, since permanent stains are left on garments; avoid contact with eyes or other sensitive areas.
8. Avoid sunlight and artificial light for 24 hours following photochemotherapy; wear full protective ultraviolet filtering glasses.
9. Follow planned schedule and family planning practices before, during, and following therapies using retinoids and methotrexate.
10. Consult with physician when needed for clarification and assistance in therapies.

Nursing diagnosis

Knowledge deficit

Related factors: Lack of information about disorder

Defining characteristics: Request for information about skin disruptions, cause, treatments, and prevention of exacerbations

OUTCOME CRITERIA

Short-term
Adequate knowledge, as evidenced by client's identification of measures to take to minimize recurrence and for compliance with skin care and medication protocols (expected within 3 days)

Long-term
Adequate knowledge, as evidenced by client's meeting requirements for changes in life-style and medical regimen to achieve optimal level of health and functioning (expected within 2 weeks)

NURSING INTERVENTIONS/INSTRUCTIONS

1. Inform family members/caretakers that condition is not contagious (first visit).
2. Inform client of cause of condition and that although it is chronic, it does not affect overall health and that control of condition is possible in most cases (first visit).
3. Instruct client in general measures to reduce recurrence (first visit).
4. Identify support systems, and refer client to psychological counseling if indicated for coping, effects on body image and self-concept, and feelings of loss, grief, or isolation (any visit).
5. Refer client to social services for assistance with occupation changes (first visit).
6. Refer client to National Psoriasis Foundation for information and support (first visit).

CLIENT AND FAMILY/CARETAKER INTERVENTIONS

1. Verbalize chronicity and limitations imposed by condition.
2. Actively employ general measures to reduce relapses/recurrences:
   - Avoid skin injury or irritation.
   - Avoid overexposure to sunlight.
   - Manage emotional stress constructively.
   - Avoid infections.
3. Consult with appropriate agencies or individuals for assistance, information, and support.

Reproductive system

◣ Mastectomy

Mastectomy, or the surgical removal of a breast, is usually done to treat breast malignancy. A radical mastectomy is the removal of an entire breast, including the pectoral muscles, the lymph nodes of the axila, and the pectoral fascia; a modified radical mastectomy does not include the pectoral muscles and pectoral fascia; a simple mastectomy is the surgical removal of an entire breast. Mastectomy may be followed by the surgical reconstruction of the breast (mammoplasty).

Home care is primarily concerned with functional maintenance of the operative side and with the psychological consequences of such a loss.

Nursing diagnosis

Body image disturbance

Related factors: Loss of body part; psychosocial effect on self-concept, sexuality

Defining characteristics: Verbalization of actual change in structure of body part, missing breast, disfigurement, significance of part in regard to sexual function and desirability, negative feelings about body, change in social involvement

OUTCOME CRITERIA

Short-term
Progressive improvement in body image and adaptation to changes in function and structure, as evidenced by client's ventilating feelings, expressing concerns, and considering prosthetic purchase, reconstructive surgery, and sexual activity alterations (expected within 1 to 2 weeks)

Long-term
Optimal acceptance of changes in body structure, with positive self-concept and body image (expected within 1 to 2 months)

NURSING INTERVENTIONS/INSTRUCTIONS

1. Assess client's mental and emotional status and ability to adapt and cope (see Psychosocial Assessment, p. 41, for guidelines) (first visit).
2. Accept feelings of mutilation, grief, depression, and anxiety as result of surgery (each visit).
3. Allow time and opportunity for client to ventilate feelings, express concerns, and ask questions. Note nonverbal as well as verbal cues for assistance to communicate feelings (each visit).
4. Explore client perception of effect of breast loss on self-concept, self-image, and sexuality (first and second visits).
5. Give specific and accurate information about sexual activity (third or fourth visit):
   • Fear of exposure, rejection, or pain is common.
   • Sexual activity may be resumed in 4 to 6 weeks with physician approval.
   • Initial use of breast prosthesis during sexual activity may be a transitory buffer.
   • Instruction in sensate focusing can increase awareness of other sensitive and erotic zones.
6. Discuss availability of a proper prosthesis; include types of prostheses, emotional readiness for fitting, clothing to be worn when shopping for prosthesis, and cost (first visit).
7. Initiate referral to counseling if appropriate (fourth or fifth visit).
8. Refer to occupational therapy as needed.

CLIENT AND FAMILY/CARETAKER INTERVENTIONS

1. Verbalize feelings and concerns; ask questions if needed.
2. Participate in personal care and grooming; select clothing that enhances body image without revealing prosthesis.
3. Initiate purchase of a breast prosthesis.
4. Consider sexual options, with gradual resumption of activity and satisfaction.
5. Consider reconstructive breast surgery; speak with others who have had this surgery.

Nursing diagnosis

Fluid volume excess

Related factors: Compromised regulatory mechanisms

Defining characteristics: Lymphedema in arm on operative side; fear/refusal to exercise arm and shoulder

OUTCOME CRITERIA

Short-term

Minimal or absence of fluid accumulation in operative arm, as evidenced by arm circumference at baseline measurements and client's compliance with postoperative mastectomy exercises (expected within 1 to 2 weeks)

Long-term

Adequate lymph drainage with absence of arm swelling, optimal fluid balance, and full range of motion in arm on operative side (expected within 1 to 2 months)

NURSING INTERVENTIONS/INSTRUCTIONS

1. Assess operative site, chest wall, posture, bilateral upper arm circumference (6 cm above elbow), and complaints of arm heaviness (each visit).
2. Assess ability of client to demonstrate hospital exercise regimen for baseline; note instructions given at discharge (first visit).
3. Encourage self-care in activities of daily living (bathing, grooming, dressing, washing and brushing hair) (first and second visits).
4. Demonstrate and establish an activity/exercise regimen as ordered (first visit)·
   - Avoid strenuous activity and heavy lifting or carrying until sutures are removed and incision is healed.
   - Begin resumption of light tasks at home and work as tolerated.
   - Exercise regularly, three or four times a day; stop when pulling or pain occurs, and resume when discomfort ceases.
   - Practice fist clenching, shoulder rotation, hand climbing up and down wall, hand swinging, and abduction exercises of arm.

- Rest affected arm above heart level; elevate arm during sleep.
5. Initiate referral to a structured postmastectomy exercise program such as that offered by a physical therapist or YWCA's Encore.

CLIENT AND FAMILY/CARETAKER INTERVENTIONS

1. Participate in self-care, including activities that involve raising the arms over the head.
2. Perform exercises three or four times per day; take analgesic before exercise if needed; stop and rest between exercises when needed.
3. Resume household, occupational, and recreational tasks and activities.
4. Participate in community-sponsored programs for rehabilitation or physical therapy.
5. Use pneumatic sleeve or elastic arm stocking to relieve edema.

Nursing diagnosis

Knowledge deficit

Related factors: Lack of knowledge about disease and postoperative care

Defining characteristics: Request for information on and instruction in postoperative care regimen and chemotherapy regimen

OUTCOME CRITERIA

Short-term
Adequate knowledge, as evidenced by client's statements about disease, treatment expectation and progression, and measures to prevent injury or infection (expected within 1 week)

Long-term
Adequate knowledge, as evidenced by compliance with treatment regimens, resulting in optimal health and return to optimal functioning (expected within 1 month).

NURSING INTERVENTIONS/INSTRUCTIONS

1. Assess life-style, ability to adapt, learning abilities, and family participation and support (first visit).
2. Assess operative site for size, color, temperature, approximation of edges of incision, presence of drainage, and need for dressing change (each visit).
3. Instruct client to notify physician of changes in incisional area or temperature elevation (first visit).
4. Assess changes in vital signs, posture, gait, balance, and use of operative side (each visit).
5. Instruct client in administration of analgesics, including dose, frequency, side effects, and food/drug/alcohol interactions; differentiate between operative and phantom breast pain, numbness and pins-and-needles sensation in area, and advise that these will eventually disappear (first visit).
6. Instruct client in measures to prevent or minimize injury or infection, to protect arm from exposure and bumping, and to have all blood pressure checks, injections, and blood withdrawals done on unaffected arm (first visit and reinforce on second visit).
7. Avoid any burns, cuts, knicks, scratches, or insect bites or stings of affected arm on operative side (first visit).
8. Instruct client to wear clothing over arm that is protective, loose, and non-restrictive and to avoid carrying purse or parcels with arm on affected side (first visit).
9. Instruct client to always cleanse all skin breaks and apply antiseptic and to notify physician if arm becomes red, hot, or swollen (first visit).
10. Discuss and provide written information about prescribed adjuvant therapy, such as chemotherapy or radiation, and inform client of protocols regarding these treatments and when to appear at clinic or agency for therapy (each visit).
11. Demonstrate and instruct client in breast self-examination (BSE) for remaining breast and to perform examination each month after menstrual period or if menopausal (third or fourth visit).
12. Instruct client to keep physician appointments and to have yearly mammogram, and ultrasound if needed, on remaining breast (fourth visit).
13. Initiate referral to support groups such as Reach for

Recovery, I Can Cope, or psychological counseling if appropriate (first visit).

CLIENT AND FAMILY/CARETAKER INTERVENTIONS

1. Monitor wound healing, and notify physician of changes at site or fever.
2. Administer analgesic for pain, and verbalize pain descriptors and causes.
3. Prevent any injury to arm on operative side; protect and support arm as needed.
4. Read and interpret written information on adjuvant therapies, and ask questions to clarify information and modify behaviors.
5. Perform monthly BSE correctly and have yearly mammogram.
6. Keep appointments with physician and for therapies and tests.
7. Pariticipate in support group and/or counseling focusing on breast diseases and surgery.

Eye, ear, nose, and throat

◢ Auditory/Visual Impairment

Auditory impairment is the inability to hear adequately as a result of the aging process (presbycusis) or other physical or psychological condition. Visual impairment is the inability to see adequately as a result of the aging process (presbyopia) or other physical or psychological condition. Each type of loss imposes life-style changes upon an individual that require the use of an aid (hearing aid or glasses) to compensate for the impairment.

Home care is primarily concerned with teaching of the use and care of sensory aids and with prevention of injury as a result of the deficit.

Nursing diagnosis

Altered sensory perception (auditory, visual)

Related factors: Chronic illness; aging; neurologic disease or deficit; altered status of sense organ; psychologic stress

Defining characteristics: Hypoxia; electrolyte imbalance; use of drugs that affect the central nervous system (stimulants or depressants, mind altering); anxiety (narrowed perceptual fields); visual and auditory distortions; change in usual response to stimuli; expressed impairment in auditory and/or visual perception

OUTCOME CRITERIA

Short-term
Adequate sensory perception, as evidenced by client's awareness of need for life-style changes to compensate for auditory or visual loss (expected within 3 to 7 days)

Long-term
Optimal sensory perception, as evidenced by incorporation of life-style changes into activities of daily living and other activities to achieve health and functioning within identified limitations (expected within 1 month)

NURSING INTERVENTIONS/INSTRUCTIONS

1. Assess sensory abilities, limitations in activities of daily living imposed by sensory loss, and need for supplementary aids (see Eye, Ear, Nose, and Throat Assessment, p. 38, for guidelines) (first visit).
2. Interact with client in well-lit, quiet room free from external distractions, and allow time to process communication and respond (each visit).
3. Use as many sensory modalities as the client is comfortable with (each visit).
4. When communicating with a hearing-impaired individual (each visit):
   • Avoid covering mouth or chewing gum when speaking.
   • Face client.
   • Speak slowly and clearly; avoid shouting; a lower-pitched voice may help.
   • Repeat instruction or conversation if client does not respond or responds inappropriately.
   • Be sure hearing aid is turned on if present or that hearing aid is used.
5. When communicating with a visually impaired individual (each visit):
   • Announce arrival and departure.
   • Use touch only if indicating that you will do so and if client does not object.
   • Include client in all conversation, and speak in moderate tone.
   • Sit directly in front of client, in a well-lit room.
   • Be sure glasses or contact lenses are used.
6. Encourage use of assistive aids or devices, such as large-print reading material or Braille, large-numbered telephone dials, amplified telephone box, and closed-caption or narrative TV (first visit).
7. Instruct client about importance of annual examination for eye or ear disorders or deficits (first visit).

8. Instruct client in administration of eyedrops, ointments, eardrops, or other prescribed treatments (first visit).
9. Support referral to community resources for assistance and information (first visit).

CLIENT AND FAMILY/CARETAKER INTERVENTIONS

1. Use communication skills that are meaningful for client with a particular sensory deficit.
2. Use supplementary and assistive aids.
3. Consult physician about changes in perception and for yearly or more frequent examinations.
4. Seek out community resources that assist hearing or visually impaired individuals and families.

Nursing diagnosis

High risk for trauma

Related factors: Poor vision or hearing; lack of safety precautions and education

Defining characteristics: Request for information on preventing falls or other injury; reluctance to engage in activities (self-care and social)

OUTCOME CRITERIA

Short-term
Absence of injury, as evidenced by compliance with safety precautions and use of assistive aids (expected within 2 days)

Long-term
Maintenance of optimal health and functioning without injury (expected within 2 weeks and thereafter)

NURSING INTERVENTIONS/INSTRUCTIONS

1. Assist client in identifying limitations and safety hazards in the environment (first visit).
2. Assess ability of client to problem solve and to resolve these threats to safety (first visit).
3. Instruct client and family to provide and maintain clear pathways, remove throw rugs and clutter, and maintain intact cords and electrical appliances (first visit).

4. Instruct family to provide constant, adequate, well-distributed, glare-free light in all rooms and to place night-light in bathroom (first visit).
5. Instruct client to take time when adjusting to changes in light intensity, especially when climbing stairs (first visit).
6. Emphasize importance of using aids at all times (first visit).
7. Supply client with a list of available supplemental aids for telephone, reading material, doorbell, and others specific to client (first visit).
8. Instruct family and client to retain furniture placement and familiarity of environment and to provide rails or objects to hold on to when moving about (first visit).

CLIENT AND FAMILY/CARETAKER INTERVENTIONS

1. Identify hazards and eliminate or modify them.
2. Allow time for all activities; seek assistance when needed.
3. Use assistive and supplemental aids.
4. Maintain familiar environment; obtain assistance from trained pet for hearing or vision if appropriate.

◣ Cataract Removal and Lens Implantation

Cataract removal is the surgical removal of a lens that has become cloudy or opaque, causing visual impairment. Cataract development may be caused by senile degeneration, congenital trauma, disease (diabetes mellitus), or drug therapy (corticosteroids). The method of removing a cataract depends on a client's particular type of cataract and particular eye, and the time for removal is determined by the extent of impairment experienced (reading, driving, participation in activities). A cataract may be removed by intracapsular extraction, in which the entire lens is removed, including the capsule that surrounds it, by touching the lens with a cold probe that freezes the lens and then removes it from the eye. Another method is extracapsular extraction, in which the back portion of the capsule is left behind to help secure an intraocular lens implant and hold the vitreous fluid in proper position inside the eye. A third method is extracapsular extraction in which the cataract is broken into small particles by ultrasound and then suctioned out of the eye. A hard or soft lens may be implanted to replace the lens that has been removed. An alternative to the intraocular lens implant is the use of cataract glasses or contact lenses.

Home care is primarily concerned with the teaching of medication regimens (eyedrops and ointment) and measures to prevent complications of infection, glaucoma, retinal detachment, or corneal damage.

Nursing diagnosis

Altered sensory perception (visual)

Related factors: Altered status of sense organ

Defining characteristics: Bandaged eye; reduced visual acuity in nonoperative eye; change in visual acuity until operative eye stabilizes

OUTCOME CRITERIA
Short-term
Improved visual acuity in operative eye, as evidenced by client's statements that vision is improving to baseline expectation and by compliance with postoperative eye medication regimen (expected within 3 days)

Long-term
Return of visual acuity and stabilization, as evidenced by return to 20/20 or 20/30 vision (expected within 4 weeks)

NURSING INTERVENTIONS/INSTRUCTIONS
1. Announce your presence when entering room while client's eye is covered; use normal tone of voice (each visit).
2. Advise client that someone should be in attendance while anesthesia is metabolized and eye is covered (first visit).
3. Inform client of activities that require assistance and determine if referral for home health aide is needed (first visit).
4. Inform client of postoperative visits to physician on first, second, and seventh postoperative days for examination of operative eye and possible suture removal (first visit).

5. Inform client of visual progression (first visit):
   - Dark glasses may be suggested to reduce glare.
   - New prescription for lens in glasses on operative eye may be secured.
   - Diplopia may result after unilateral correction.
   - Use of interim glasses will result in clear central vision only, and head must be turned to bring peripheral objects into central vision.
   - Depth perception will be affected if one eye covered or implant not performed
   - Contact lenses may be used in some instances and require fewer adaptations.
   - If lens is not implanted, permanent lenses in glasses will be prescribed 4 to 12 weeks postoperatively.
   - Gradual adaptation and full adjustment occur for optimal vision.

CLIENT AND FAMILY/CARETAKER INTERVENTIONS

1. Participate in activities of daily living (ADL) and other activities (driving, reading, TV) within 1 week of surgery with physician recommendation.
2. Wear corrective lenses as prescribed.
3. Notify physician if vision changes or decreases.
4. Comply with postoperative physician visits until discharged.

Nursing diagnosis

Knowledge deficit

Related factors: Lack of exposure to information about postoperative care

Defining characteristics: Request for information about medication regimen to prevent infection, prevent increased intraocular pressure, and reduce inflammation and about protection of eye from trauma

OUTCOME CRITERIA

Short-term

Adequate knowledge, as evidenced by client's stating responsibilities to be carried out postoperatively to prevent complications (expected within 2 to 3 days)

Long-term
Adequate knowledge, as evidenced by absence of infection, glaucoma, or trauma of operative eye and by compliance with treatment regimen (expected within 4 weeks)

NURSING INTERVENTIONS/INSTRUCTIONS

1. Inspect eye after dressing removed; note color, and check for edema and presence of purulent drainage (each visit).
2. Assess for return of vision and increased acuity (each visit).
3. Assess for headache or pain and severity; instruct client to notify physician if pain sharp and sudden and not relieved (first visit).
4. Instruct client in eye care (cleansing from inner to outer area), hand washing, and administration of eyedrops and eye ointment (steroids, antibiotics, mydriatics), and include dose, technique, frequency, side effects, and implications for activity (first visit).
5. Instruct client to protect eye with shield during sleep for 1 week after physician removes initial dressing and shield (first visit).
6. Instruct client to avoid lifting, stooping, straining, bending, rubbing or bumping eye, or sneezing; instruct client to use stool softener and/or cough suppressant if needed (first visit).
7. Instruct client in positioning during sleep: rest on back or on nonoperative side; avoid lying flat; use small pillow or raise head of bed with foam rubber wedge (first visit).
8. Instruct client to ambulate carefully to avoid bumping or jostling (first visit).
9. Instruct client to use eye medications until entire amount is administered or to follow physician's instructions for length of therapy (first visit).

CLIENT AND FAMILY/CARETAKER INTERVENTIONS

1. Perform medical asepsis procedures before eye care and medication administration.
2. Use warm compress to remove discharge from operative eye.
3. Protect eye with shield, glasses, or both.
4. Avoid activities that will cause injury or increase intraocular pressure.

5. Participate in ADL with assistance if needed or independently.
6. Instill eyedrops or apply eye ointment correctly and safely, as instructed and prescribed.
7. Rest and sleep in optimal position without placing pressure on eye.
8. Report any sudden pain or change in vision to physician immediately.

Psychiatric care plans

◣ Alcohol/Drug Abuse

Alcohol or drug abuse is a progressive disorder that affects all body systems. It can precipitate cirrhosis of the liver, esophageal varicies, coma, and death. Several theories describe the alcoholic or drug abuser as having a fixed outlook, retarded emotional development, poor impulse control, chronic low self-esteem, and low frustration tolerance and as being highly dependent. Serious family dysfunction can contribute to alcohol or drug abuse.

Home care primarily focuses on the teaching of a medication regimen and on life-style changes

Nursing diagnosis

Altered thought process

Related factors: Physiologic changes; impaired judgment

Defining characteristics: Inaccurate interpretation of environment; distractibility; egocentricity; hypervigilance or hypovigilance

OUTCOME CRITERIA

Short-term
Adequate thought process, as evidenced by client's identifying correctly activities happening in his or her environment and by client's being oriented to surroundings after prompting by health care worker (expected in 3 days)

Long-term
Adequate thought processes, as evidenced by client verbalizing that alcohol or drugs have caused alteration in thought (expected in 2 months)

NURSING INTERVENTIONS/INSTRUCTIONS

1. Assess for memory deficits (long, short) by asking questions about the past and the present (first visit).
2. Provide an unhurried, patient, reassuring approach to the client that is both positive and empathetic (each visit).
3. Assist in helping the client to order recent events according to time sequence. Provide support for correct answers (each visit).
4. Explore with the client his or her perception of self; reinforce reality when appropriate (each visit).
5. Plan and implement a consistent approach to the client's care (each visit).
6. Repeat for the client instructions or information; ask the client to restate information in his or her own words (each visit).
7. Use patterns of recall (each visit).
8. Limit sensory input and choices to decrease distractions and frustrations (each visit).
9. Ask the client to make realistic commitments, and hold the client accountable for fulfillment of commitments (any visit).

CLIENT AND FAMILY/CARETAKER INTERVENTIONS

1. Maintain calm, caring attitude during treatment; stay with client.
2. Attempt to prevent or discourage stressful situations.
3. Develop and use effective coping skills that decrease anxiety.

Nursing diagnosis

Ineffective individual coping

Related factors: Personal vulnerability; difficulty handling new situations; previous ineffective or inadequate coping skills; inadequate coping skills, with substitution of alcohol, anxiety, fear

Defining characteristics: Verbalization of inability to cope or inability to ask for help; inability to meet role expectations;

inability to meet basic needs; inability to problem solve; alteration in societal participation; destructive behavior toward self or others; inappropriate use of defense mechanisms; change in usual communication patterns; verbal manipulation

OUTCOME CRITERIA

Short-term
Effective individual coping, as evidenced by client's attending support group (such as Alcoholics Anonymous) and verbalizing relationship of alcohol or drug abuse to difficulty in present life situation (expected within 7 days)

Long-term
Effective individual coping, as evidenced by client's making necessary life-style changes (expected within 2 months)

NURSING INTERVENTIONS/INSTRUCTIONS

1. Assess for psychosomatic symptoms: sleep, eating, bowel problems (each visit).
2. Assess support system, how the system functions, and if it is adequate (first visit).
3. Establish rapport, show acceptance of the person, and establish a positive relationship with him or her (each visit).
4. Reduce the number of decisions that the client must make, including the need to problem solve (first visit).
5. Allow client sufficient time to make decisions; start with decisions that have only two options (first and second visits).
6. Discuss alternative ways of coping; allow these new coping techniques to be tried in a safe, nondestructive environment (each visit).
7. Use positive rather than negative reinforcement during the testing of new coping mechanisms (each visit).
8. Allow client time to verbalize feelings of denial, anger, guilt, or grief regarding crisis situation (each visit).
9. Acknowledge the validity of fear and other feelings (each visit).
10. Encourage client to talk about the changes the crisis will cause (each visit).
11. Listen and clarify the client's perception of the crisis situation (each visit).

12. Assist client to sort out the facts concerning the crisis (any visit).
13. Assist client in seeking and accepting help, and provide referral to psychiatrist or psychologist if needed (each visit).
14. Identify defense mechanisms used and whether they are being used positively or negatively. Reinforce positive coping mechanisms that have been successfully used in the past but that are not being used now (any visit).

CLIENT AND FAMILY/CARETAKER INTERVENTIONS

1. Include the family in sorting out information regarding the crisis.
2. Discuss with the family the need to avoid judgments regarding the client's behavior.
3. Refer to Al-Anon or other support group for family.

Nursing diagnosis

Knowledge deficit

Related factors: Lack of recall; misinterpretation of information; cognitive limitation; lack of interest in learning

Defining characteristics: Verbalization of the problem; inappropriate or exaggerated behavior (e.g., hysterical, hostile, agitated, apathetic); inaccurate follow-through of instructions; inaccurate performance on test

OUTCOME CRITERIA

Short-term
Adequate knowledge, as evidenced by client's explaining needed life-style changes and medication regimen and by client's ability to verbalize the effects of substance abuse and its affects on therapies (expected within 5 days)

Long-term
Adequate knowledge, as evidenced by client's demonstrating change in life-style, following through with medication regimen and rehabilitation, and verbalizing the advantages of abstaining from alcohol or drug abuse (expected within 1 month)

NURSING INTERVENTIONS/INSTRUCTIONS

1. Assess client's strengths and weaknesses through interviewing, and determine previous interests or areas of success (first visit).
2. Assess client's knowledge regarding Antabuse therapy: action, side effects, and response if patient drinks while on Antabuse (first visit).
3. Assess client's developmental level, educational level, vocabulary level, and past decisions regarding health practices (first visit).
4. Assess information client has about life-style change that is needed by asking specific questions (first visit).
5. Discuss what needs to be taught and who needs to be taught, including family members who may be responsible for health care (first and second visits).
6. Provide positive feedback for participation and adequate information (each visit).
7. Demonstrate techniques using several sessions; increase difficulty at each session; require return demonstration after each session.
8. Evaluate teaching plan (any visit).

CLIENT AND FAMILY/CARETAKER INTERVENTIONS

1. Determine progress with the client, and revise schedules on the basis of observed progress.
2. Use available resources for health maintenance and delivery, with client's input.
3. Institute appropriate referrals and use of support systems through community agencies.

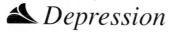

Depression

Depression is an affective disorder characterized by an altered mood with symptoms of poor self-esteem, sadness, guilt, hopelessness, emptiness, and despondency. Views about the cause of depression include environmental, societal, genetic, and biomedical theories.

Home care is primarily concerned with the teaching of medication regimens and life-style changes that may be needed, providing a safe environment (frequently after hospitalization), and maintenance of daily well-being.

Nursing diagnosis

Hopelessness

Related factors: Prolonged activity restriction, creating isolation; failing or deteriorating physiologic condition; long-term stress; abandonment; lost belief in transcendent values (i.e., God)

Defining characteristics: Passivity, decreased verbalization; decreased affect; verbal cues (despondent content); turning away from speaker; closing eyes; decreased appetite; increased sleep; lack of initiative; decreased response to stimuli

OUTCOME CRITERIA

Short-term
Decreased hopelessness, as evidenced by decreased negative verbalization and increased eye contact with health care provider (expected within 3 days)

Long-term
Decreased hopelessness, as evidenced by increased involvement in care and activities (expected within 1 month)

NURSING INTERVENTIONS/INSTRUCTIONS

1. Assess for isolation (physical, emotional, spiritual), chronic stress, and poor physical health (first visit).
2. Assess for defense mechanisms used: denial, isolation, regression (first visit).
3. Assess for nonverbal and verbal indicators of hopelessness: poor eye contact, slumped posture, flat affect, monotone speech, retarded speech (first visit).
4. Discuss how life used to be and activities performed when client was happy (first visit).
5. Allow client to take as much responsibility as possible in own care (each visit).
6. Assist client to set realistic goals in areas of life that he or she can control (first and second visits).

7. Discuss how life has changed and what would make life satisfying again (any visit).
8. Provide referral to appropriate groups, depending on client's condition (any visit).

CLIENT AND FAMILY/CARETAKER INTERVENTIONS

1. Include family in planning, including referrals to outside agencies for help.
2. Attempt to prevent or discourage stressful situations.
3. Develop and use effective coping skills that decrease depression.

Nursing diagnosis

Ineffective individual coping

Related factors: Personal vulnerability; difficulty in handling new situations; previous ineffective or inadequate coping skills; inadequate coping skills, with substitution of alcohol, anxiety, fear

Defining characteristics: Verbalization of inability to cope or inability to ask for help; inability to meet role expectations; inability to meet basic needs; inability to problem solve; alteration in societal participation; destructive behavior toward self or others; inappropriate use of defense mechanisms; change in usual communication patterns; verbal manipulation

OUTCOME CRITERIA

Short-term
Effective individual coping, as evidenced by client's statement of life-style changes that relieve depression (expected within 5 days)

Long-term
Effective individual coping as evidenced by client's achievement of necessary life-style changes and by client's understanding of relationship between feelings and antecedent event (expected within 1 month)

NURSING INTERVENTIONS/INSTRUCTIONS

1. Assess for psychosomatic symptoms: sleep problems, eating problems, bowel problems (first visit).
2. Assess support system and how the system functions (first visit).
3. Encourage and assist client to identify feelings and relationship between feelings and event/stressor when event is known (each visit).
4. Establish rapport, show acceptance of the person, and establish a positive, concerned relationship with him or her (each visit).
5. Reduce the number of decisions that the patient must make, including the need to problem solve (first and second visits).
6. Allow client sufficient time to make decisions; start with decisions that have only two options (first and second visits).
7. Discuss alternative ways of coping; allow these new coping techniques to be tried in a safe, nondestructive environment (any visit).
8. Use positive rather than negative reinforcement during the testing of new coping mechanisms (each visit).
9. Allow client time to verbalize feelings of denial, anger, guilt, or grief regarding crisis situation (each visit).
10. Acknowledge the validity of fear, hostility, and anxiety (any visit).
11. Encourage the client to talk about the changes the situation has caused (any visit).
12. Listen to and clarify the client's perception of the situation (any visit).
13. Assist the client to sort out the facts concerning the situation (any visit).
14. Identify defense mechanisms used, and determine whether they are being used positively or negatively. Reinforce positive coping mechanisms that have been successfully used in the past but that are not currently being used (any visit).
15. Avoid giving false reassurance (each visit).
16. Assist the client to recognize early symptoms of depression and ways to alleviate them (first visit).

CLIENT AND FAMILY/CARETAKER INTERVENTIONS

1. Seek and accept help, and utilize referral to day care, crisis center, psychiatrist, or psychologist, if needed.
2. Sort out and analyze information from the family regarding the crisis.
3. Avoid judgments regarding the client's behavior.

Nursing diagnosis

Impaired social interaction

Related factors: Knowledge/skill deficit about ways to enhance mutuality; communication barriers; absence of available significant others or peers; limited physical mobility; therapeutic isolation; sociocultural dissonance; environmental barriers; altered thought processes

Defining characteristics. Verbalized or observed discomfort in social situation; verbalized or observed inability to receive or communicate a satisfying sense of belonging, caring, interest, or shared history; observed use of unsuccessful social interaction behaviors; dysfunctional interaction with peers, family, and/or others; family report of change of style or pattern of interaction

OUTCOME CRITERIA

Short-term
Adequate socialization, as evidenced by client's communicating with significant others and requesting other people to interact with him or her (expected within 1 week)

Long-term
Adequate socialization, as evidenced by client's expressing interests that are appropriate to developmental age or stage, use of eye contact while interacting, and absence of hostility in voice and behavior (expected within 1 month)

NURSING INTERVENTIONS/INSTRUCTIONS

1. Assess for limited social contacts, preoccupation with own thoughts and feelings, and number of social contacts per week (first visit).
2. Assess for positive feelings that occur from contact with others (first visit).

3. Discuss being alone, amount of time needed, and how client feels during this time (any visit).
4. Acknowledge feelings of loneliness, and discuss feelings of rejection, hostility, and insecurity (any visit).
5. Identify cultural norms, and discuss how isolation occurs when social norms are not followed (any visit).
6. Identify behaviors that are not considered socially acceptable to dominant culture; acknowledge and reinforce acceptable behaviors (any visit).
7. Discuss frequent testing of relationships and how testing may lead to social isolation (any visit).
8. Encourage verbal communication, eye contact, and involvement in community functions (any visit).

CLIENT AND FAMILY/CARETAKER INTERVENTIONS

1. Attempt to prevent or discourage interactions with negative individuals.
2. Develop and use effective coping skills that decrease isolation.

Nursing diagnosis

Knowledge deficit

Related factors: Lack of exposure to information; lack of recall; misinterpretation of information; cognitive limitation; lack of interest in learning; unfamiliarity with information resources

Defining characteristics: Verbalization of the problem; inappropriate or exaggerated behavior (e.g., hysterical, hostile, agitated, apathetic); inaccurate follow-through of instructions; inaccurate performance on test

OUTCOME CRITERIA

Short-term
Adequate knowledge, as evidenced by client's ability to explain reasons for depression (expected within 3 days)

Long-term
Adequate knowledge, as evidened by client's ability to demonstrate needed life-style changes, participate in treatment programs, and identify resources (expected within 1 month)

NURSING INTERVENTIONS/INSTRUCTIONS

1. Assess strengths and weaknesses through interviewing, and determine previous interest areas of success (first visit).
2. Assess developmental level, educational level, vocabulary level, age, and past discussion regarding health practices (first visit).
3. Assess extent of client's information about depression by asking specific questions (first visit).
4. Provide information about drug therapy, potential side effects, precautions, and benefits, and emphasize that client is not to stop drug suddenly (first visit).
5. Refer client to support agencies and resources (any visit).
6. Discuss progress with the client, and revise schedules based on observed progress (any visit).
7. Provide written instructions as well as verbal instructions (each visit).

CLIENT AND FAMILY/CARETAKER INTERVENTIONS

1. Administer drug therapy correctly and consistently, and note progress to report or need for change in therapy.
2. Use available resources for health maintenance and delivery.

◣ *Physical/Emotional Abuse*

Physical abuse is considered to be a destructive act or injury inflicted by a caregiver. Emotional abuse includes threats and acts of degradation that are damaging to a person's self-worth.

Home care is primarily concerned with the teaching aspects of symptoms of abuse and with adequate prevention, evaluation, and reporting of abuse.

Nursing diagnosis

High risk for trauma

Related factors: Interactive conditions between individual and environment that pose a risk to the defensive and adaptive resources of the individual

Defining characteristics: Internal environment: weakness; poor vision; balancing difficulties; lack of safety or drug education; lack of proper precautions; cognitive or emotional difficulties. External environment: people or provider.

OUTCOME CRITERIA

Short-term
Absence of trauma, as evidenced by client's statement that trauma has not occurred (expected within 1 week)

Long-term
Absence of trauma, as evidenced by absence of falls, injuries, or death from abuse (expected within 2 months)

NURSING INTERVENTIONS/INSTRUCTIONS

1. Assess client, situation, and environment for potentially abusive situation (first visit).
2. Identify and remove actual dangers in the environment (see Defining Characteristics) (each visit).

CLIENT AND FAMILY/CARETAKER INTERVENTIONS

1. Increase awareness of the possibility of abuse by family and caregivers.
2. Provide for respite care of client to relieve caregiver.

Nursing diagnosis

Altered family processes

Related factors: Situational transition or crisis; developmental transition or crisis

Defining characterstics: Family system unable to meet physical needs of its members; family system unable to meet emotional needs of its members; family system unable to meet spiritual needs of its members; inability to express or accept wide range of feelings; inability to express or accept feelings of members; family unable to meet security needs of its members; inability of family members to relate to each other for mutual growth and maturation; family uninvolved in community activities; inability to accept or receive help appropriately; rigidity in function and roles; family not demonstrating respect for individuality and autonomy of its members; family unable to adapt to change or deal with traumatic experience constructively; family failing to accomplish current or past developmental tasks; unhealthy family decision-making process; failure to send and receive clear messages; inappropriate boundary maintenance; inappropriate or poorly communicated family rules; rituals, symbols; unexamined family myths; inappropriate level and direction of energy

OUTCOME CRITERIA

Short-term
Family allows for individual differences of its members (expected within 1 week)

Long-term
Family allows for all individuals to be involved in the decision-making process; all family members state that basic needs (physical, emotional, spiritual) are being met within the family (expected within 3 months)

NURSING INTERVENTIONS/INSTRUCTIONS

1. Assess decision-making or problem-solving techniques used in the family (who influences the decisions in the family, who makes the final decision, all persons involved in the process) (first visit).
2. Assess the developmental stage of the family and of each member (are there developmental lags in any one of the members) (first visit).
3. Assess for coalitions in the family (who takes whose side during arguments), triangling, and scapegoating) (first visit).
4. Assess the realistic view of the crisis (first visit).
5. Assess the availability of support systems outside the family (any visit).
6. Identify ineffective coping mechanisms used; acknowledge and encourage positive coping mechanisms (each visit).
7. Discuss ambivalence, hostility, guilt, and anxiety and how these emotions affect the family; discuss verbalizing these feelings and emotions (each visit).
8. Assist the family to identify the major stressors in the family (each visit).
9. Allow client and family to verbalize about situational or maturational crises that are occurring within the family; determine whether family crises are occurring at the same time as individual crises (each visit).

10. Discuss the concept of tolerance and how a nonjudgmental attitude leads to feelings of security in the family (first visit).
11 Identify the family's need for further professional help, and refer them to appropriate agencies (any visit).

CLIENT AND FAMILY/CARETAKER INTERVENTIONS

1. Family involved in decision making related to the client.
2. Avoid severe stressors in the family, and develop more appropriate coping mechanisms.

Nursing diagnosis

Impaired home maintenance management

Related factors: Disease or injury of family member; insufficient family organization or planning; insufficient finances; unfamiliarity with neighborhood resources; impaired cognitive or emotional functioning; lack of knowledge; lack of role modeling; inadequate support systems

Defining characteristics: Household members express difficulty in maintaining their home in a comfortable fashion; household requests assistance with home maintenance; household members describe outstanding debts or financial crises; disorderly surroundings; unwashed or unavailable cooking equipment, clothes, or linens; accumulation of dirt, food wastes, or hygienic wastes; offensive odors; inappropriate household temperature; overtaxed family members (e.g., exhausted, anxious); lack of necessary equipment or aids; presence of vermin or rodents; repeated hygienic disorders; infestations, or infections

OUTCOME CRITERIA

Short-term
Absence of dirt, food wastes, or hygienic waste; absence of offensive odors; washed or available cooking equipment, clothing, linens; absence of hygienic disorders, infestations, infections; absence of vermin (expected within 1 week)

Long-term
Household members state ease in maintaining home in comfortable fashion (expected within 3 months)

NURSING INTERVENTIONS/INSTRUCTIONS

1. Assess mental status, including orientation, affect, and level of consciousness (first visit).
2. Assess mobility (ambulation, equipment needed) (first visit).
3. Assess self-care abilities (hygiene, dressing, eating) (first visit).
4. Assess housekeeping skills (first visit).
5. Assess ability to organize housekeeping activities (first visit).
6. Provide referral for outside help or preparation of meals if needed (any visit).
7. Discuss making an organizational plan to be followed daily; include all family members (first visit).
8. Discuss rotation of household chores (first visit).
9. Discuss preparation of meals for 2 days or the entire week (any visit).

CLIENT AND FAMILY/CARETAKER INTERVENTIONS

1. Reorganize family chores.
2. Utilize family and persons in the community who may help with home maintenance.

Nursing diagnosis

Knowledge deficit

Related factors: Lack of exposure to information; lack of recall; misinterpretation of information; cognitive limitation; lack of interest in learning; unfamiliarity with information resources

Defining characteristics: Verbalization of the problem; inappropriate or exaggerated behavior (e.g., hysterical, hostile, agitated, apathetic); inaccurate follow-through of instructions; inaccurate performance on test

OUTCOME CRITERIA

Short-term
Adequate knowledge, as evidenced by client's ability to verbalize definition of signs and symptoms of abusive behavior (expected within 3 days)

Long-term
Adequate knowledge, as evidenced by client's ability to report
abuse (expected in 2 weeks)

NURSING INTERVENTIONS/INSTRUCTIONS

1. Assess strengths and weaknesses of relationship between
   caretaker and client (first visit).
2. Assess information known about abuse; ask specific questions (first visit).
3. Discuss what needs to be taught (first visit).
4. Discuss abuse, symptoms, and prevention (any visit).

CLIENT AND FAMILY/CARETAKER INTERVENTIONS

1. Use available resources for prevention of abuse; use
   client's input.
2. Institute appropriate use of support systems and referrals to
   community agencies.

◣ *Schizophrenia*

A group of disorders about which little is known, schizophre-
nias are characterized as psychoses. Symptoms include looseness of associations, ambivalence, autistic thought, and disturbances of affect. A break with reality also occurs, leading to
severe problems with communication, day-to-day functioning,
and personal relationships. Schizophrenia may be categorized
as catatonic, paranoid, undifferentiated, or residual.

**Home care primarily focuses on the teaching of a med-
ication regimen, activities of daily living, and establishing
rapport with one caregiver.**

Nursing diagnosis

Ineffective individual coping

Related factors: Personal vulnerability; difficulty handling new situations; previous ineffective or inadequate coping skills; inadequate coping skills with substitution of anxiety, fear

Defining characteristics: Inability to meet role expectations; inability to meet basic needs; inability to problem solve; alteration in societal participation; destructive behavior toward self or others; inappropriate use of defense mechanisms; change in usual communication patterns

OUTCOME CRITERIA

Short-term

Adequate individual coping, as evidenced by client's answering questions appropriately and absence of pacing (expected within 1 week)

Long-term

Adequate individual coping, as evidences by client's ability to participate in own care and activities of daily living (expected within 3 months)

NURSING INTERVENTIONS/INSTRUCTIONS

1. Reduce stimulation in the client's area; remove client from noise and bright light (first visit).
2. Assist client with activities that relieve overactivity, such as walking, pacing, or jogging (any visit).
3. Make clear-cut statements, omit details, and repeat statements as necessary (all visits).
4. Do not ask the client to make decisions because this will cause confusion (all visits).
5. Identify simple activities that the client can complete in a short time (any visit).
6. Instruct client in administration of antianxiety and neuroleptic medications as ordered (all visits).

CLIENT AND FAMILY/CARETAKER INTERVENTIONS

1. Include the family in sorting out information regarding the client's illness.

2. Discuss with the family the importance of avoiding judgments regarding the client's behavior.

Nursing diagnosis

High risk for violence directed at others

Related factors: Antisocial character; panic states; rage reactions

Defining characteristics: Body language: clenched fists, tense facial expressions, rigid posture, tautness indicating effort to control; hostile, threatening verbalizations: boasting about prior abuse of others; increased motor activity: pacing, excitement, irritability, agitation; overt aggressive acts: goal-directed destruction of objects in environment; substance abuse or withdrawal; suspicion of others, paranoid ideation, delusion, hallucinations

OUTCOME CRITERIA

Short-term
Absence of violence, as evidenced by absence of verbal abuse and absence of hostile posture (clenched fists, pacing agitation, rigidity, threatening verbal communication) (expected within 1 week)

Long-term
Absence of violence, as evidenced by absence of verbal threats or actions (expected within 3 months)

NURSING INTERVENTIONS/INSTRUCTIONS

1. Address the feeling responsible for the aggression (any visit).
2. Approach the client in a calm, reassuring way (all visits).
3. Look for early clues to aggression, such as pacing, muttering, or slapping fists, and try to intervene early (all visits).

CLIENT AND FAMILY/CARETAKER INTERVENTIONS

1. Deal with client's escalating behaviors.
2. Avoid placing emotional pressure on the client that may lead to violence.

Nursing diagnosis

Sensory/perceptual alteration

Related factors: Altered sensory reception, transmission, and/or integration; psychological stress

Defining characteristics: Restlessness; irritability; altered communication patterns; hallucinations

OUTCOME CRITERIA

Short-term
Controlled hallucinations (expected within 1 week)

Long-term
Absence of hallucinations (expected within 3 months)

NURSING INTERVENTIONS/INSTRUCTIONS

1. Observe for listening pose (tilting head, nodding) that indicates hallucination (all visits).
2. Establish reality during hallucinations by stating the client's name and present situation (all visits).
3. Ask the client to share the content of the hallucination, not to reinforce it but to prevent harm to himself or others (any visit).
4. Gear interactions with the client to feelings rather than thoughts (all visits).
5. Observe for specific activities or subjects that initiate hallucinations (any visit).

CLIENT AND FAMILY/CARETAKER INTERVENTIONS

1. Intervene when the client is hallucinating.
2. Distract the client when he or she is hallucinating.

Nursing diagnosis

Knowledge deficit

Related factors: Lack of recall; misinterpretation of information; cognitive limitation; lack of interest in learning

Defining characteristics: Inappropriate or exaggerated behavior (e.g., hysterical, hostile, agitated, apathetic); inaccurate follow-through of instructions; inaccurate performance on test

OUTCOME CRITERIA

Short-term
Adequate knowledge, as evidenced by client's explaining needed life-style changes and medication regimen (expected within 5 days)

Long-term
Adequate knowledge, as evidenced by client's demonstrating change in life-style and following through with medication regimen and rehabilitation (expected within 1 month)

NURSING INTERVENTIONS/INSTRUCTIONS

1. Assess client's strengths and weaknesses through interviewing, and determine previous interests or areas of success (first visit).
2. Assess client's developmental level, education level, vocabulary level, and past decisions regarding health practices (first visit).
3. Discuss what needs to be taught; include in the discussion family members who may be responsible for health care (first visit).
4. Provide positive feedback for participation and adequate information (any visit).
5. Demonstrate techniques using several sessions; increase difficulty at each session; require return demonstration after each session.
6. Evaluate teaching plan (any visit).

CLIENT AND FAMILY/CARETAKER INTERVENTIONS

1. Revise schedules on the basis of observed progress.
2. Use available resources for health maintenance and delivery; use client's input.
3. Institute appropriate referrals and support systems through community agencies.

General care plans

◣ Chemotherapy and External Radiation Therapy

Chemotherapy and radiation therapy are treatment modalities that are used to cure, control, or palliate cancer. Radiation therapy may be administered alone or in combination with surgery or chemotherapy. Chemotherapy protocols include alkylating agents, antimetabolites, antitumor antibiotics, plant alkaloids, nitrosureas, corticosteroids, hormones, and unclassified miscellaneous and investigational drugs. These agents are given in combination for prescribed periods of time and frequency, depending on the malignancy being treated. They may be administered by oral, intramuscular, intravenous, intrathecal, intraarterial, intracavity, subcutaneous, topical, intraperitoneal, or perfusion routes, depending on tumor site.

Home care is primarily concerned with administration of chemotherapy, teaching of the physical and emotional effects and resulting care and needs during administration of chemotherapy and/or radiation therapy, and assessment and treatment of side effects.

Nursing diagnosis

Ineffective individual coping

Related factors: Multiple life changes; inadequate coping methods

Defining characteristics: Verbalization of inability to cope or ask for help; inability to problem solve; chronic worry and anxiety; inappropriate use of defense mechanisms

OUTCOME CRITERIA

Short-term
Improved coping, as evidenced by client's statement of under-standing of need for adaptations in life-style and positive coping strategies (expected within 1 week)

Long-term
Optimal coping, as evidenced by client's participation in and adaptation to altered life-style and by client's compliance with medical regimen to maintain optimal health and functioning (expected within 1 to 2 months)

NURSING INTERVENTIONS/INSTRUCTIONS

1. Assess for developmental level and dependency needs, mental status, behavioral and emotional changes, use of defense mechanisms and their effectiveness, and ability to problem solve (first visit).
2. Establish a trusting relationship and facilitate an open discussion to explore options and develop skills in coping and problem solving (each visit).
3. Help client to identify coping skills that work, and encourage positive feeling about success of any adaptation or changes (each visit).
4. Include client in all planning and formulation of realistic goals; assist if requested to do so (each visit).
5. Provide accepting, nonjudgmental attitude and environment when teaching and discussing needs and changes to be made in life-style (each visit).
6. Encourage expressions of fears, concerns, and questions regarding therapy and effects (each visit).
7. Initiate social services and counseling referrals (any visit).

CLIENT AND FAMILY/CARETAKER INTERVENTIONS

1. Develop coping for long-term treatment and possible outcome.
2. Share feelings, fears, concerns with caretaker, family.
3. Plan and participate in own care and health promotion.
4. Set goals and strategies for coping with life-style changes.
5. Participate in support group with those who have similar conditions.
6. Utilize social services, counseling, and clergy as needed.

Nursing diagnosis

Altered nutrition: less than body requirements

Related factors: Inability to ingest and absorb nutrients because of biologic factors (chemotherapy/radiation therapy)

Defining characteristics: Anorexia; lack of interest in food; weakness; fatigue; weight loss; inadequate nutritional intake; stomatitis; vomiting; altered taste perception; mucositis of bowel

OUTCOME CRITERIA

Short-term
Adequate nutrition, as evidenced by intake of prescribed dietary regimen and stabilization of weight without anorexia, nausea, and vomiting (expected within 1 to 2 weeks)

Long-term
Adequate nutritional status, as evidenced by intake of required nutrients for optimal health and functioning during and after therapy (expected within 1 month and ongoing)

NURSING INTERVENTIONS/INSTRUCTIONS

1. Assess nutritional status, including food preferences, cultural and religious restrictions, caloric requirements, and effect of different medications on food intake (first visit).
2. Calculate ideal weight for size, sex, frame, and height; instruct client in measuring weight weekly (first visit).
3. Assess for diarrhea, nausea, vomiting, anorexia, weight loss, fatigue, malaise, and reactions to meals (each visit).
4. Instruct client to schedule rest periods after meals and to have 6 to 8 hours of sleep per night (first visit).
5. Inform client of measures to facilitate eating, including eliminating odors; relaxed atmosphere; quiet environment; eating smaller, more frequent attractively prepared meals; taking antiemetics ½ hour before meals (first visit).
6. Inform client of newer antiemetics and success in controlling nausea and vomiting, and instruct in administration (first visit).
7. Instruct client to maintain a food diary for one week that includes type and amount of food consumed and method of preparation (first and second visits).

8. Instruct and include client in food selections for a high-protein, high-carbohydrate, high-caloric diet and to avoid hot, spicy foods; incorporate assessment data and food diary into menu planning (first and second visits).

9. Provide information for caloric and vitamin supplements (first visit).

10. Suggest oral hygiene before each meal (first visit).

11. If client's appetite is poor, suggest eating more frequent meals in smaller amounts and increasing amounts slowly as tolerated (first visit).

12. Initiate referral to nutritionist if needed (any visit).

13. Refer home health aide to assist with feeding and meal preparation as needed.

CLIENT AND FAMILY/CARETAKER INTERVENTIONS

1. Maintain or gain weight as determined.

2. Participate in planning and ingestion of well-balanced diet with restrictions as determined.

3. Promote pleasant environment, preferred food preparation, and dietary pattern that enhances intake.

4. Weigh weekly using same scale, at same time of day, wearing same amount of clothing, and record in a log.

5. Maintain a 7-day food diary listing types and amounts of all foods eaten.

6. Eat a high-protein, high-carbohydrate, high-calorie diet; to assist with meal preparation, secure a cookbook for cancer clients.

7. Use high-calorie supplements as needed.

8. Take daily vitamins.

9. Administer antiemetic 30 minutes before meals.

Nursing diagnosis

Diarrhea

Related factors: Inflammation or irritation of bowel; malabsorption of bowel (chemotherapy/radiation therapy)

Defining characteristics: Abdominal pain; cramping; increased frequency; loose, liquid stools; urgency; mucus in stool; increased frequency of bowel sounds; mucositis

OUTCOME CRITERIA

Short-term

Return of baseline bowel pattern, as evidenced by decrease in the frequency of bowel eliminations and by stool characteristics within baseline parameters (expected within 1 week)

Long-term

Minimal or absence of diarrheal bowel eliminations, as evidenced by soft formed stools eliminated according to baseline pattern (expected within 2 weeks)

NURSING INTERVENTIONS/INSTRUCTIONS

1. Assess bowel elimination patterns and stool characteristics (see Gastrointestinal System Assessment, p. 17, for guidelines) (first visit).
2. Instruct client to maintain a record of bowel movements, including number and when they occur and characteristics such as color, amount, consistency, odor, and presence of mucus, blood, or pus (first visit)
3. Monitor medication administration, and instruct in intake and output, antidiarrheals, and anticholingerics, monitor intake and output ratio with increased fluid intake (each visit).
4. Instruct client to notify physician if diarrhea becomes more severe or frequent, if bleeding is noted, or if fatigue or weakness is noted (first visit).

CLIENT AND FAMILY/CARETAKER INTERVENTIONS

1. Administer antidiarrheal correctly as needed.
2. Report diarrhea that is not controlled or reveals blood, pus, or mucus.
3. Adjust diet and avoid foods irritating to bowel.
4. Monitor fluid intake and output, and increase fluid intake up to 3000 ml/day as needed.

Nursing diagnosis

Altered oral mucous membrane

Related factors: Medication (chemotherapeutic agents)

Defining characteristics: Stomatitis, oral lesions or ulcers, oral pain or discomfort

OUTCOME CRITERIA

Short-term
Minimal changes in oral mucous mumbrane, as evidenced by decreased inflammation and oral pain and by intact mucous membrane (expected wtihin 4 to 7 days)

Long-term
Oral mucous membrane maintained intact, as evidenced by absence of stomatitis and associated signs and symptoms (expected within 1 to 2 weeks and ongoing during therapy)

NURSING INTERVENTIONS/INSTRUCTIONS

1. Assess oral cavity for redness, pain, ulcerations, dysphagia, and dryness (each visit).
2. Instruct client to provide mouth care after meals, to rinse mouth with saline, hydrogen peroxide or sodium bicarbonate solution, or viscous lidocaine every 2 hours or as needed and to avoid commercial mouthwashes or alcohol (first visit).
3. Instruct client to avoid mouth breathing, smoking, and hot and spicy or irritating foods (first visit).
4. Instruct client to avoid using a hard toothbrush and to remove dentures except for meals (first visit).
5. Instruct client to apply petroleum jelly or cocoa butter to lips and artificial saliva preparation to oral cavity; instruct client to use topical anesthetic and fungal antibiotic if prescribed (first visit).
6. Instruct client to take cool beverages, popsicles, and ice cream to soothe oral cavity (first visit).

CLIENT AND FAMILY/CARETAKER INTERVENTIONS

1. Assess oral cavity for stomatitis, and report condition that deteriorates in spite of treatments.
2. Perform oral care using soft brush, unwaxed floss, soft-tipped applicator, and mouth wash consisting of acceptable solution.
4. Apply topical preparations for dryness.
5. Avoid commercial products for mouth care and irritants to oral cavity, such as hot, spicy foods, alcohol, and tobacco, and ingest cool fluids and bland, smooth foods.

Nursing diagnosis

Impaired skin integrity

Related factors: Internal factor of medication (chemotherapy); external factor of radiation

Defining characteristics: Disruption of skin surfaces; dryness; pruritis; blistering, allergic rashes; hyperpigmentation; irritation and excoriation of perianal area from diarrhea

OUTCOME CRITERIA

Short-term
Skin intact, as evidenced by absence of irritation, dryness, rash, or breaks (expected within 1 week)

Long-term
Skin integrity maintained, as evidenced by absence of skin disruption and by skin protection to achieve optimal condition during treatments (expected ongoing during treatments)

NURSING INTERVENTIONS/INSTRUCTIONS

1. Assess for skin condition at irradiation site, itching, irritation at perianal area; assess skin for dryness, pruritis, rashes; review skin care protocol for clients receiving chemotherapy and/or radiation therapy (each visit).
2. Instruct client to cleanse skin with mild soap and warm water and pat dry; avoid using soap, lotions, or deodorants or washing or removing marks of any kind placed on skin at irradiation site (first visit).
3. Instruct client to avoid any massage, scratching, adhesive tape, pressure, or sun exposure to skin, to wear soft, loose clothing, and to use a sun screen for a year following treatment (first and second visits).
4. Instruct client to expose irradiation site to the air and to apply only prescribed preparations to skin twice a day, such as A & D Ointment for dryness, cornstarch to absorb moisture, and hydrocortisone cream to reduce inflammation (first visit).
5. Instruct client to cleanse and dry perianal area after each bowel elimination and to apply A & D Ointment or karaya gel to area (first visit).

6. Instruct client to assess for skin breakdown and to report any open areas to physician (first visit).

CLIENT AND FAMILY/CARETAKER INTERVENTIONS

1. Perform measures to protect skin integrity during chemotherapy and/or radiation therapy.
2. Provide safe cleansing and protection to skin.
3. Avoid exposure of skin to harmful pressure, rubbing, or irritants.
4. Apply ointments to prevent or treat dryness, itching, or irritation of skin.
5. Preserve markings placed on skin by x-ray personnel.
6. Report skin breakdown to physician.

Nursing diagnosis

Altered protection

Related factors: Abnormal blood profile (chemotherapy/radiation)

Defined characteristics: Leukopenia from bone marrow depression; thrombocytopenia from bone marrow depression; anemia from bone marrow depression; proneness to bleeding, infection, fatigue, weakness

OUTCOME CRITERIA

Short-term
Control of bleeding or infection tendency, as evidenced by absence of bleeding or infection at any site (expected within 1 week)

Long-term
Absence of bleeding or infectious process, with blood profile within acceptable parameters during therapy (expected for duration of therapy)

NURSING INTERVENTIONS/INSTRUCTIONS

1. Assess for bleeding, including petechiae, ecchymoses, oozing or frank bleeding from any orifice or skin site, or blood in stool or urine; assess joints for pain and swelling; assess for increased weakness and fatigue (each visit).

2. Assess for fever; chills; decreased breath sounds, dyspnea with or without exertion; cough; chest pain; cloudy, foul-smelling urine; and frequency, burning, and urgency in urinary elimination (each visit).

3. Assess, as available, white blood cells, red blood cells, hematocrit, hemoglobin, platelets, and urine or sputum culture results, and compare to levels at which bleeding or infection is probable (any visit).

4. Instruct client to avoid any trauma to skin and to take measures to prevent falls or other injury in home environment (first visit).

5. Instruct client to avoid exposure to others with infections or illnesses that might be transmitted (first visit).

6. Instruct client in hand-washing technique, to wear mask if needed, and to avoid sharing utensils or articles such as linens or clothing (first visit).

7. Instruct client to avoid use of safety razor, hard toothbrushing, blowing nose hard, or straining at defecation (first visit).

8. Inform client of importance of having laboratory tests done as scheduled to determine bone marrow function and possible effects (first visit).

9. Instruct client to report any persistent symptoms to physician (each visit).

CLIENT AND FAMILY/CARETAKER INTERVENTIONS

1. Take and record temperature, respirations, and pulse as needed.

2. Adapt activities of daily living and other activities to physical tolerance, and rest when feeling fatigued.

3. Assess daily for bleeding or infectious process, and report any findings to physician.

4. Avoid trauma to skin or mucous membranes resulting from straining or using harsh implements.

5. Administer stool softeners and vitamin K as prescribed; avoid aspirin or aspirin products.

6. Avoid exposure to persons with infections, crowded places, and use of or exposure to contaminated articles.

7. Provide protective isolation measures based on laboratory results.

8. Report for all appointments for laboratory tests and physician follow-up.
9. Secure and transport blood, urine, and sputum specimens to laboratory.

Nursing diagnosis

Body image disturbance

Related factors: Biophysical effect of chemotherapy/radiation

Defining characteristics: Alopecia; negative feeling about body; physical changes caused by therapy or surgery

OUTCOME CRITERIA

Short-term
Improved body image, as evidenced by client's statement of reason for change and measures to take to disguise the change (expected within 2 to 3 days)

Long-term
Enhanced body image, as evidenced by client's verbalization of more positive feelings about appearance and the temporary state of the changes caused by chemotherapy/radiation (expected within 2 to 4 weeks and duration of therapy)

NURSING INTERVENTIONS/INSTRUCTIONS

1. Before therapy, inform client of potential for hair loss and instruct client to prepare with purchase of a wig or to use a scarf, turban, or large hat (first visit).
2. Allow client to express, in an accepting and nonjudgmental environment, feelings about hair loss, weight loss, nail changes, skin discoloration, and surgical scarring (each visit).
3. Instruct client to use a mild shampoo and to avoid use of curlers, dryers, hair spray, hot iron, or harsh brushing of hair (first visit).
4. Inform client that hair will grow back after treatment regimen but may be coarser and a slightly different color (first visit).
5. Inform of clothing with high necks, loose fit, long sleeves, or leg covering (slacks) to select to cover exposed surgical areas or prostheses (first visit).

CLIENT AND FAMILY/CARETAKER INTERVENTIONS

1. Secure wig, hairpiece, scarf, or other clothing to deal with concerns such as hair loss, thinness, skin discoloration, scarring, or prosthesis.
2. Use makeup to cover discoloration of skin.
3. Express feelings about appearance and coping skills to maintain life-style and improved body image.
4. Avoid actions that injure hair, skin, or nails.

Nursing diagnosis

Knowledge deficit

Related factors: Lack of information about therapy

Defining characteristics: Expressed need for information about chemotherapy/radiation therapy and effects and about health maintenance needs

OUTCOME CRITERIA

Short-term

Adequate knowledge, as evidenced by client's statement of therapy regimen and of its temporary effect on health status (expected within 2 to 3 days)

Long-term

Adequate knowledge, as evidenced by client's compliance with medical protocol and actions to maintain optimal health and functioning during therapy (expected for duration of therapy)

NURSING INTERVENTIONS/INSTRUCTIONS

1. Assess client's life-style, ability to adapt, and learning ability and interest, family participation and support, and availability of community agencies that offer information and support (first visit).
2. Assess client's knowledge of reason for therapy and what effects can be expected (first visit).
3. Instruct client in administration of each chemotherapeutic drug, including what action the drug has on the malignant cells, route of administration, dosage, frequency, and combination protocols, with length of time given, side effects, and treatments given to prevent or control them; provide

client with a written protocol and check-off sheet to take to physician for administration of chemotherapy (first and second visits).

4. Instruct client in radiation site, effect of radiation, frequency of treatment, length of therapy, and protecton of irradiated area (first visit).

5. Inform client that fatigue and other effects of therapy begin during first week and gradually disappear 2 to 4 weeks after therapy ends (first visit).

6. Inform client of medications administered to counteract toxic effects of therapy and those given to treat complications of therapy (first visit).

7. Assist client to plan for fluid, nutritional, activity, rest, and sleep requirements and to modify them according to effects of therapy (each visit).

8. Instruct client to notify physician of any severe side effects and to keep all follow-up appointments for medications, treatments, and laboratory tests (first visit).

9. Initiate referral to community agencies and social and economic services to assist with transportation, meals, homemaking, shopping, economic problems, medical equipment and supplies, information, and psychological support (any visit).

CLIENT AND FAMILY/CARETAKER INTERVENTIONS

1. Meet fluid, dietary, exercise, and sleep requirements on the basis of assessment and abilities.

2. Verbalize chemotherapy and/or radiation protocol and measures to take to promote desired effect.

3. Maintain positive attitude regarding effect and result of treatment.

4. Administer medications as instructed to treat side effects of therapy.

5. Report uncontrolled side effects to physician.

6. Keep all appointments during therapy.

7. Contact American Cancer Society or other agencies as appropriate to needs.

◢ *Hospice Care*

Hospice care is a concept of holistic care that provides compassion, concern, support, and skilled care for the terminally ill client. It includes physical, psychological, social, and spiritual care by a medically supervised interdisciplinary team of professionals and volunteers. Hospice care in the home is based on client and family need and may be part time, intermittent, scheduled on a regular basis, or provided on a 24-hour on-call basis. Support for grieving before and after the death of the client is included in the care plan for client and family.

Home care is primarily concerned with the control of symptoms and promotion of comfort through palliative care.

Nursing diagnosis

Chronic pain

Related factors: Chronic physical disability; progressive invasion of malignant tumor

Defining characteristics: Altered ability to continue previous activities; long-term pain that becomes progressively more severe; tumor metastasis and pressure as mass becomes larger

OUTCOME CRITERIA

Short-term
Pain decreased, as evidenced by client's statement that severity has been reduced with appropriate analgesic therapy (expected within 1 week)

Long-term
Pain absent or controlled with continuous or intermittent analgesic therapy administered intramuscularly, intravenously, or subcutaneously and based on need (expected for duration of terminal state)

NURSING INTERVENTIONS/INSTRUCTIONS

1. Assess status of pain and client's ability to tolerate pain (each visit).

2. Administer intravenously or intramuscularly analgesic of choice that will achieve pain control, or instruct client in subcutaneous self-administration with a pump device (first and second visits).
3. Provide a quiet, restful environment, and reduce stimuli to a minimum (first visit).
4. Instruct client to place self in position of comfort and to change positions gently and carefully to prevent additional pain (first visit).
5. Instruct client in guided imagery or relaxation techniques and provide music if these actions are appropriate (any visit).

CLIENT AND FAMILY/CARETAKER INTERVENTIONS

1. Administer analgesic therapy as needed to relieve or control pain.
2. Maintain quiet, well-ventilated, temperature-controlled, and restful environment.
3. Avoid any stressful or anxiety-provoking situations.
4. Provide music or other desirable diversions as appropriate.

Nursing diagnosis

Ineffective family coping: compromised

Related factors: Situational crisis of dying family member

Defining characteristics: Significant persons preoccupied with personal reactions of fear, grief, guilt, and anxiety regarding client's condition

OUTCOME CRITERIA
Short-term
Improved coping, as evidenced by client and family's acknowledgement of terminal state of illness and ability to grieve and support palliative treatment of family member (expected within 1 week)

Long-term
Optimal coping abilities and support of family members to facilitate client's comfort and care (expected during hospice experience)

NURSING INTERVENTIONS/INSTRUCTIONS

1. Assess family interactions, ability to cope, strengths and inner resources, ability to support family member who is terminally ill, and presence of or need for an advance directive in compliance with the Self-Determination Act (each visit).
2. Inform family that care and concern extend to all family members according to their needs (first visit).
3. Provide accurate information to family about treatment and goal of hospice care and about what can and cannot be changed; allow for questions and clarifications (each visit).
4. Provide client with written information about right to know what treatment is planned and right to decide in advance what treatment is wanted or not wanted under special or serious conditions, in order to control medical treatment decisions. Inform client of right to execute advance directives through a Living Will or a Durable Power of Attorney for Health Care according to state laws (first visit).
5. Encourage family to discuss strengths and options for use of coping skills that are helpful (each visit).
6. Include family members in as much care of client as they feel ready and able to perform; allow family to plan client's needs around family routines if possible (each visit).
7. Allow for family members to grieve in an accepting and nonjudgmental environment; assist family to identify grieving behaviors (each visit).
8. Inform family of government and community agencies and referral to interdisciplinary caregivers as needed and as available for hospice care (any visit).
9. Encourage family to accept social services, counseling from clergy, and psychotherapy as needed (first visit).

CLIENT AND FAMILY/CARETAKER INTERVENTIONS

1. Complete an advance directive stating choice for health care, or name someone to make these choices if unable to make decisions about medical treatment.
2. Support and perform care if possible.
3. Verbalize concerns and feelings about client's condition during terminal stage of illness.
4. Cope with the imminent loss of a loved one.
5. Participate in planning and assisting with care.

6. Seek assistance from other professionals as needed.
7. Progress through grieving process.
8. Prepare for death of family member.
9. Maintain an open, honest approach and communication among family members and client.

Nursing diagnosis

Fatigue

Related factors: Overwhelming psychological or emotional demands; state of physical discomfort

Defining characteristics: Weakness; inability to maintain and perform usual routines and activities of daily living

OUTCOME CRITERIA

Short-term
Minimal fatigue, as evidenced by client's obtaining needed assistance in personal care (expected within 1 to 2 weeks)

Long-term
Optimal level of energy maintained and fatigue level minimized during terminal phase of illness (expected during length of hospice care)

NURSING INTERVENTIONS/INSTRUCTIONS

1. Provide assistance or complete care, including bathing, grooming, personal hygiene, toileting or urinary and bowel elimination care, feeding and drinking as appropriate, and gown changing (each visit).
2. Provide position changes, skin care, and aids to prevent pressure on susceptible areas (each visit).
3. Provide clean linens, massage with lotion, glycerin to lips, and mouth care with rinses or glycerin swabs (each visit).
4. Perform range-of-motion exercises for all joints, and maintain body alignment without compromising comfort (each visit).
5. Provide necessary assistance and care for all body processes as needed, support all body parts, and provide for every physical need without causing additional fatigue to client (each visit).
6. Anticipate needs of client and family, and pace activities

according to energy level of client and family (each visit).
7. Utilize touch to exhibit caring (each visit).
8. Provide all interventions on a continuous basis.

CLIENT AND FAMILY/CARETAKER INTERVENTIONS

1. Accept total physical care and support of all failing systems on a continuous basis.
2. Promote quality of life with comfort and support to client.
3. Conserve client's energy, and preserve client's emotional and physical status.
4. Comply with legal/ethical issues regarding terminal care (witholding basic needs, nonresuscitation).

◣ *Neoplasms (Malignant)*

Malignant neoplasms, or cancer, is a term used to identify disease processes characterized by unregulated cell changes that are capable of metastasis, or spread to other organs of the body. Cancer is classified according to the type of tissue involved; lymphomas originate in the lymphatic or infection-preventing system organs; leukemias originate in the blood-forming organs; sarcomas originate in connective tissue, bone, or muscle; and carcinomas originate in the epithelial cells of organs. Metastasis occurs via the vascular system or the lymphatic system or by implantation from the primary site of the tumor. In addition to the classification of cancer by anatomic site or tissue of origin, the cells are graded by appearance and differentiation, from grade I through grade IV, and the extent of the disease is described by staging, from stage 0 through stage IV. Typing, grading, and staging are used as a basis to determine treatment modalities, whose goal may be cure, control, or palliation of the disease. There are at least 200 diseases in this group, and this care plan for clients with malignant conditions is presented to assist with the problems common to all or most of these clients who receive care in the home. Since treatment for this condition consists of surgical intervention, chemotherapy, and/or radiation therapy, the Postoperative and Chemotherapy/External Radiation care plans should be used in conjunction with this one for a comprehensive approach to care of the client with cancer.

Home care is primarily concerned with the teaching and caring aspects of the client's physical and emotional needs and with implementation of the medical protocol to preserve and maintain optimal physical health and function.

Nursing diagnosis

Anxiety

Related factors: Threat of death; threat to or change in health status

Defining characteristics: Apprehension; uncertain outcome; increased tension and helplessness; fearfulness; poor prognosis; possible early death; changes in life-style and temperament; powerlessness; depression; withdrawal

OUTCOME CRITERIA

Short-term
Decreased anxiety, as evidenced by client's statement of reduced fear, worry, and apprehension regarding change in health status and possible poor prognosis (expected within 1 to 3 weeks)

Long-term
Management or control of anxiety level, as evidenced by adaptation to change in life-style and by compliance with and acceptance of treatment regimen to achieve desired goal of medical protocol (expected within 1 to 2 months and ongoing)

NURSING INTERVENTIONS/INSTRUCTIONS

1. Assess client's mental and emotional status regarding life-threatening illness (see Psychosocial Assessment, p. 41, for guidelines) (first visit).
2. In an accepting environment, encourage expressions of fears and concerns and questions regarding therapy and its effects (each visit).
3. Assist client to identify needed changes in life-style and methods to make necessary changes (first visit and reinforce each visit).
4. Inform client of all activities, treatments and tests, and

effects to expect; reinforce information about the disease and client condition given by the physician (each visit).

5. Allow client to direct own care and make own choices when possible regarding treatment regimen and plan of care (each visit).

6. Initiate referral to counseling, support group, and agencies that may assist with social services and economic and health care needs (first visit).

7. Instruct client in relaxation exercises, music therapy, or imagery, or introduce other techniques to reduce anxiety (first and second visits).

CLIENT AND FAMILY/CARETAKER INTERVENTIONS

1. Develop coping methods for long-term treatment and possible outcome.
2. Maintain manageable level of anxiety.
3. Seek information that will reduce anxiety.
4. Express fears and concerns about necessary changes in life-style.
5. Contact and consult with support services available.

Nursing diagnosis

Anticipatory grieving

Related factors: Perceived potential loss of physiopsychosocial well-being

Defining characteristics: Expression of distress at potential loss; anger; guilt; denial of potential loss; sorrow; choked feelings; changes in sleep, eating, and activity patterns

OUTCOME CRITERIA

Short-term
Progress in grieving, as evidenced by attitude and behavior changes manifested by stage in process (expected within days)

Long-term
Grief process resolving, as evidenced by resumption of life-style with or without changes as needed and by integration of grieving stage into life-style and activities (expected within 2 to 3 months and ongoing)

NURSING INTERVENTIONS/INSTRUCTIONS

1. Assess degree and stage of grief (each visit).
2. Inform client of stages of grieving process and that behavior is acceptable for specific stage, that progress goes back and forth, and that resolution will be final stage (first visit).
3. Allow expression of feelings and perception of effects of therapy, potential loss, and death in a nonjudgmental environment (each visit).
4. Initiate referral for psychological and spiritual counseling as appropriate (any visit).

CLIENT AND FAMILY/CARETAKER INTERVENTIONS

1. Progress through grief process to resolution.
2. Seek counseling as needed.
3. Verbalize stages and behaviors during grief process.

Nursing diagnosis

Knowledge deficit

Related factors: Lack of information about disease

Defining characteristics: Expressed need for information, at understandable level, about cancer, treatment modalities, and limitations imposed by the disease

OUTCOME CRITERIA

Short-term
Adequate knowledge, as evidenced by client's statement of disease process and type of cancer, diagnostic and classification methods, proposed treatment, and expected results (expected within 1 week)

Long-term
Adequate knowledge, as evidenced by client's understanding of and compliance with treatment protocol to achieve optimal physical and functional status within identified therapeutic goal (expected within 2 to 3 months and ongoing, depending on disease progression)

NURSING INTERVENTIONS/INSTRUCTIONS

1. Assess client's life-style, ability to adapt, learning ability and interest, family participation and support, and need

for reinforcement of information given by physician (first visit).

2. Inform client of disease process, possible causes, reasons for signs and symptoms, and changes in body appearance and function (first visit).

3. Inform client of importance of maintaining all follow-up care and appointments with physician, laboratory testing, and scheduled chemotherapy and/or radiation therapy during treatment protocol (first visit and reinforce second visit).

4. Provide client with accurate information about the benefits of proven therapies and fallacies of unproven methods of cancer treatment, which might include chemicals or drugs, dietary supplements, and occult or mechanical devices or techniques (first visit).

5. Outline treatment protocol, length of therapy, expected discomforts and results, and side effects in honest, under standable terms (each visit).

6. Inform client of any limitations or restrictions to follow during therapy, including performance of activities of daily living within energy tolerance, avoiding sun exposure and alcohol intake, and arranging for leaving work or loss of work during therapy.

7. Inform client of common problem of fear associated with the disease and methods of coping with and reducing it after diagnosis and during the initial phases of treatment (first visit).

8. Inform client of and refer to hospice care if appropriate, and explain the availability of this care in the future if appropriate (any visit).

9. Refer client to American Cancer Society for information, support groups, and equipment or supplies as needed (any visit).

10. In a realistic manner, inform client of importance of a hopeful attitude about the disease and the progress that has been made in curing the disease (any visit).

CLIENT AND FAMILY/CARETAKER INTERVENTIONS

1. Verbalize information about the disease and important factors that contribute to its effect on the body.

2. Verbalize needed changes in life-style to accommodate treatment regimen.

3. Establish and maintain hope.
4. Adapt to presence of cancer, and comply with scheduled follow-up appointments.
5. Avoid unproven therapies and methods of controlling disease.
6. Contact and utilize community agencies for information and support.
7. Participate in goal setting and decisions regarding care.

◢ *Postoperative Care Following Inpatient or Outpatient Surgery*

Postoperative care involves the physical and emotional care of a client following surgery and discharge from the hospital or care of a client after surgery done in an outpatient surgical unit and discharge to home on the day of surgery. Outpatient surgery usually involves minor procedures that are done with administration of local anesthetics and/or short-acting inhalation anesthetics.

Home care is concerned with the teaching of safety management and preservation of health and function following outpatient surgery and with maintenance and reinforcement of the hospital discharge teaching for follow-up care at home.

Nursing diagnosis

High risk for infection

Related factors: Inadequate primary defenses; invasive procedure

Defining characteristics: Surgical wound (broken skin) with redness, swelling, pain, drainage; respiratory changes (stasis of secretions) with decreased breath sounds, shortness of breath; urinary changes (stasis of body fluids) with cloudy, foul-smelling urine with or without indwelling catheter

OUTCOME CRITERIA

Short-term

Reduced risk of infectious process following surgery, as evidenced by client's compliance with postoperative measures to prevent bacterial contamination (expected within 1 to 2 weeks)

Long-term

Absence of infectious process, as evidenced by wound healing without complication and by absence of postoperative complications, with return of optimal health and functional status (expected within 1 to 2 months)

NURSING INTERVENTIONS/INSTRUCTIONS

1. Assess, and instruct client to assess, wound site(s) for edge approximation and healing; drainage device for characteristics and amount of wound drainage; changes in color, temperature, or drainage; presence of swelling at surgical site; and increased pain (each visit).

2. Assess urine for characteristic changes and for catheter patency if one is in place; assess for respiratory changes in rate, depth, and ease and for change in sputum to yellow or other color (each visit).

3. Instruct client in hand washing technique and to perform before direct care, before meals, and after using bathroom (first visit).

4. Instruct client in continued use of incentive spirometry, coughing and deep breathing exercises, and assist client to plan daily schedule for times and frequency (first visit).

5. Instruct client in wound care and dressing change using sterile technique; how to care for and dress wound drains and device; how to remove dressing and application of smaller dressing; reporting pain, redness, or swelling at site; allow for return demonstration (first visit and reinforce on second visit).

6. Instruct client in need to void every 2 hours and to report any change in color or odor; teach client how to care for catheter and prevent entry of bacteria into the bladder (first visit).

7. Instruct client to monitor temperature and note chilling or elevation to over 100° F and to report to physician (first visit).

8. Instruct client in administration of antibiotic therapy to pre-

vent or treat infection, whether oral or topical (ointment, drops), including route, dose, time, frequency, side effects, and drug and food interactions, and to instruct client to complete entire prescription (first visit).
9. Instruct client to avoid exposure to people with upper respiratory infections or who are ill (first visit).

CLIENT AND FAMILY/CARETAKER INTERVENTIONS
1. Administer antibiotic therapy correctly and as prescribed.
2. Provide care to surgical site as needed, using sterile technique.
3. Monitor temperature and condition of site(s).
4. Assess respiratory and urinary function, and report signs and symptoms of infection.
5. Utilize hand-washing technique when appropriate.
6. Avoid exposure to persons with infections or touching wound site.

Nursing diagnosis

Self-care deficit (bathing/hygiene, dressing/grooming, toileting)

Related factors: Pain; discomfort with movement; intolerance to activity

Defining characteristics: Decreased strength and endurance; inability to perform or complete activities of daily living (ADL) independently; reluctance to attempt movement and activity; fear of injury to incision

OUTCOME CRITERIA
Short-term
Improvement in self-care performance, as evidenced by progressive participation in ADL and increased activity within prescribed limitations (expected within 1 to 2 weeks)

Long-term
Independence in ADL, as evidenced by client's meeting requirements for self-care within limitations or restrictions for optimal postoperative health and function and return to work (expected within 2 months, depending on surgical procedure)

NURSING INTERVENTIONS/INSTRUCTIONS

1. Assess client's ability to perform ADL, fatigue level, pain on movement or during activity, and need for special procedures or treatments before, during, or after ADL (see Functional Assessment, p. 43, for guidelines) (each visit).
2. Instruct client to assist with ADL as needed without compromising client independence or progressive self-care (first visit)
3. Allow client to develop own plan of progressive care and goals to achieve during convalscence and to revise plan as needed (each visit).
4. Instruct client to accept assistance when needed until weakness and fatigue diminish (first visit).
5. Instruct client to avoid strenuous activity or activities (first visit).
6. Instruct client in use of energy-saving devices and techniques for ADL (first visit).
7. Instruct client in administration of analgesics for pain on the basis of assessment before activities (first visit).
8. Instruct client to rest after activity, pace activities, and set limits if needed (first visit).
9. Refer home health aide to assist in ADL as needed.

CLIENT AND FAMILY/CARETAKER INTERVENTIONS

1. Schedule rest and activity on the basis of individual needs and condition.
2. Participate in ADL within set limits, with goals for daily or weekly progress toward independence.
3. Assist with any activity requiring support; ask for assistance when needed until independence achieved.
4. Use energy-saving devices or aids in ADL.
5. Administer analgesics when needed, based on assessment, to allow for optimal activity and ADL performance.

Nursing diagnosis

Knowledge deficit

Related factors: Lack of information about follow-up postoperative care

Defining characteristics: Expressed need for information about postoperative activity restrictions, nutrition and fluid needs, bowel and urinary elimination, and prevention of complications

OUTCOME CRITERIA

Short-term
Adequate knowledge, as evidenced by client's statement of postoperative medical regimen requirements and performance of postoperative procedures and treatments (expected within 1 to 2 weeks)

Long-term
Adequate knowledge, as evidenced by client's compliance with postoperative care regimen to achieve return to optimal health and functioning (expected within 4 to 6 weeks)

NURSING INTERVENTIONS/INSTRUCTIONS

1. Assess client's life-style, ability to adapt, learning ability and interest, and family participation and support (first visit).
2. Assess knowledge of surgical procedures, reason for surgical intervention for correction of problem, and where procedure performed (hospital or outpatient unit), and provide information needed or reinforce information already received if necessary (first visit).
3. Instruct client in medication administration as ordered, including times, dosage, frequency, side effects, and food and drug interactions (first and second visits).
4. Inform client of bowel and bladder elimination changes and causes and about use of stool softener, fluid intake, and exercising to assist in return to normal pattern (first visit).
5. Inform client of importance of compliance with activity/exercise regimen proposed, and instruct client to avoid activities that place stress on operative area (changing position, lifting, pushing, pulling, stooping) and to avoid heavy lifting, carrying, or straining (first visit).
6. Instruct client in incision care and in protecting it during bathing with a plastic cover taped to skin on the sides in shape of a picture frame (first visit).
7. Instruct client in appropriate amount of daily fluids, up to 3 liters per day, and inclusion of protein and vitamin C in dietary planning; offer food lists and sample menus, and

assist client to coordinate with food and fluid preferences (first and second visits).

8. Inform client of time to resume work schedule and activities to avoid (any visit).
9. Instruct client to report incisional pain, increased drainage, elevated temperature, or any discomfort or changes in other body areas (first visit).
10. Instruct client to comply with follow-up schedule to see physician as advised after surgery or hospital discharge (first visit).

CLIENT AND FAMILY/CARETAKER INTERVENTIONS

1. Administer all medications accurately; use check-off sheet as a reminder and to avoid errors.
2. Establish and maintain bowel and urinary elimination patterns.
3. Report adverse effects of medications, treatments, and surgical intervention if appropriate.
4. Participate in approved activites, and avoid those that place stress on incisional area.
5. Provide and ingest fluids and nutrients to facilitate health.
6. Maintain a written daily plan for compliance with postoperative requirements.
7. Return to work, or seek occupational rehabilitation or retraining if appropriate.

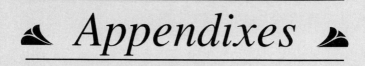

Appendixes

◢ Index of Nursing Diagnoses*

*Derived from Taxonomy I, revised 1992 with official nursing diagnoses, presented by the North American Nursing Diagnosis Association (NANDA).

Fluid volume deficit, high risk for
Fluid volume excess
Gas exchange, impaired
Grieving, anticipatory
Grieving, dysfunctional
Growth and development, altered
Health maintenance, altered
Health seeking behaviors (specify)
Home maintenance management, impaired
Hopelessness
Hyperthermia
Hypothermia
Incontinence, functional
Incontinence, reflex
Incontinence, stress
Incontinence, total
Incontinence, urge
Individual coping, ineffective
Individual management of therapeutic regimen, ineffective
Infection, high risk for
Injury, high risk for
Knowledge deficit (specify)
Noncompliance (specify)
Nutrition: less than body requirements, altered
Nutrition: more than body requirements, altered
Nutrition: high risk for more than body requirements, altered
Oral mucous membrane, altered
Pain
Pain, chronic
Peripheral neurovascular dysfunction, high risk for
Personal identity disturbance
Physical mobility, impaired
Poisoning, high risk for
Post-trauma response
Powerlessness
Protection, altered
Rape-trauma syndrome
Rape-trauma syndrome: compound reaction
Rape-trauma syndrome: silent reaction
Role performance, altered
Self-care deficit (bathing/hygiene, feeding, dressing/grooming, toileting)

Self-esteem, chronic low
Self-esteen, situational low
Self-esteem disturbance
Sensory/perceptual alterations (specify) (visual, auditory,
    kinesthetic, gustatory, tactile, olfactory)
Sexual dysfunction
Sexuality patterns, altered
Skin integrity, impaired
Skin integrity, high risk for impaired
Sleep pattern disturbance
Social interaction, impaired
Social isolation
Spiritual distress
Suffocation, high risk for
Swallowing, impaired
Thermoregulation, ineffective
Through processes, altered
Tissue integrity, impaired
Tissue perfusion, altered (specify) (renal, cerebral, cardiopul-
    monary, gastrointestinal, peripheral)
Trauma, high risk for
Unilateral neglect
Urinary elimination, altered
Urinary retention
Violence, high risk for: self-directed or directed at others

◣ *Psychosocial Nursing Diagnoses Related to Home Care Planning*

The NANDA-approved nursing diagnoses here are listed with possible relationships; these diagnoses may be used in home care plans included in this book. Nursing diagnoses may be selected on the basis of medical diagnoses and individual client and family assessments that include nursing history and physical examination data.

ADJUSTMENT, IMPAIRED

Related factors: Disability requiring change in life-style; inadequate support systems; impaired cognition; sensory overload; assault to self-esteem; altered locus of control; incomplete grieving

ANXIETY

Related factors: Unconscious conflict about essential values/goals of life; threat to self-concept; threat of death; threat to or change in health status; threat to or change in socioeconomic status; threat to or change in role functioning; threat to or change in environment; threat to or change in interaction patterns; situational/maturational crises; interpersonal transmission/contagion; unmet needs

BODY IMAGE DISTURBANCE

Related factors: Biophysical; cognitive/perceptual; psychosocial; cultural or spiritual

CAREGIVER ROLE STRAIN

Related factors: Severity of illness of care receiver; client discharged with significant home care needs; caregiver health impairment; unpredictable illness course or instability in receiver's health; addiction or codependency; psychological or cognitive problems in care receiver; caregiver not developmentally ready for role; developmental delay of caregiver or receiver; marginal family adaptation or dysfunction prior to caregiving situation; marginal caregiver's coping patterns; poor relationship between caregiver and receiver; disruptive, bizarre behavior of care receiver

DECISIONAL CONFLICT (SPECIFY)

Related factors: Unclear personal values/beliefs; perceived threat to value system; lack of experience or interference with decision making; lack of relevant information; support system deficit; multiple or divergent sources of information

DEFENSIVE COPING

Related factors: Superior attitude toward others; difficulty in establishing/maintaining relationships; hostile laughter or ridicule of others; difficulty in reality testing of perceptions; lack of follow-through or participation in treatment or therapy

DENIAL, INEFFECTIVE

Related factors: Conscious or unconscious attempt to disavow knowledge or meaning of an event; refusal to admit fear of death, illness, or invalidism; refusal to admit impact of illness on life pattern

DIVERSIONAL ACTIVITY DEFICIT

Related factors: Environmental lack of diversional activity, as in long-term hospitalization or frequent lengthly treatments

FAMILY COPING: COMPROMISED, INEFFECTIVE

Related factors: Inadequate or incorrect information or understanding by a primary person; temporary preoccupation by a significant person who is trying to manage emotional conflicts and personal suffering and is unable to perceive or act effectively in regard to client's needs; temporary family disorganization and role changes; other situational or developmental crises or situations the significant person may be facing; little support provided by client, in turn, for primary person; prolonged disease or disability progression that exhausts supportive capacity of significant people

FAMILY COPING: DISABLING, INEFFECTIVE

Related factors: Significant person with chronically unexpressed feelings of guilt, anxiety, hostility, despair, etc.; dissonant discrepancy of coping styles for dealing with adaptive tasks by the significant person and client or among significant people; highly ambivalent family relationships; arbitrary handling of family's resistance to treatment, which tends to solidify defensiveness as it fails to deal adequately with underlying anxiety

FAMILY COPING: HIGH RISK FOR GROWTH

Related factors: Needs sufficiently gratified and adaptive tasks effectively addressed to enable goals of self-actualization to surface; family members attempt to describe growth impact of crisis on their own values, priorities, goals, or relationships;

family member is moving in direction of health-promoting and enriching life-style that supports and monitors maturational processes, audits and negotiates treatment programs, and generally chooses experiences that optimize wellness; individual expresses interest in making contract on a one-to-one basis or on a mutual-aid group basis with another person who has experienced a similar situation

FAMILY PROCESSES, ALTERED

Related factors: Situational transition and/or crises; developmental transition and/or crises

FEAR

Related factors: Natural or innate origins—sudden noise, loss of physical support, weight, pain. Learned response—conditioning, modeling from, or identification with others; separation from support system in a potentially threatening situation (hospitalization, treatments, etc.); knowledge deficit or unfamiliarity; language barrier; sensory impairment; phobic stimulus or phobia; environmental stimuli.

GRIEVING, ANTICIPATORY

Related factors: Perceived potential loss of significant other; perceived potential loss of physiopsychosocial well-being; perceived potential loss of personal possessions

GRIEVING, DYSFUNCTIONAL

Related factors: Actual or perceived object loss (object loss is used in the broadest sense); objects may include: people, possessions, a job, status, home, ideals, parts and processes of the body; thwarted grieving repsonse to a loss; absence of anticipatory grieving; chronic fatal illness; lack of resolution of previous grieving response; loss of significant others; loss of physiopsychosocial well-being; loss of personal possessions

GROWTH AND DEVELOPMENT, ALTERED

Related factors: Inadequate caretaking; indifference, inconsistent responsiveness, multiple caretakers; separation from significant others; environmental and stimulation deficiencies; effects of physical disability; prescribed dependence

HOPELESSNESS

Related factors: Prolonged activity restriction, creating isolation; failing or deteriorating physiologic condition; long-term stress; abandonment; lost belief in transcendent values/God

INDIVIDUAL COPING, INEFFECTIVE

Related factors: Situational crises; maturational crises; personal vulnerability; multiple life changes; inadequate relaxation; inadequate support system; unmet expectations; work overload; unrealistic perceptions; inadequate coping method; too many deadlines

PERSONAL IDENTITY DISTURBANCE

Related factors: Unable to distinguish between self and nonself

POST-TRAUMA RESPONSE

Related factors: Disasters, wars, epidemics, rape, assault, torture, catastrophic illness or accident

POWERLESSNESS

Related factors: Health care environment; interpersonal interaction; illness-related regimen; life-style of helplessness

ROLE PERFORMANCE, ALTERED

Related factors: Disruption in perception of one's role performance; role conflict

SELF-ESTEEM, CHRONIC LOW

Related factors: Long-standing negative feelings about self and capabilities

SELF-ESTEEM, SITUATIONAL LOW

Related factors: Episodic negative feelings about self and capabilities in response to a crisis, loss, or change

SELF-ESTEEM DISTURBANCE

Related factors: Negative feelings about self and capabilities directly or indirectly expressed

SOCIAL INTERACTION, IMPAIRED

Related factors: Knowledge/skill deficit about ways to enhance mutuality; communication barriers; self-concept disturbance; absence of available significant others or peers; limited physical mobility; therapeutic isolation; sociocultural dissonance; environmental barriers; altered thought processes

SOCIAL ISOLATION

Related factors: Factors contributing to the absence of satisfying personal relationships, such as: delay in accomplishing developmental tasks; immature interests; alterations in physical appearance; alterations in mental status; unacceptable social behavior; unacceptable social values; altered state of wellness; inadequate personal resources; inability to engage in satisfying personal relationships

SPIRITUAL DISTRESS (DISTRESS OF THE HUMAN SPIRIT)

Related factors: Separation from religious/cultural ties; challenged belief and value system, e.g., as a result of moral/ethical implications of therapy or as a result of intense suffering

VIOLENCE, HIGH RISK FOR: SELF-DIRECTED OR DIRECTED AT OTHERS

Related factors: Antisocial character; battered women; catatonic excitement; child/elder abuse; manic excitement; organic brain syndrome; panic states; rage reactions; suicidal behavior; temporal lobe epilepsy; toxic reactions to medication

---

◢ *Guidelines for Medication Administration*

Medications commonly administered in the home include those given orally, sublingually, topically, intramuscularly, subcutaneously, and by inhalation that are prescribed by the physician to treat one or more conditions and are scheduled for regular administration or in response to client request when needed. The nursing implications of medication administration in the home are focused on the teaching aspects of self-administration by the client to ensure safe, effective results from the therapy. This includes instruction in dosage, route, frequency, time, form, side effects to report, methods of administration, and safe storage.

ASSESSMENT

1. Age, weight
2. Medications taken, either prescribed or over the counter
3. Drug allergies
4. Compatibility of medications being taken; compatibility with foods
5. Past dependency or risk for present dependency on drugs
6. Use of alcohol, caffeine-containing beverages, herbal products, and tobacco
7. Daily routines and best times for medication administration
8. Information about each drug and special recommendations for administration
9. Ability to swallow tablets
10. Cognitive, mental capacities
11. Expiration dates of medications; where medications are kept and if kept separate from other drugs in home

INTERVENTIONS

1. Prepare medications in labeled containers; water, food, or whatever needed to administer; and pill crusher if appropriate and if medication does not need to be swallowed whole.
2. Check medications for correct name, dosage, route, and time, and formulate a checklist for client to use that includes time schedules that revolve around daily routines.
3. Check drug dosage before, during and after administration to ensure accuracy; compare with checklist or drug container.
4. Prepare drug(s) by pouring liquids, placing tablet in cup or in hand or crushing and mixing with water or in food such as applesauce, or uncapping ointment and squeezing small amount to discard.

5. Offer to client with a glass of water or other fluid to swallow or mixed in food to swallow, or to drink from measured cup; or to apply to affected area with applicator; or to place under tongue or in the cheek.
6. Document administration of medication(s) on checklist.
7. Note any side effects and instruct client to report any to the physician.
8. Store medications in safe area away from children.
9. Follow special instructions in administering a medication, such as taking before or after a meal or using a straw.
10. Follow special instructions for metered-dose inhalant administration that are included in the insert.
11. Suggest and instruct client in use of reminder devices with compartments for drugs that match administration times and how to refill daily.
12. Inform client that if drug is forgotten, wait until next dosage time unless dose can be taken within 1 hour after scheduled time (this will depend on frequency of dosage).

EVALUATION

1. Client uses checklist and administers drug(s) accurately.
2. Client uses reminder devices effectively and refills daily.
3. Client knows drug action, dosage, frequency, route, form, side effects, and incompatibilities with foods and other drugs.
4. Client takes preventive measures and stores drugs safely.
5. Client reports side effects to physician; stops medication until physician is notified.

◣ *Infection Control Guidelines: Universal Precautions*

Universal precautions are those actions taken to prevent transmission of microorganisms from one person to another. They include care of hands, care of inanimate objects or articles used, and use of barriers and techniques to protect against transmission to client or caretaker.

HANDS

1. Always wash hands before contact with client or performance of a procedure, even if gloves are worn; wash hands after completion of a procedure even if gloves are worn, and wash immediately if bare hands are exposed to blood or body secretions or excretions.
2. Wear gloves if possibility exists of touching blood, body fluids, secretions, or excretions on any item or article or specimen exposed to these fluids.
3. Avoid contact with body fluids or contaminants if skin on hands has breaks, rashes, or any eruptions.

PROTECTIVE WEAR

1. Always wear disposable gloves in presence of possible contamination by body fluids, whether from skin, clothing, or supplies/equipment.
2. Wear mask, gown, and eye goggles during direct or close contact, if soiling of clothing is likely, coughing is present, or spattering of body fluids is possible.

EQUIPMENT/SUPPLIES

1. Used linens and bathing articles should be laundered with detergent and hot water; disposable contaminated articles should be double-bagged and incinerated.
2. Dishes should be cleansed in dishwasher or detergent and hot water or disposed of after use if a disposable type (double-bagged and incinerated if contaminated).
3. Tissues from upper respiratory infection secretions should be bagged and disposed of by incineration; disposable supplies bagged and incinerated after use; reusable supplies disinfected with commercial solution or 1:10 bleach solution, rinsed, and allowed to air dry; spills of body fluids cleansed and treated with 1:10 bleach solution; disposable breathing bag used for CPR and discarded after use.
4. Wear gloves to draw blood or administer intravenous or parenteral injections, and take precautions to prevent accidental sticks to hands.
5. Label specimens of blood or body fluids for special precau-

tions that are needed for laboratory personnel; place specimen in a bag and label before transport to lab.

6. Needles and syringes should be disposed of in a hard container (coffee can or jar); refrain from recapping, cutting, or bending needles.

DISINFECTION

1. Moist heat by boiling in water in a covered container for 10 minutes after water has been boiled for 1 hour

2. Dry heat by placing cloth-wrapped article on a flat pan and baking in oven at 350° for 1 hour.

3. Commercial solutions diluted according to instructions and articles submerged for 10 minutes, rinsed well, and air dried.

4. Home-prepared solution of white vinegar 1:3 or bleach 1:10; used for submersion of articles or cleansing of contaminated areas.

▲ *Medicare, Medicaid, and Private Insurance Payment Guidelines*

1. Usually all clients who are over 65 years of age, disabled for 2 years or more, or on renal dialysis receive Medicare benefits for health care. They also may have supplemental private health insurance that covers expenses that Medicare does not pay; these plans vary and benefits are policy specific.

2. Medicaid is a government assistance plan that differs from state to state. Coverage is reserved for a segment of the population whose economic status complies with the payment standards set by government regulations (usually 50% federal and 50% state funded).

3. CHAMPUS insurance benefits and coverage are reserved for government employees eligible to receive these payments via past or present employment or service to the government.

4. Private health insurance may be individually owned and paid for or part of a group policy sponsored and paid for completely or in part by the client's employer.

5. Private long-term care insurance may include home care benefits following a hospitalization or long-term facility stay, or it may be for home care exclusively as a single policy or as a rider to a long-term nursing home policy.

6. Requirements and benefits for government and private insurance change periodically; major areas of coverage usually include client assessment, teaching, and performing complex procedures, with hours or number of visits allowed depending on acuity and type of skilled care needed; skilled care is needed before a home health aide will be paid.

7. Medicare, Medicaid, and third-party payors require documentation of homebound status and skilled care need (varies from state to state), with specific, detailed functional limitations included in the medical diagnoses; for example: acute exacerbation of rheumatoid arthritis on _____ (date) with inability to move from bed to chair. They also require a medical plan of care and medical orders for home care.

8. The medical diagnosis should include an appropriate adjective for a better description; for example: "uncontrolled diabetes." Give the most acute diagnosis as the principal diagnosis, and include the dates of onset.

9. Care plans are initially developed by a nurse after an appropriate nursing history and assessments of client are completed, or they may be developed by physical, occupational, or speech therapist.

10. Discharge must be considered if nursing interventions are not needed for up to 3 weeks and no problems exist or recur for which Medicare benefits would apply.

11. Specific nursing diagnoses that identify nursing problems, as opposed to medical diangoses, which identify medical conditions, are required; for example:

    Diabetes mellitus   Knowledge deficit related to subcutaneous administration of insulin

12. Goals must be written as "outcomes," which are to be achieved in a specific period of time (e.g., short-term and long-term). The examples that follow are goals for client and for nurse:

- Client states purpose of insulin, action, dosage, time, and side effects (expected within 3 days or during second visit).
- Teach client insulin administration (expected within 10 days or by end of fourth visit).

13. Goals must reflect nursing diagnosis and specify actions expected to solve the problems stated in the diagnosis; this may vary with Medicare requirements.

14. Interventions are the stated actions that the nurse, client, and family or caretaker complete to achieve the goals. Specific skilled care and teaching that relate to the diagnosis and physician orders should be delineated. A list of specific personnel performing interventions should be included with the activities in the care plan.

15. Nursing diagnoses and interventions are listed in order of priority. Medicare and insurance plans do not pay for maintenance care except in the case of a private insurance plan that is specifically for long-term care, although Medicaid will sometimes pay for skilled management for short term.

16. The review or evaluation includes dates when goals are expected to be achieved or not achieved.

17. The frequency of paid visits depends on the diagnosis, the acuteness of the condition, client or caretaker ability to learn, presence of a caretaker to teach, stability of client's condition, and multiple medical diagnoses. Parameters may or may not be given as a basis for the number of visits that would be acceptable. Start with a higher frequency of visits; then taper down if possible and schedule for 2 or 3 times per week; daily visits are usually allowed only for an acute phase or teaching; however, proper documentation will allow for daily or twice daily visits to be covered by Medicare.

18. The nurse assesses need for physical therapy, but physician order is needed for this referral.

19. The physical therapy, occupational therapy, and referral for social worker are ordered by the physician.

20. A home health aide may be placed in the home if no one is able to perform personal care for the client; this care by an aide is allowed only if skilled care is also needed for the client for Medicare or Medicaid benefits.

21. At least two of the following skilled care interventions are necessary for Medicare payment:

- Assessment and evaluation
- Hands-on care and procedures
- Teaching

SUGGESTED SCHEDULE FOR VISITS

Visits would be determined by individual need and agency policy, physician orders, homebound status, insurance criteria, and need for skilled care and intermittent care.

Nurse (RN)

Discharge: 1 mo	*Discharge: 1½–2 mo*	*Discharge: 2–3 mo*
×1–2/wk: 1–2 wk	×3/wk: 1–2 wk	×3/wk: 1–2 wk
q2wk: ×1–2	×2/wk: 1 wk	×2/wk: 2–3 wk
	×1/wk: 1–2 wk	×1/wk: 2–4 wk
	q2wk: ×1–2	q2wk: ×1

Physical Therapist (PT)

Discharge of 1–2 mo

×3/wk: 2–3 wk	×2–3 wk: 6–8 wk
×2/wk: 1–2 wk	*or*
×1/wk: 1–2 wk	×1–2 wk: 2–3 wk

Occupational Therapist (OT)
×1–2/wk: 2–3 wk
×1/wk: 3–4 wk
×2–3 wk: 6–8 wk

Social Worker (MSW)
×2–3 visits; repeat and document as needed for additional monthly visits

Speech Therapist (ST)
×3/wk: 3–4 wk
×2–3/wk: 3–4 wk
×2/wk: 2–3 wk

Home Health Aide (HHA)
×3–4/wk; frequency and length of visits depend on medical necessity for personal care, i.e., bedbound, extreme weakness, severe exertional dyspnea

COVERAGE

Usually Covered
1. New diabetic condition requiring insulin administration and glucose monitoring
2. New colostomy, ileostomy, ileal conduit, or similar surgery

3. Hypertension and other cardiac conditions (unstable and requiring medication changes)
4. Intramuscular or intravenous injections or infusions
5. Foley catheter changes; disimpaction
6. Nasogastric, gastrostomy, and tracheostomy tube changes
7. Mechanical ventilation
8. Skilled foot care
9. Dressing changes
10. Assessments and teaching functions
11. Claims for first 3 weeks after hospital discharge or initial claims the first month of service

Not Usually Covered (Unless Family Cannot Understand Instructions)

1. Vital signs, medication, fluid intake and output
2. Repetition and reinforcement of instruction
3. Positioning of client in bed
4. Provision of emotional support
5. Provision of active or passive range-of-motion exercises
6. Check of fecal impaction and for catheter changing unless appropriately documented
7. Prevention of pressure areas after initial teaching
8. Setup of medications and administration of eyedrops (limited to 3 visits for Medicare) or ointments
9. Assessment of chronic obstructive pulmonary disease for intermittent positive-pressure breathing (IPPB) treatment and frequency
10. Medications given by injection if not medically necessary
11. Stable client who continues to be monitored
12. Procedures performed by person usually not considered skilled
13. Preventive care, especially if previously taught

Problem Areas for Coverage

1. Frequent physician contacts with no new orders
2. Chronic diagnosis with no change in treatment plan by physician
3. Too few or too many visits
4. Medical necessity for procedure
5. Procedures not corresponding with diagnoses
6. Rehabilitative claims of more than 3 months unless properly documented
7. Repeated instruction
8. Custodial care

9. Not homebound; will vary in different areas
10. Unskilled or intermittent care
11. Daily visits of more than 3 weeks unless estimated time of healing and necessity of teaching are documented.

◣ *Tips on Documentation*

BASIC CONSIDERATIONS

1. Documentation done weekly should indicate that client is homebound, with specific notation of physical, mental, or emotional limitations or restrictions that would not allow leaving home. Homebound status is determined by state for Medicaid or third-party payor; Medicare allows leaving home for short periods of time if infrequent. Notes should not indicate activities done outside the home except for physical or laboratory appointments, providing the frequency would not indicate the possibility of outpatient care. Some situations indicating homebound treatment follow:
   a. Fractures or disabilities that prevent ambulation without assistance or use of assistive aids or that prevent weight bearing or the use of arms to open doors, etc.
   b. Shortness of breath with slight exertion, as in chronic obstructive pulmonary disease or chronic heart failure
   c. Weakness as the result of surgery or illness or client being easily fatigued
   d. Dizziness, weakness, poor balance, or unsteady gait
   e. Incision, draining wound, or dressing changes
   f. Indwelling catheter
   g. Wheelchair or bed bound
   h. Sensory deficiencies such as visual or auditory impairment or aphasia
   i. Paraplegia, quadriplegia, hemiplegia, numbness of extremities, paresis, or impaired peripheral circulation
   j. Mental confusion, extreme anxiety, or paranoia
   k. Obesity if mobility is compromised
   l. Severe pain
   m. Inability to communicate effectively

    n. Unstable blood glucose levels causing weakness, dizziness

2. List all medical diagnoses on the care plan because care may be needed for more than one condition; document the most acute diagnosis as the principal diagnosis, using onset or exacerbation date.
3. Indicate a date for each problem or nursing diagnosis in the care plan.
4. Document goals and goal achievement with dates at least weekly on the plan, with procedures or activites that meet the goals, and include the frequency and persons responsible for the activities.
5. Document in the care plan the exact services being provided that require skilled, professional nursing care.
6. Indicate in the care plan the time frames in which care will be provided, such as two to three times per week or less, depending on condition and insurance parameters; plan for and provide the more frequent visits at the beginning of the home care.
7. Documentation should be succinct, descriptive, and relevant. Omit items or words that do not relate or contribute to the necessary information.
8. Each note should contain why the visit was needed; use specific information from assessment to affirm medical necessity and specific care given.
9. Omit words describing care given, such as:
   a. Use of *chronic* for *acute exacerbation*
   b. Use of *monitor* for *assess* or *evaluate* if condition has stabilized
   c. Use of *reinforce* or *repeat instruction* instead of *reinstruct* for instruction
   d. Use of *discussed* instead of *instructed*
   e. Use of *check* instead of *assess*
   f. Use of *observe* instead of *assess*
   g. Use of words such as *stabilized* or *reviewed* instead of *responding to treatment*
   h. Use of *provide emotional support* instead of *making a referral*
   i. Use of *prevent* if instruction has already been given to a client
10. Document what is wrong with the client, not only client's

progress or what is right with him or her. Indicate need for care, not that care is no longer needed; for example:

Incorrect: respirations improving in rate, depth, and ease

Correct: respirations remaining at 28 per minute with use of accessory muscles and presence of dyspnea

11. Document information in a factual, objective manner. Avoid injecting subjective information; for example:

    Incorrect: general weakness

    Correct: able to ambulate only 10 feet without fatigue, dizziness, and shortness of breath

    Incorrect: reddened area on right heel

    Correct: reddened area on right heel, measuring 1 cm in diameter

12. Document all care that relates to medical diagnoses and orders. Be specific and include all care and skills performed; for example: instruct client to draw insulin into syringe, using sterile technique.

13. Qualify diagnoses when possible, such as unstable diabetes, newly diagnosed diabetic, uncontrolled hypertension, acute exacerbation of chronic obstructive pulmonary disease.

14. Document unstable states that require interventions such as medication or catheter changes, sterile irrigations, pulmonary physiotherapy, and others that need skilled nursing care; document response to medication and treatment changes. Make sure that skilled care matches the diagnoses and physician orders.

15. Document exercise or other regimens that are performed to restore function lost because of condition being treated and described by the medical diagnoses.

16. Document any obstacles or debilitated states that need to be overcome to achieve optimal health and functioning, such as mental deficiencies.

ADDITIONAL CONSIDERATIONS

1. Do not document the following:
   a. Private sitter or companion
   b. Client trips
   c. Medications reviewed
   d. Repetitive teaching unless client has limited intelligence or increased anxiety

   e. Lack of progress when progress should be seen; instead document inability to participate in therapy as a result of mental or physical disabilities
   f. Maintenance care
2. Do document the following:
   a. Why client or family cannot be taught a procedure
   b. Poor comprehension of client or family
   c. Specific signs and symptoms of disease taught to client
   d. Therapeutic diet taught, with sample menus
   e. Return demonstrations by client to evaluate level of completence
   f. Medications taught; teach one each visit related to the disease
   g. Wound measurement, color, drainage
   h. Activity/exercise instruction
3. Requirements for documentation of supervision visits:
   a. Supervision for licensed vocational nurse (LVN) or home health aide (HHA) specific to payment source, including notation about client and family expression of satisfaction with care; comprehension of care plan by HAA, support given and encouragement in ADL progression with or without assistance, and responses; continuation or withdrawal of LVN or HHA
   b. Assigning registered nurse, physical therapist, occupational therapist, or other professional to provide care; removal when care completed
   c. Summary of care plan for past 2 to 3 weeks
   d. Client and family responses regarding care
   e. Evaluation of care and needs provided by LVN or HHA
   f. Care plan revision if needed or restatement of the existing plan
   g. When to review plan, usually in 2 to 4 weeks (every 2 weeks for Medicare, every 4 weeks for Medicaid and third-party payors)
   h. Signature and date

EXAMPLES OF NURSING NOTES

First Visit
S ubjective
   Age and sex
   Brief medical history
   Nursing history

Anxiety level

Discharge instructions

Understanding of medical problems

Ability of client and family to adapt

Family support and participation; safety issues

O bjective

Physical assessment

Physical abilities/limitations in ADL

Home assessment

A ctions

Formulate care plan and nursing diagnoses; formulate contingency plan if no professional caretaker is available

Develop short- and long-term goals

Develop nursing and client and family interventions

Instruct client and family in interventions

P lanning

Assess need for other personnel for care

Assess need for supplies or equipment

Decide what to do during next visit

Assess need for long-term planning prior to discharge

Assess need to refer to other community resources

Discharge Visit

S ubjective

Statement of feelings of client

Progress toward health and functioning

O bjective

Physical assessment findings

Independence in ADL, limitations, and restrictions

Goals not achieved; goals achieved

A ctions

Formulate discharge instructions (written)

Develop nursing and client and family interventions

P lanning

Provide client and family with resources in community

Notify physician of discharge; provide summary or report

Notify agency of case closing date

◣ *Guidelines for Client Self-Determination**

The Patient Self-Determination Act requires Medicare- and Medicaid-certified hospitals, long-term facilities, home care agencies, and other health care providers and organizations to give patients information about their right to make their own health care decisions, including the right to accept or refuse medical treatment. It also includes requirements for providers to educate their staffs on issues related to advance directives. The act was incorporated into the Omnibus Budget Reconciliation Act of 1990 (OBRA 1990) and took effect on December 1, 1991.

PROVISIONS OF THE LAW

1. Provide all adult individuals with written information about their rights under state law to make health care decisions, including the right to execute advance directives. State law will be developed at the state level, and the federal law does not override any state law that would allow a health care provider to object on the basis of conscience to implementing an advance directive.

2. Inform patients, residents, and clients about the facility or agency policy on implementing advance directives. Written information required by law must be given out at the time of the individual's admission as an inpatient by a hospital, as a resident by a nursing facility, or as an outpatient by a home health care provider, by prepaid health plans when an individual is enrolled, and by hospices at the time of initial receipt of hospice care.

3. Document in the patient's medical record whether he or she has executed an advance directive.

4. Do not discriminate against an individual on the basis of whether he or she has executed an advance directive.

5. Provide staff and community education on advance directives.

*Adapted from Health Care Financing Administration Fact Sheets, Department of Health and Human Services, November 1991.

DEFINITION OF ADVANCE DIRECTIVE

A written statement, which one completes in advance of serious illness, about how one wants medical decisions made. It allows one to state choices for health care or to name someone to make those choices if one is unable to make decisions about medical treatment now or in the future. It allows one to say "yes" to treatment wanted or "no" to treatment not wanted.

TYPES OF ADVANCE DIRECTIVES

1. Living Will: A written form approved by a state that specifies the kind of medical care the client wants or does not want if he or she becomes unable to make his or her own decisions. A Living Will may be initiated by using a form developed by the state, completing and signing a preprinted form available in the community, developing one's own form, or writing a statement of treatment preferences. Advice may be solicited from an attorney or physician to ensure that one's wishes are understood and followed.
2. Durable Power of Attorney for Health Care: A signed, dated, and witnessed paper naming another person, such as a spouse, daughter, son, or close friend, as the client's agent or proxy to make medical decisions for the client if he or she should become unable to make them for himself or herself. May include instructions about any treatment the client wishes to avoid. Some states have specific laws allowing for health care power of attorney and provide printed forms.

Some state laws make it better to have one or the other, and it may be possible to have both or to combine the two types (describes treatment choices in situations and names someone to make decisions for the client when necessary). Either of these may be changed or canceled at any time. Some states allow a change by oral statement.

An advance directive should be signed and dated, with copies given to the physician and others as needed. A copy should be given to the client's attorney if he or she has a durable power of attorney, a copy should be given to the physician to become a part of the permanent record, and a copy should be put in a safe place where it can be found easily if needed. A card should be placed in the client's purse or wallet that states the existence of an advance directive, where it is located, and the name of the client's agent or proxy if appropriate.

◣ *Selected Common Laboratory Values**

Test	Conventional Range	SI Range
BLOOD		
Acetoacetate plus acetone	Negative	
Aldolase	1.3–8.2 U/L	22–137 nmol·sec^{-1}/L
Ammonia	12–55 µmol/L	12–55 µmol/L
Amylase	4–25 units/ml	4–25 arb. units
Arterial blood gases		
pH	7.35–7.45	Same
PCO$_2$	35–45 mm Hg	4.7–6.0 kPa
PO$_2$	75–100 mm Hg (age dependent in room air)	10.0–13.3 kPa
Bilirubin	Direct: up to 0.4 mg/100 ml; total: up to 1.0 mg/100 ml	Up to 7 µmol/L
Calcium	8.5–10.5 mg/100 ml	2.1–2.6 mmol/L
Chloride	100–106 mEq/L	100–106 mmol/L
Complement, total hemolytic	150–250 U/ml	
C3	83–177 mg/100 ml	0.83–1.77 g/L
C4	15–45 mg/100 ml	0.15–0.45 g/L

*From Scully RE, editor: Case records of the Massachusetts General Hospital, *N Engl J Med* 314:39–49, January 2, 1986. Reprinted by permission of The New England Journal of Medicine.

Test	Conventional Range	SI Range
Complete blood count		
Hematocrit	Female: 37%–48%	0.37–0.48
	Male: 45%–52%	0.45–0.52
Hemoglobin	Female: 12–16 g/100 ml	7.4–9.9 mmol/L
	Male: 13–18 g/100 ml	8.1–11.2 mmol/L
Leukocyte count	4300–10,800/cu mm	$4.3–10.8 \times 10^9$/L
Erythrocyte count	4.2–5.9 million/cu mm	$4.2–5.9 \times 10^9$/L
Creatine kinase	Female: 10–79 U/L	167–1317 nmol·sec^{-1}/L
	Male: 17–148 U/L	283–2467 nmol·sec^{-1}/L
Creatinine	0.6–1.5 mg/100 ml	53–133 μmol/L
Digoxin	1.2 ± 0.4 mg/ml	1.54 ± 0.5 nmol/L
	1.5 ± 0.4 mg/ml	1.92 ± 0.5 nmol/L
Erythrocyte sedimentation rate	Female: 1–20 mm/hr	1–20 mm/hr
	Male: 1–13 mm/hr	1–13 mm/hr
Folic acid		
Normal	>3.3 ng/ml	>7.3 nmol/L
Borderline	>2.5–3.2 ng/ml	>5.75–7.39 nmol/L
Glucose	Fasting: 70–110 mg /100 ml	3.9–5.6 mmol/L
Immunoglobulins		
IgG	639–1349 mg/100 ml	6.39–13.49 g/L
IgA	70–312 mg/100 ml	0.7–3.12 g/L
IgM	86–352 mg/100 ml	0.86–3.52 g/L
Iron	50–150 μg/100 ml	9.0–26.9 μmol/L
Lipase	2 units/ml or less	Up to 2 arb. units

Test	Conventional Range	SI Range
Lipids		
Cholesterol	120–220 mg/100 ml	3.10–5.69 mmol/L
Triglycerides	40–150 mg/100 ml	0.4–1.5 g/L
Magnesium	1.5–2.0 mEq/L	0.8–1.3 mmol/L
Partial thromboplastin time (activated)	25–38 sec	25–38 sec
Phenytoin	5–20 µg/ml	20–80 µmol/L
Phosphatase (alkaline)	13–39 U/L	217–650 nmol·sec^{-1}/L
Phosphorus (inorganic)	3.0–4.5 mg/100 ml	1.0–1.5 mmol/L
Platelet count	150,000–350,000/cu mm	150–350 × 10^9/L
Potassium	3.5–5.0 mEq/L	3.5–5.0 mmol/L
Protein		
Total	6.0–8.4 g/100 ml	60–84 g/L
Albumin	3.5–5.0 g/100 ml	35–50 g/L
Globulin	2.3–3.5 g/100 ml	23–35 g/L
Prothrombin time	Less than 2 sec deviation from control	Less than 2 sec deviation from control
Reticulocyte count	0.5%–2.5% red cells	0.005–0.025
Salicylate (therapeutic)	20–25 mg/100 ml	1.4–1.8 mmol/L
Sodium	135–145 mEq/L	135–145 mmol/L
Total triiodothyronine (T$_3$)	75–195 ng/100 ml	1.16–3.00 nmol/L
Total thyroxine (T$_4$) by RIA	4–12 µg/100 ml	52–154 nmol/L
Transaminase, SGOT (asparate amino-transferase, AST)	7–27 U/L	117–450 nmol·sec.$^{-1}$/L
Transaminase, SGPT (alanine aminotransferase, ALT)	1–21 U/L	17–350 nmol·sec $^{-1}$/L

Test	Conventional Range	SI Range
Urea nitrogen	8–25 mg/100 ml	2.9–8.9 mmol/L
Uric acid	3.0–7.0 mg/100 ml	0.18–0.42 mmol/L
URINE		
Acetone plus acetoacetate	0	0 mg/L
Creatinine	15–25 mg/kg body weight/day	0.13–0.22 mmol·kg^{-1}/day
Protein	≤150 mg/24 hr	<0.15 g/day
Sugar	0	0 mmol/L
Urobilinogen	Up to 1.0 Ehrlich U	To 1.0 arb. unit
STOOL		
Fat	Less than 5 g in 24 hr or less than 4% of fat intake in 3 days	<5 g/day
Occult blood	0	0

◢ Selected Home Care Resources

American Federation of Home Health Agencies
1320 Fenwick Lane, Suite 500
Silver Spring, MD 20910
(301) 588-1454

American Hospital Association
Division of Ambulatory and Home Care Services
840 North Lake Shore Drive
Chicago, IL 60611
(312) 280-6000

Council of Community Health Services
National League for Nursing
10 Columbus Circle
New York, NY 10019
(212) 582-1022

Foundation for Hospice and Home Care
519 C Street, NE
Washington, DC 20002
(202) 547-1022

National Association for Home Care
519 C Street, NE
Washington, DC 20002
(202) 547-7424

National Health Publishing
99 Painters Mill Road
Owings Mills, MD 21117

Other

Alzheimer's Disease and Related Disorders
360 Michigan Avenue
Chicago, IL 60602
(312) 853-3060

American Association of Retired Persons
1909 K Street, NW
Washington, DC 20049
(202) 872-4700

American Cancer Society
90 Park Avenue
New York, NY 10016
(212) 599-8200

American Council of the Blind
1211 Connecticut Avenue, NW, Suite 506
Washington, DC 20036
(202) 833-1251 or 1-800-424-8666

American Diabetes Association
2 Park Avenue
New York, NY 10016
(212) 683-7444

American Dietetic Association
430 North Michigan Avenue
Chicago, IL 60611
(313) 280-5012

American Heart Association
7320 Greenville Avenue
Dallas, TX 75231
(214) 750-5300

American Red Cross
Local Offices

Arthritis Foundation
1314 Spring Street, NW
Atlanta, GA 30309
(404) 872-7100

Cystic Fibrosis Foundation
6000 Executive Boulevard
Rockville, MD 20852
(301) 881-9130

Meals on Wheels
Local Offices

Medic-Alert
P.O. Box 1009
Turlock, CA 95381-1009
(209) 668-3333
1-800-344-3226

National Easter Seal Society
2023 West Ogden Avenue
Chicago, IL 60612
(312) 243-8400

National Information Center of Deafness
Gallaudet College
Kendall Green
Washington, DC 20002
(202) 651-5109

National Institute on Aging
National Institutes of Health
Building 31, Room 5C35
Bethesda, MD 20205
(301) 496-1752

National Institute of Arthritis, Diabetes and Digestive and Kidney
    Diseases
National Institutes of Health
Westwood Building, Room 403
Bethesda, MD 20205
(301) 496-7495
    or
1555 Wilson Boulevard, Suite 600
Rosslyn, VA 22209
(301) 496-9707

National Institute of Mental Health
Public Inquiries
5600 Fishers Lane,
Room 11A-21
Rockville, MD 20857
(301) 443-2403

National Kidney Foundation
2 Park Avenue
New York, NY 10016
(212) 889-2210

United Ostomy Association
2001 West Beverly Boulevard
Los Angeles, CA 90057
(213) 413-5510

United Way
Regional/Local Offices

Veterans Administration
810 Vermont Avenue, NW
Washington DC 20420

Mail Order Equipment/Supplies
Listings in local telephone yellow pages and:

Anik, Inc.
P.O. Box 3232
San Rafael, CA 94912
(415) 461-1477

Brookstone Co.
Vose Farm Road
Peterborough, NH 03458
(603) 924-9511

Comfortably Yours
Aids for Easier Living
53 West Hunter Avenue
Maywood, N.J. 07670
(201) 368-0400

Fashion-Able
5 Crescent Street
Rocky Hill, NJ 08553
(609) 921-2563

Independent Living Aids, Inc.
11 Commercial Court
Plainview, NY 11803

Travenol Home Therapy
1 Baxter Parkway
Deerfield, IL 60015
(312) 948-2000

◢ BIBLIOGRAPHY

Aukamp V, Shaw R: *Nursing care plans for adult home health clients: nursing diagnoses and interventions,* East Norwalk, Conn, 1989, Appleton & Lange.

Bedrosian CA.: *Home health nursing diagnoses and care plans,* East Norwalk, Conn, 1988, Appleton & Lange.

Bowyer CK: *The complex care team: meeting the needs of high technology nursing at home, Home Health Care Nurse* 4:24, Jan–Feb 1986.

Burrell LO: *Adult nursing in hospital and community settings,* East Norwalk, Conn, 1992, Appleton & Lange.

Department of Health and Human Services: Health Care Financing Administration Fact Sheets, November 26, 1991.

Dolan MB: *Community and home health care plans,* Springhouse, Penn, 1989, Springhouse Publishing Co.

Gould EJ: *Standardized home health nursing care plans: a quality assurance tool, QRB* 11:334, Nov 1985.

Haddad AM, Kapp MB: *Ethical and legal issues in home health care,* East Norwalk, Conn, 1990, Appleton & Lange.

Humphery CJ, Milone-Nuzzo P: *Home care nursing: an orientation to practice,* East Norwalk, Conn, 1991, Appleton & Lange.

Kim MJ et al: *Pocket guide to nursing diagnoses,* ed 4, St Louis, 1991, Mosby-Year Book.

Martinson IM, Widmer A, editors: *Home health care nursing,* Philadelphia, 1989, WB Saunders.

North American Nursing Diagnosis Association: *Official nursing diagnoses: proceedings of the Tenth Conference,* St Louis, 1992, Mosby–Year Book.

Pokalo, C: Understanding of the patient self-determination act, *J Gerontol Nurs* 18(3):47, March 1992.

Scherman SL: *Community health nursing care plans: a guide for home health care professionals,* ed 2, Albany, NY, 1990, Delmar Publishers.

Scully RE, editor: Case records of the Massachusetts General Hospital, *N Engl J Med* 314:39, Jan 2, 1986.

Shannon MT, Wilson BA: *Govoni and Hayes' drugs and nursing implications,* ed 7, East Norwalk, Conn, 1992, Appleton & Lange.

Swearingen PL: *Manual of nursing therapeutics: applying nursing diagnoses to medical disorders,* ed 2, St Louis, 1990, Mosby-Year Book.

Walsh J et al: *Manual of Home Health Care Nursing,* Philadelphia, 1987, JB Lippincott.

Zastocki DK, Rovinski CA: *Home care: patient and family instruction,* Philadelphia, 1989, WB Saunders Co.

Index